FUCHS'S
RADIOGRAPHIC EXPOSURE, PROCESSING AND QUALITY CONTROL

Figure 1. *Frontispiece.* X-ray film has been prepared in many sizes for medical work. The largest film (32 by 72 inches) used was for the entire body radiography of a woman, aged thirty-three, exhibiting hip pathology. The radiograph was made with a one-second exposure, 75 kVp, 150 mA, 12 feet target-film distance, fast screens, and tissue-compensating filtration.

FUCHS'S RADIOGRAPHIC EXPOSURE, PROCESSING AND QUALITY CONTROL

Sixth Edition

By

QUINN B. CARROLL, M.Ed., R.T.

Director
Radiography Department
Midland College
Midland, Texas

CHARLES C THOMAS · PUBLISHER, LTD.
Springfield · Illinois · U.S.A.

Published and Distributed Throughout the World by

CHARLES C THOMAS • PUBLISHER, LTD.
2600 South First Street
Springfield, Illinois 62794-9265

© *1998 by* CHARLES C THOMAS • PUBLISHER, LTD.

ISBN 0-398-06830-5

Library of Congress Catalog Card Number: 97-36977

First Edition, 1955
Second Edition, 1958
Third Edition, 1985
Fourth Edition, 1990
Fifth Edition, 1993
Sixth Edition, 1998

With THOMAS BOOKS *careful attention is given to all details of manufacturing
and design. It is the Publisher's desire to present books that are satisfactory as to their
physical qualities and artistic possibilities and appropriate for their particular use.*
THOMAS BOOKS *will be true to those laws of quality that assure a good name
and good will.*

Printed in the United States of America
SM-R-3

Library of Congress Cataloging in Publication Data
Carroll, Quinn B.
    Fuchs's radiographic exposure, processing, and quality control /
Quinn B. Carroll. -- 6th ed.
            p.   cm.
    Includes index.
    ISBN 0-398-06830-5 (cloth)
    1. Radiography, Medical. I. Fuchs, Arthur W. (Arthur Wolfram),
1895-   . II. Title.
        [DNLM: 1. Radiography. 2. Techology, Radiologic. WN 160 C319f
        1998]
    RC78.C35   1998
    616.07'572--dc21
    DNLM/DLC
    for Library of Congress   97-36977
                                                                        CIP

To
WOLFRAM CONRAD FUCHS
Roentgen Pioneer
1865-1907

and

ARTHUR WOLFRAM FUCHS
(1895-1962)

CONTRIBUTING AUTHORS

EUCLID SEERAM, RTR, BSc, MSc
British Columbia Institute of Technology
Burnaby, British Columbia, Canada

WILLIAM S. HEATHMAN, BS, RTR
Midland College
Midland, Texas

PREFACE TO THE SIXTH EDITION

ARTHUR W. FUCHS was a man who understood and believed in experiential learning. The philosophy is that learning obtained through hands-on experience is more likely to be understood, retained and applied than are notes from lectures. Thus, the first edition had a format of illustrated experimentation. It focused upon the real considerations of the daily practice of medical radiography rather than on physical theory. For this reason, I am honored to be able to associate my name with his in producing this updated and expanded edition on radiographic imaging.

If other educators in radiography have experienced the same kinds of frustrations in finding a comprehensive and practical text as I have, it is hoped that this edition will fill that void. While there are several excellent physics texts in the field, some of which claim by their titles to be technique books, texts on practical technique are few and far between.

It should be noted at the outset that this edition is intended to complement radiographic physics texts rather than duplicate them. It picks up where they leave off, bridges the gap between theory and practice, and therefore assumes some basic knowledge of physical principles upon which the concepts of practical technique can be built. Care was taken to include only those physics topics which directly relate to the manipulation of equipment in controlling the outcome on the image. Hence, although there is an early chapter on atomic interactions upon which much of

the subsequent chapters build, there is no treatment of electricity or mechanics. This book addresses the questions of which variables must be manipulated to control image qualities and why, nothing more.

This volume also attempts to bridge the gap between quality control and technique. These two subjects have been taught and written about separately for too long. All of the concepts and rules of technique are completely dependent upon quality control for their validity. Many students have struggled with apparent contradictions in the principles of technique they have been taught simply because they were working with poorly calibrated equipment. Although some instructors cover quality control in a different course or semester, by finding these concepts alongside practical technique in the same text the student can recognize that there are scientific explanations for techniques that do not always produce results with exactness.

Mr. Fuchs also realized that it is easier to assimilate information in small bits than in large amounts at a time. Consequently, he organized his book variable by variable, rather than image quality by image quality. There are only six essential qualities to an image. There are well over twenty fundamental variables which affect image quality. This edition holds true to the original, presenting the effects of each variable upon the six image qualities in each chapter, rather than inundating the student with twenty factors to learn about in each chapter. However, since technique courses are frequently organized by image qualities, a chapter has been added on "Analyzing the Radiographic Image," which reviews all of the material in this manner.

Unique additions to the book include chapters on technique by proportional anatomy, constructing technique charts from scratch, and how to solve multiple technique problems similar to those presented on certification examinations in radiography. Chapters covering automatic and programmed exposure controls, automatic processors, sensitometry and dark-room quality control have been added. The early chapter covering image qualities ensures that the student obtains a clear and complete concept of each of the six image components before proceeding to the effects of each variable upon them. It is easy to confuse a higher contrast image for a sharper image or a fogged image for an overexposed image. This chapter helps prevent these types of misconceptions as more and more advanced and complicated topics are presented.

The Fifth Edition was expanded in accordance with a survey of educators using the text, and contributing authors were instrumental in making improvements. Chapters have been added on pathology and casts, scattered radiation, analyzing the image, minimizing patient dose, equipment quality control, special image processing systems (daylight systems and PACS), along with mobile, fluoroscopic and digital imaging. Material has been added to many other chapters, and most importantly, the chapters on technique by proportional anatomy, technique charts and automatic exposure controls have been expanded to include more detailed information. Review questions and suggested laboratory demonstrations have been added at the ends of chapters.

Changes in the Fifth Edition were also

intended to make the text even more "user-friendly" for students. An important table on radiographic terminology has been added to Chapter 1, helping students translate between terms used in the text, other terms widely used by educators, and terms used on the certifying examination of the American Registry of Radiologic Technologists. Additional material helping students with mathematical calculations has been included in Chapters 5, 6, 18, and 30 (mAs, kVp, distance changes and multiple technique problems).

The Sixth Edition significantly expanded Chapter 14 on intensifying screens and Chapter 28 on Automatic Exposure Controls, not only bringing the material up to date in these essential areas of modern radiography, but presenting one of the most thorough practical treatments of these topics available. Terminology and abbreviations were brought in line with ARRT standards and current conventions, and additional effort was invested in making the text yet more student-friendly, with clear, concise explanations, plentiful examples, ample illustrations and practice exercises to reinforce mathematical concepts.

A considerable effort was made to cover all material suggested by the ASRT curriculum guide, without duplicating typical physics texts and maintaining a focus on practical application.

It is sincerely hoped that this text will contribute to the competency and fulfillment of radiographers in their career, to the professionalism and cost effectiveness of radiology departments, and ultimately to the enhancement of patient care in medical radiography.

Q.B.C.

ACKNOWLEDGMENTS

I WISH TO EXPRESS my thanks to the professional staff of Charles C Thomas, Publisher for their valuable help in developing, illustrating, and producing the text.

Special thanks to Euclid Seeram and William Heathman for their valuable contributions to a text which remains a classic in the field, and to all of my professional colleagues who have offered suggestions for improvements, assisted with corrections and shared their expertise and association over the years.

I am grateful to Jason, Melissa, Chad, Tiffani, Brandon, and Tyson for their patience when I am writing.

Above all, I wish to express my gratitude to my wife Margaret for her unwavering support and confidence in all that I do and for her belief in what each human being can do.

CONTENTS

Part I
PRODUCING THE RADIOGRAPHIC IMAGE

Part II
VISIBILITY FACTORS

Part III
GEOMETRICAL FACTORS

Part IV
COMPREHENSIVE TECHNIQUE

Part V
SPECIAL IMAGING METHODS

Part VI
PROCESSING THE RADIOGRAPH

FUCHS'S
RADIOGRAPHIC EXPOSURE, PROCESSING AND QUALITY CONTROL

Part I

PRODUCING THE RADIOGRAPHIC IMAGE

Chapter 1

X-RAYS AND RADIOGRAPHIC VARIABLES

A SATISFACTORY UNDERSTANDING of exposure and processing terms requires at
least a limited knowledge of x-rays and their
characteristics. X-rays are a form of invisible radiant energy and were discovered by
Wilhelm Conrad Röntgen on November 8,
1895. They are quite similar to light in their
general properties since they travel at the
same speed and obey many of the same
laws. A distinguishing feature of x-rays,
however, is their extremely shortwave
length–only about one ten-thousandth the
wave length of *visible* light. It is this property that is responsible for the x-rays' ability to
penetrate materials that ordinarily would
absorb or reflect light.

GENERATION OF X-RAYS

The generation of x-rays is a complex
process. Fortunately, a knowledge of only
a few of the principles is necessary. The
essential feature of x-ray production is the
striking of matter by high speed electrons;
this may occur within or outside a vacuum.
Basically, the device in which x-rays are
generated is the x-ray tube.

X-rays are produced in an x-ray tube
when electrons, traveling at great speed in
a high vacuum, under stress of high voltage, collide with a metallic target of high
molecular weight such as tungsten. The
efficiency of production of x-rays is very
small, for only about one part in a thousand
of electron energy at average kilovoltages is
converted into x-rays that are penetrating
enough to make a radiograph; the balance
of energy is dissipated as heat.

The x-ray tubes employed by the early
workers contained gas under low pressure.
These tubes were known as Crookes or
Hittorf tubes. Röntgen's early tubes (Figure
2) were of the Crookes type which consisted of a pear-shaped glass tube filled with air
under reduced pressure. An aluminum
cathode was installed in the small end of
the tube and, through a stem of glass on the
side of the tube was inserted an aluminum
anode.

When a high voltage current was passed
between the cathode and anode, the residual gas in the tube became ionized and a
stream of electrons was repelled by the
cathode. Many of these electrons were
attracted to the anode because of its location in the tube, but the majority of the
electrons were bombarded against the glass
at the end of the tube. The sudden stop-
page of the electrons against the glass produced x-rays.

When the Jackson *focus* tube was made,
the electron stream was focused on to a
metal anode inclined at an angle so that a
larger amount of radiation could be concentrated on a particular area.

Maintenance of a constant pressure in
the early gas tubes was almost impossible

Figure 2. Photograph of the gas discharge tubes employed by Roentgen in his experiments that led to his discovery of the x-rays.

for the pressure would vary with each use of the tube. These early tubes were quite erratic. The advent of the Coolidge hot cathode x-ray tube made possible the generation of a constant source of x-rays that could be easily duplicated at will. This tube was invented by Dr. W. D. Coolidge of the General Electric Company and announced December 27, 1913 (Figure 3).

X-RAY TUBE

The modern x-ray tube consists of a highly evacuated glass bulb into which are sealed two electrodes–the cathode, or *negative* electrode (the source of electrons), and the anode, or *positive* electrode (the source of x-rays). The degree of vacuum of the x-ray tube and the arrangement of the electrodes are such that no electrical discharge

between the cathode and the anode is possible until the filament in the cathode is heated (Figures 4 and 5).

Thermionic Electron Emission

Employing the principle that all *hot* bodies emit electrons, a spiral, incandescent filament of tungsten wire is incorporated in the cathode of the usual form of x-ray tube. This filament is heated by a current of low amperage from a low voltage step-down transformer. The temperature of the filament, as governed by the amount of current that passes through it, controls the number of electrons emitted–the higher the filament temperature, the greater the electron emission. Because of its small mass an electron rapidly develops greater speed in an electric field. Surrounding the filament tube electrodes by a high-voltage transformer. This voltage, which may be varied at will, regulates the *speed* with which the electrons cross the gap between the cathode and the anode. Thousands of volts (kilovolts) are normally used for this purpose. The stream of electrons forms a conducting path for the high voltage current to reach the anode. Upon impact with the focal spot of the tube, the electrons produce a stream of x-rays which are emitted over a 180° angle from the focal spot of the target.

Figure 3. Photograph of an early Coolidge stationary anode tube in which the electrons originate in heated tungsten filament.

is a shield that serves to focus the electron stream from the heated filament to the *focal spot* on the tungsten target located at the end of the anode. The stream of electrons from cathode to anode constitutes the tube current and is measured in milliamperes. The electron stream is propelled by high-voltage electricity impressed on the

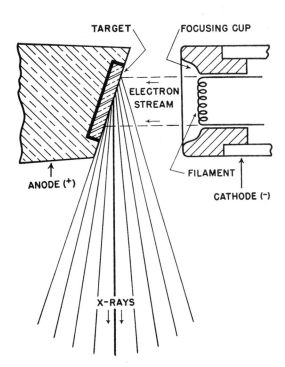

Figure 4. Diagram of the essential elements of an x-ray tube wherein electrons generated by a heated filament in the cathode are bombarded against a tungsten-rhenium target in the anode, resulting in x-ray production.

Rotating Anode Tube

The Coolidge tube was still limited in the quantity of x-rays it could produce.

Figure 5. Photograph of a modern x-ray tube with the cathode visible to the lower left, the rotating anode disc in the middle, and the rotor which rotates the anode disc on the right half.

With the enhanced electron emission of a hot cathode, the stationary anode plate could be melted from the intense bombardment of electrons. To prevent this destruction of the anode surface, a better way of dissipating the heat had to be devised. In 1936, the *rotating anode tube* was developed (Figure 5).

The rotating anode is shaped like a disc and composed of a metal with good heat-conducting and electron-conducting characteristics, usually molybdenum. The front surface of the disc is coated with an alloy of tungsten and rhenium. These two elements are made of "large" atoms with many orbital electrons, and are very effective at stopping the electron beam emitted from the cathode. With their high melting points, tungsten and rhenium are ideal metals for the "target" surface of the anode.

The anode disc is connected to a rotor shank (Figure 5) which is actually part of a motor. Whenever the "rotor" switch is depressed on an x-ray machine, this shank spins at the same time that the cathode filament is heated. By spinning the anode disc, the target surface struck by the electron beam is constantly changing. The heat is distributed across a greater surface area, and the anode is less likely to melt.

Thus, the three most essential components to the modern x-ray tube can be described as (1) the vacuum tube, (2) the heated cathode, and (3) the rotating anode.

X-ray Wave Length

Despite the enormous energy in the electron stream, only a small portion is converted to x-rays; the bulk is dissipated as heat at the anode. The greater the force of impact of the electrons on the anode, the shorter is the wave length of the x-rays produced and the more readily do they penetrate the object being examined. In other words, the higher the voltage, the greater is the speed of the electrons striking the anode. The result is a decrease in wave length of the x-rays emitted and an increase in both their intensity and penetrating power. Wave lengths are measured in *ångstrom (Å) units*; an ångstrom unit is equal to 10^{-8} centimeter. The useful range of wave lengths for medical radiography is approximately *0.10 to 0.50 ångstrom units.*

INTERACTIONS IN THE ANODE

The wave lengths and the energy levels of x-rays in the beam are determined by the specific interactions of the electrons with the atoms in the anode. Atoms with a high atomic number will have much larger nuclei as well as many more orbital electrons with which the high-speed electrons from the cathode may interact. This means that more interactions will occur, and that those which do occur will result in higher-energy x-rays being produced. This is the reason why tungsten and rhenium (atomic number 74 and 75, respectively) are used as target material on the anode.

When a high-speed electron strikes an atom in the anode, it must interact either with the nucleus of the atom or with an orbital electron in one of the electron shells.

BREMSSTRAHLUNG

If the electron passes near the atomic nucleus, the positive attraction of the nucleus will cause it to *brake* or slow down. This deceleration in the speed of the electron represents a loss of kinetic energy, and that energy lost is emitted as an x-ray *photon* (Figure 6). The word "photon" is often used to denote a single x-ray. X-rays produced by this interaction are called *bremsstrahlung* (braking radiation) and they account for about 85 per cent, on average, of the total x-ray beam.

High-speed electrons may pass by the nucleus at various distances from it. The closer an electron approaches the nucleus, the greater will be its deceleration, and the higher will be the energy (KeV) of the emitted x-ray. Bremsstrahlung, occurring at various distances from the atomic nucleus,

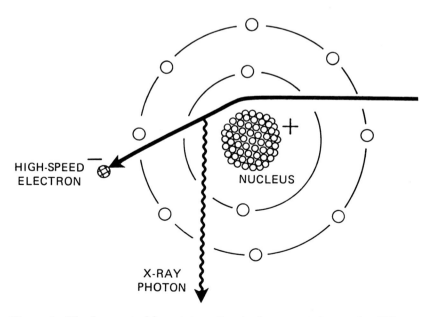

Figure 6. The bremsstrahlung interaction in the x-ray tube anode. When a high-speed electron is attracted to a nearby atomic nucleus, it decelerates and changes direction, losing energy. The lost energy is emitted as an x-ray.

produces a wide range of x-ray energies and is thus responsible for the heterogeneous or poly-energetic nature of the x-ray beam. Heterogeneity contributes to the differential absorption of x-rays within the patient which provides *subject contrast* and makes the radiographic image possible. If all of the x-rays were of the same energy, the image would be extremely poor. Subtle differences between tissues only show up on the radiograph when a variety of x-ray energies result in a wide range of differential absorption and subject contrast.

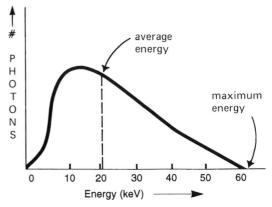

Figure 8. Graph of the actual bremsstrahlung x-ray beam spectrum with filtration present and the kVp set to 60. X-rays with the lowest energies are absorbed by the glass, oil, and filters through which they pass. The average energy is about 20 keV, one-third of the kV peak.

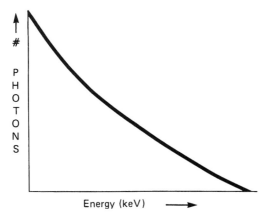

Figure 7. Graph of the bremsstrahlung x-ray beam spectrum as it would appear with no filtration. Most x-rays are generated at lower energy (keV) levels. Very few are produced at the highest energies.

The distance at which an electron will pass a nucleus is a function of statistical probability. It is more likely that it will pass farther away from the nucleus, where greater areas are involved, than that it will pass very near the nucleus. Hence, more x-rays are produced at low energies than at higher energies. A plot of this relationship between energy levels and the numbers of x-rays produced would look like Figure 7. However, because inherent filtration in the x-ray tube stops the x-rays with the lowest energies, the remaining bremsstrahlung

portion of the beam is graphed like Figure 8.

Reviewing Figure 8, note that there are very few x-rays emitted from the x-ray tube at very low energies, because of filtration. There are also very few x-rays emitted at high energies. This is because of the statistical distribution of the bremsstrahlung interaction. (It is more likely that an electron will pass the nucleus at a large distance than that it will pass very close to the nucleus.) The *total* number of x-rays produced by bremsstrahlung is represented by the *total area* under the beam spectrum curve on the graph. Bremsstrahlung x-rays are produced at many different energies, making the beam *heterogeneous. Note that the average energy of these x-rays is about one-third of the maximum energy.*

CHARACTERISTIC RADIATION

The second possibility for the high-speed electron is that instead of interacting with the nucleus, it will interact with one of the orbital electrons in the atomic shells. When it passes near an orbital elec-

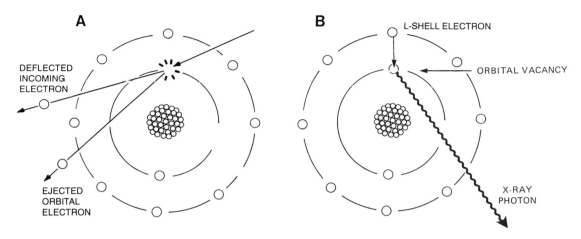

Figure 9. The characteristic interaction in the x-ray tube anode. In step *A*, an incoming electron from the filament collides with and dislodges an orbital electron from the atom. In step *B*, the atom "pulls" down an electron from a higher orbit to fill the vacancy left. As this electron drops into a lower orbit, it loses energy which is emitted as an x-ray.

tron, its repulsive force will eject the orbital electron out of its orbit, leaving a vacancy in the electron shell of the atom. The atom, left with a net positive charge, will pull in another electron, usually from an outer shell, to fill the vacancy. Energy is lost when an electron falls from an outer orbit into an inner orbit, and that energy is emitted as a characteristic x-ray (Figure 9). Characteristic radiation makes up about 15 per cent of the average x-ray beam.

Characteristic x-rays depend entirely on the difference in energy levels between orbits in the atom. Since we know what the energy levels for each orbit in the atoms of each element are, we can predict accurately what characteristic x-ray energies will be for the tungsten and rhenium in the anode. X-rays will be emitted at distinct energies, rather than over a range of energies like bremsstrahlung. A graph of the characteristic spectrum would appear as Figure 10.

In tungsten atoms, characteristic x-rays will be produced in the innermost electron shell having 57, 66 and 69 kilovolts of energy. The second orbital shell will produce x-rays of 10 and 12 KeV, and the third shell

will produce x-rays with about 2 KeV. Inherent beam filtration will remove virtually all of the 2-kV x-rays, so these do not show on the graph in Figure 10. Filtration also removes most of the 10- and 12-kV x-rays, thus, the graph plots them but

Figure 10. Graph of the characteristic x-ray beam spectrum for tungsten. X-rays are emitted only at discrete energy levels based upon the difference between binding energies of orbital shells in the atom. Electrons falling from various outer shells into the *K-Shell* emit x-rays having 57, 67, and 69 keV of energy. The lines to the far left represent *L-Shell* x-rays.

showing a reduced number. Those characteristic x-rays having 57, 66 and 69 kV escape the x-ray tube and are considered part of the useful beam. These show up on the beam spectrum graph as tall spikes.

Adding the predominant bremsstrahlung to the characteristic x-rays, a complete graph of the spectrum of the total x-ray beam appears as Figure 11. This graph illustrates how homogeneous characteristic radiation (the spikes) combines with heterogeneous bremsstrahlung (the bell curve) to produce a total filtered x-ray beam which is generally heterogeneous in nature and in which most of the x-rays have about one-third of the maximum energy produced.

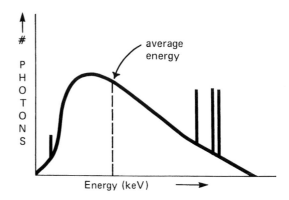

Figure 11. Shape of the complete diagnostic x-ray beam spectrum, representing both bremsstrahlung and characteristic interactions, with filtration present.

X-RAY BEAM SPECTRA

Graphs of the x-ray beam spectrum will be used in later chapters to demonstrate the effects of various changes, and the student must have a clear understanding of the interpretation of a spectrum such as that in Figure 11. An x-ray beam spectrum curve plots the *amount* of x-rays against their *energy*. Recall that an x-ray beam is heterogeneous, having a mixture of x-rays of many different energy levels. The spectrum curve depicts how many x-rays there are each energy. The energy is usually measured in kilovolts.

This is similar to drawing a graph of a graduating high school class, plotting the number of graduates against their height. There would be a few very tall graduates, and a few very short ones, but most of them would be of medium height, in an average

range. The height distribution curve would be graphed in a "bell" shape, just as the x-ray spectrum curve is. The total number of all high school graduates would be represented by the total area under the curve.

In a similar fashion, the heterogeneous x-ray beam includes a few x-rays of very low kilovoltage (energy), and a few with very high kilovoltage, but *most* of the x-rays in the beam will have some intermediate kilovoltage. On the graph, a higher curve would indicate more x-rays. A shift in the position of the spectrum curve to the right would indicate higher kilovoltages of energy, and a shift to the left would indicate lower energy levels. Thus, the height and position of the x-ray beam spectrum curve represent both the quantity and the quality of the x-ray beam.

PROPERTIES OF X-RAYS

Although x-rays exhibit all of the properties of visible light, and many similarities between light and x-rays may be readily noted, the effects produced are so different that it is preferable to consider the properties of x-rays separately from other types of radiation. For example, light is refracted by glass and, consequently, is capable of being focused by a lens in such instruments as cameras, microscopes, etc. X-rays can also be refracted, but to such a very slight degree that it requires the most refined apparatus to detect this phenomenon. Hence, the use of any kind of lens is quite out of the question.

An outstanding characteristic of the x-rays is their ability to penetrate matter of any kind. They are also able to expose photographic film, which makes radiography possible. When lengthy exposures are employed, x-rays have the power to change the color of many chemicals. Another important characteristic is the ability of x-rays to excite fluorescence in many substances, such as barium platino-cyanide, zinc sulfide, calcium tungstate, and many others. This fact makes possible the use of fluoroscopic and intensifying screens made with these substances for fluoroscopy, or for reducing the x-ray exposure in radiography. X-rays are a powerful agent in the treatment of cancer and other diseases. Air can be ionized by x-rays–a principle employed in the R-meter or ionization chamber used for measuring various kinds of x-radiation.

THE X-RAY BEAM

The x-ray beam may be likened to the *reflected* light from an object that passes through the lens of a camera to expose a photographic film. The x-ray beam, however, *passes through* the human body or object to expose the x-ray film.

The x-ray beam (Figure 15) may be divided into two parts, the *primary* beam and the *remnant* beam.

Primary Radiation

The primary radiation is confined to the portion of the x-ray beam emitted from the x-ray tube. It is not materially altered in its quality as it passes toward the object being examined.

Remnant Radiation

The remnant radiation is that radiation that emerges from the body tissues to expose the x-ray film and record the radiographic image. It is the *image-forming* radiation. The remnant radiation also contains secondary radiation emitted by the tissues, the amount depending upon its wave length and the manner in which it is controlled.

At average diagnostic kilovoltage levels, about 5 per cent or less of the primary radiation traverses completely through the patient's body, without interacting with any of the atoms in the patient, and strikes the film. In addition, about 15 per cent of the primary radiation interacts with atoms resulting in the production of secondary photons which make it out of the patient and strike the film. The remaining 80 per cent of the primary beam is totally absorbed within the patient.

Therefore, the total intensity of the remnant beam striking the film is about one-fifth or 20 per cent of the intensity of the primary beam. Further, it may be said that at least 75 per cent, 15 out of the 20 (the actual range is 75%-90%), of the remnant radiation striking the film is secondary radiation produced in the patient.

ATTENUATION

Absorption, properly called *attenuation,* actually refers to the reduction in x-ray intensity that occurs as the x-ray beam traverses the body part. Absorption is influenced by the atomic number and density of the tissue traversed as well as its thickness and the wave length of the radiation employed. Organic tissue offers no particular penetration problem but it necessitates; control over the large amounts of secondary radiation that often are emitted. Inorganic tissue (such as bone) contains such a large quantity of mineral matter that extreme absorption of radiation may occasionally constitute a problem. High tissue density is often associated with large tissue thicknesses and special procedures are required to secure satisfactory radiographs.

ABSORPTION BY HOMOGENEOUS OBJECT

A homogeneous object is one in which the material composing it is structurally uniform such as a block of aluminum.

To demonstrate the absorption character of an object of homogeneous consistency but unequal in thickness, an aluminum step-wedge (Figure 12) may be employed. X-ray absorption by an aluminum step-wedge is diagrammatically shown in Figure 13. The portion of the x-ray beam passing through the first step of the wedge is slightly absorbed and the remnant radiation produces a high film exposure to represent this step. The absorption by the second step of the wedge is greater than that of the first step because it has twice the thickness; the intensity of the remnant radiation is thereby further reduced and a lesser film exposure is produced; and, so on for the remainder of the steps. As the thickness of the object increases with each step of the wedge, the intensity of the primary beam is reduced so that less and less radiation emerges to expose the film. The image, therefore, consists of a graduated scale of gray shades. These gray shades are called *densities.*

Figure 12. Photograph of an aluminum "step wedge" penetrometer used for experimental purposes in radiography.

Absorption-Density Relation

It may be seen from the above that the difference in x-ray absorption of each step of aluminum had a direct relationship to its respective radiographic density. Since each step of the wedge was homogeneous, and uniform in its x-ray absorption, radiographic densities varying in tone value representative of each step resulted. The

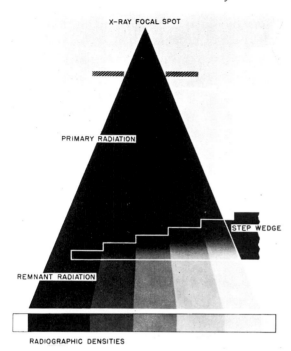

Figure 13. Diagram showing passage of x-rays through a homogeneous material (step wedge) that has steps of varying thickness.

image density of each step was directly related to the intensity of the remnant radiation reaching the film.

ABSORPTION BY BODY PART

When x-rays pass through human tissue, each type of tissue absorbs its proportion of radiation according to its own tissue density and thickness. For example, as x-rays pass through one thickness of flesh, then through a thickness of bone and finally through another thickness of flesh, the total absorption is the sum of the various degrees of absorption exercised by the different tissues (Figure 14). Radiographic delineation of human tissues cannot be predicated upon their thicknesses alone. Their physical state (tissue density and atomic number) is of the greatest importance from the standpoint of x-ray absorption. Absorption by various tissue compo-

nents introduces the element of *subject contrast* which is of major importance.

Subject Contrast

Tissue differences–sometimes called subject contrast–represent the differences in x-ray absorption occurring in an anatomical part. The greater the x-ray absorption of a tissue with relation to adjacent tissue, the greater the subject contrast; the lower the tissue absorption, the lower the contrast. For example, greater subject contrast is exhibited between bone and surrounding soft tissues than between kidney tissue and muscle. Also, the selective absorption of each tissue component within the leg causes different intensities within the remnant beam to produce variations in the image densities. As illustrated by the

Figure 14. Diagram illustrating the penetration and absorption of an x-ray beam as it traverses a body part (leg) whose components absorb the x-rays in varying degree depending upon their thickness and tissue density.

wedge (Figure 13), it was possible to differentiate between the various thicknesses of metal simply by comparing the value of one density with another. The same situation in a measure holds true with the leg, but, in addition, the composite absorption of x-rays by superimposed tissues of different types at different planes materially affects the image. Variation in thickness and composition is often evidenced as small differences in radiographic density. Since these differences are to be interpreted by the radiologist as anatomic details, they should be easily visible and translucent when viewed on the x-ray illuminator.

X-RAY BEAM NOMENCLATURE

Figure 15 illustrates various components of the x-ray beam and their abbreviations, with which the beginning radiography student must become familiar.

The focal spot, abbreviated *FS*, refers to the specific area on the target surface of the x-ray tube anode which is bombarded by high speed electrons. All of the x-rays produced emanate from this small area. It is so small (about the size of a pinhead) that in describing an x-ray beam the focal spot is considered to be a *point* from which all x-rays emerge. X-rays are actually emitted in all directions from this point, but only a small portion are allowed to escape the x-ray tube housing in a controlled direction, forming a fan-shaped beam (Figure 15). (X-rays traveling into the anode are absorbed by the anode material itself, and most of the remainder are absorbed by a lead housing around the x-ray tube. Those traveling in the desired direction are allowed to escape through a "window.")

Primary Radiation (PR) refers to the beam projected from the focal spot or "source" to the object (OB), prior to any absorption taking place. Remnant Radiation (RR) describes the beam emanating from the object and exposing the radiographic film.

The central ray (CR) is the center of the x-ray beam. The term is employed in describing the direction of the x-rays in a given projection. The course of the central ray may be considered to extend from the focal spot of the x-ray tube to the x-ray film.

The entire distance traversed by the cen-

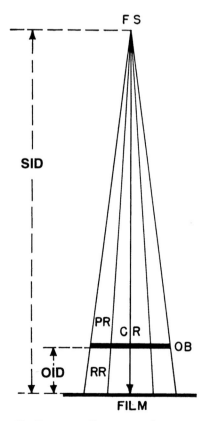

Figure 15. Diagram illustrating the various components of an x-ray beam with relation to an object and an x-ray film.

tral ray is known as the source-image receptor distance (SID). The distance from the object or body part to the x-ray film is known as the object-image receptor distance (OID) (Figure 15).

Some electrical terms in constant use are also abbreviated. The first of these is milliamperage (mA). The milliampere is the unit for measuring the flow rate of electricity passing through the x-ray machine and across the x-ray tube. The exposure time (s) delineates the amount of time in seconds during which the x-ray tube is activated for a particular exposure. The total exposure to an x-ray film is controlled by the product of the milliamperage and the exposure time, called milliampere-seconds, and abbreviated mAs, (mA X s), and pronounced like "mass" in daily usage.

Finally, the *kilovoltage-peak* refers to the energy level or "pressure" with which the electricity is being forced through the machine and across the x-ray tube. In simple terms, it controls the speed of the electricity and ultimately determines the penetrating power of the x-rays produced. Kilovoltage-peak is abbreviated *kVp*.

The Roentgen

Defined and adopted in 1937, the *roent-gen* is the international unit of quantity for both x-rays and gamma rays. It is designated by the symbol *R*.

THE PRIME FACTORS

Four of the variables to be studied in the following chapters are considered to be under the immediate and direct control of the radiographer. These are the milliamperage (mA), the exposure time (s), the kilovolt-peak (kVp) and the source-image receptor distance (SID). These have come to be known as the four *prime factors* of radiography.

The prime factors are combined below with x-ray beam nomenclature to form a list of terms and their abbreviations. These should be thoroughly memorized.

Term	*Symbol*
1. Central ray . . . . .CR	
2. Focal spot . . . . .FS	
3. Source-image receptor distance . . . . . . .SID	
4. Kilovolts peak .kVp	
5. Milliamperes . . . . .mA	
6. Milliampere-seconds . . . . .mAs	
7. Object-image receptor distance . . . . .OID	
8. Primary radiation . . . . .PR	
9. Remnant radiation . . . . .RR	
10. Secondary radiation . . . . .SR	
11. Time of exposure in seconds . . . . .s	
12. Roentgen . . . . .R	

TYPES OF RADIOGRAPHIC VARIABLES

The remainder of this book will deal with the many variables which affect the radiographic image and how they are controlled and manipulated to optimize image quality. An overview of these variables is provided by categorizing them into six general types:

1. *Electrical variables*: Electric variables include machine phase, kilovoltage, milliamperage and exposure time—anything controlled by the technological equipment in producing the x-ray beam.

2. *Geometrical variables*: Geometrical variables include the various distances, areas, focal spot size, angles and alignment of the x-ray beam, the part of interest and the image receptor (film). Positioning of the patient is actually a geometrical variable dealing with alignment, angles, centering and distances.

3. *Patient Status*: The condition of the patient, including sex, age and body habitus, as well as diseases and other conditions of the tissues in the patient, can cause alterations in image quality. The patient's ability and cooperation in obtaining optimum inspiration on chest radiographs, breathing or controlled movement on autotomographic procedures, and immobilization are essential to image quality.

4. *Image Receptor System*: The image receptor system includes anything which alters the condition of the remnant beam of rays after it has passed through the patient, and the recording medium for the image. Grids, Potter-Bucky diaphragms, intensifying screens or film holders, radiographic films, television cameras and monitor tubes, spotfilming devices, image intensifier tubes and mirror systems, computers and cine cameras are some examples. These devices are used in a number of possible combinations to provide the optimum image in the desired format.

5. *Processing Variables*: All images must be processed in some manner to be made permanent. Chemical concentrations, temperature and processing time, film storage and handling considerations are essential to the quality of the final image recorded. In computer systems, images are processed electronically to optimize quality before transferring them to a permanent medium.

6. *Viewing Conditions*: Even after the permanent image is recorded, variables affecting the visibility of that recorded image must be considered each time it is viewed for diagnosis. Ambient lighting, peripheral lighting around the film, adequate illumination through the x-ray film itself and various artifacts such as smudges or dirt on the illuminator or film must be controlled on an ongoing basis.

Every facet of radiography described in this book falls within one of these six categories of radiographic variables. It is the endeavor of the radiographer to manipulate and control them for optimum diagnosis.

SUMMARY

1. The three main components of the modern x-ray tube are the vacuum tube, the heated filament, and the rotating anode. X-rays are produced when high-speed electrons from the filament strike the anode and decelerate, losing energy.

2. Most of the x-ray beam is produced by *bremsstrahlung* interactions in the anode. The resulting *heterogeneous* energies in the beam allow *subject contrast* to be produced.

3. *Subject contrast* is the differential absorption between different types of tissues, each one absorbing a different percentage or portion of the x-ray beam.

4. A portion of the beam is produced by *characteristic* interactions in the anode. These rays have discrete energies at 10, 12, 57, 66 and 69 keV.

5. The *remnant beam* which exposes the film has about one-fifth the intensity of the primary beam and carries *subject contrast*. About three-fourths of the remnant beam consists of *secondary radiation* produced in the patient.

6. The *prime factors* for radiography include exposure time, mA, kVp and SID.

7. All *variables* affecting radiographic image quality may be classified into six categories: Electrical factors, geometry, patient status, image receptor systems, processing, and viewing conditions.

REVIEW QUESTIONS

1. Name the type of tube which first used a heated cathode filament wire to "boil off" a constant source of electrons:

2. As a source of free electrons with which the anode will be bombarded to produce x-rays, the cathode filament wire is heated to "boil" them off. Name this process:

3. Why are x-rays produced when electrons are slowed down or stopped in the anode?

4. Describe the Bremsstrahlung interaction:

5. Sketch the characteristic interaction in two parts: 1st, the ionization of an anode atom, 2nd, the resulting orbital electron shift causing the x-ray:

6. What must you know about the orbital electron shells in an atom to be able to predict the energy of a characteristic x-ray photon produced there?

7. Why is Bremsstrahlung absolutely essential for there to be any subject contrast to produce an image?

8. Draw in the graph below a beam spectrum curve for an x-ray beam with filtration, set at 68 kVp and having characteristic interactions occur at 59 kVp:

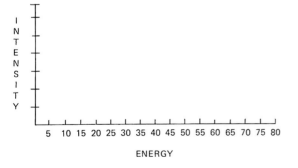

9. The intensity or amount of radiation in the remnant beam is what fraction or percentage of that in the primary beam?

10. What fraction or percentage of remnant beam reaching the film is actually primary radiation which did not interact with any atoms in the patient?

11. Define Primary Beam:

12. List the six general types of variables which affect the quality of the radiographic image:

13. X-rays are generally similar to light, but their wavelength is much _____, which enables them to penetrate materials that light cannot.

14. What are the three main components of the modern x-ray tube?

15. Why do modern x-ray tubes use rotating anodes?

16. Why are tungsten and rhenium used to coat the anode surface?

17. The average energy of a heterogeneous x-ray beam is about what fraction of its peak energy?

18. If the number of x-rays in the beam were doubled, how would it change the appearance of a graph of the x-ray beam spectrum—would the position of the curve shift to the right or left, would the amplitude shift higher or lower?

19. The difference in x-ray absorption properties between different types of tissues in the body is called _____.

20. The distance from the x-ray tube to the film cassette is abbreviated as _____.

21. List the four "prime factors" of radiography.

Chapter 2

RECORDING THE PERMANENT IMAGE

BEGINNINGS OF PHOTOGRAPHY

IN THE EARLY 18th century it became known that some silver compounds blackened when exposed to light; thus began the art of photography. In 1727, a German chemist, John H. Schultz, discovered that a paste of silver carbonate or chloride mixed with chalk became dark when it was exposed to light in a glass tube. After stencils of letters were placed on the tube and the material exposed to sunlight, black lettered images were seen when the stencils were removed. However, these images were only transient; since he knew of no way to make them permanent, the areas originally protected from light eventually darkened.

A crude camera was made in 1816 by Joseph N. Niepce from a jewel box in which a lens from a microscope was inserted. With this device, he secured an image. None of the images obtained could be made permanent. It was one thing to produce an image by exposing a silver salt to light. It was quite another to treat the image so that it would become permanent.

William Henry Fox Talbot, an Englishman, exposed silver chloride paper in a camera obscure to secure a visible image which was made permanent by treatment with sodium chloride. Talbot made an important discovery in 1840, when he found that he could develop a latent image after exposure of the silver layer. He obtained a negative image and by printing on sensitized paper was able to obtain positive images. Talbot became the inventor of the *negative-positive* method of photography. It is interesting to note that Sir John Herschel, an outstanding scientist of the period, wrote Talbot under the date of February 28, 1839, using the coined word "photography"–drawing with light–in referring to Talbot's work. He also coined the term *negative* and *positive* in reference to the photographic images. The word "photography" then was acquired by the vocabulary of all languages.

The Frenchman, Louis J. J. Daguerre, recorded images (1839) on plates covered with a silver salt that had been fumed with iodine to form a layer of silver iodide. Long exposures of these plates in a camera produced faint, unsatisfactory visual images. One day he placed one of the exposed plates in his cupboard. Upon removing the plate at a later date, he found that there was a well-defined positive image on the plate. Some mercury had been spilled in the cabinet and its fumes had "developed" the image completely. The unexposed silver iodide was removed by a solution of sodium chloride. Daguerre thereby discovered the phenomenon of development.

The invention of the gelatin silver bromide *dry* plate (September 8, 1871), by Richard L. Maddox of England served as the basis for modern photography. At first, dry plates were coated with silver by hand. The first mechanically coated glass plates were made in 1879 by George Eastman who had invented a plate-coating machine. Another product called *American Film* was introduced by Eastman in 1885. This was a stripping film which used paper as a temporary support for the emulsion. After exposure and processing, the paper was stripped away leaving a thin transparent "film" from which prints could be made. At this time also, Eastman began the manufacture of paper sensitized with an emulsion for use in cameras and called Eastman *Negative Paper.* After exposure and development, the paper was made transparent for printing by chemical treatment. In 1889, this firm introduced a flexible transparent base of nitrocellulose coated with a sensitive silver halide emulsion. This product served to advance photography greatly. Thenceforth, photosensitive materials became progressively more efficient as more knowledge concerning the science of photography accrued. Thus, the stage was set for one of man's most important discoveries wherein the photographic emulsion was to play a dominant role.

BIRTH OF RADIOGRAPHY

On November 8, 1895, Wilhelm Conrad Röntgen proved the existence of x-rays by exposing and processing a dry plate, thus opening to the world a vast new field of endeavor—radiography.

The moment of the actual discovery of the x-rays proved it to be the beginning of a new era. The very nature of the x-rays was such that the whole scientific and lay world would become absorbed in it, not alone by its very spectacular nature but also by the possibility that these new rays would open the door of knowledge to the ultimate nature of matter—something that had perplexed the best scientific minds. It was the dawn of the atomic age.

After the first few months of wild exaggeration and rumor, the discovery was stripped of its sensationalism and left to the conservative experimenter who rejoiced in the possibilities of this new discovery, for it opened to him a new field in which the reward of virgin labors could be obtained. These efforts he later found were based upon the sensitive dry plate which not alone proved the presence of the x-rays but also became the biggest factor in the ultimate development of the science of radiology.

Early Plates

At first the dry plate was used to record x-ray images but the exposures required were exceedingly long. Soon, manufacturers made plates that were more sensitive to the exposure effect of the x-rays—but they were still exceedingly slow and lacked the qualities now found in modern x-ray film. Another disadvantage of the dry plate used in those early days was that the glass of which they were made was easily broken. The development of an x-ray intensifying screen by Thomas Edison, which was composed of calcium tungstate fluorescent crystals, and its first use by Professor Michael Pupin of Columbia University, in 1896, served to augment the exposure effect of the x-rays when using glass plates, thereby extending the usefulness of the radiographic method in medicine. Until 1917, however, radiography was largely performed with fast photographic plates that were specially designed for x-ray work.

Early X-ray Film

During World War I, x-ray film was produced, but the sensitive emulsion coated only on one side of a sheet of cellulose nitrate caused excessive curl. It was also highly inflammable. The objectionable curl was shortly eliminated by coating the emulsion on *both* sides of the cellulose support. This treatment of the film gave it greater speed, and *two* x-ray intensifying screens could then be employed to further reduce the time of exposure. The quality of the film was also improved. In 1924, *safety* x-ray film was introduced. The film base upon which was coated the silver emulsion was made of cellulose acetate, a material that has the same slowburning properties of a like quantity of newsprint. Since that time, the quality and uniformity of film has been greatly enhanced. It is a far cry from the days of 1896 when a radiograph of a hand required an x-ray exposure of over an hour to the present time when only a fraction of a second is required.

MODERN X-RAY FILM

X-ray film is manufactured today with a remarkable consistency as to uniformity and quality so that its exposure and processing may be standardized. If you ever go through a film manufacturing plant, notice the utmost cleanliness and fine housekeeping that exists wherever film is made, handled and inspected. X-ray film consists of an *emulsion* of finely precipitated silver bromide crystals suspended in gelatin that is coated on *both* sides of a transparent blue-tinted polyester support called the *base*.

The emulsion coating is glued onto the film base with a thin layer of adhesive material. The emulsion is the functional part of the x-ray film, and consists of crystals of silver bromide suspended in *gelatin*. The properties of the gelatin are very important: It must be capable of suspending the crystals in a relatively even distribution, without allowing them to clump together or to settle out at the bottom layer. It must also be flexible and porous enough to allow processing chemicals to penetrate into it and reach the crystals. But, it must also not become too soft during processing or it will come off of the film base.

Figure 16. Diagram of the component layers of radiographic film: The polyester base, emulsion on either side, adhesive coats and protective T-coats.

Finally, the emulsion is protected from scratches by a thin coating of varnish called the supercoat or T-coat (tough-coating). The four component layers of the radiographic film are illustrated in Figure 16. Most film is *duplitized* or coated with emulsion on both sides, as shown in Figure 16. This is done so that it may be effectively used in screen cassettes which usually have screens on both the front and back covers of the cassette. Special "extremity" cassettes sometimes have only one screen. These are best used with single-emulsion film. When single emulsion film is loaded into such a cassette, the film emulsion must be facing and in contact with the screen. In the dark room lighting, the radiographer can recognize the emulsion side of the film as the *dull* surface. The glossy, shiny side of the film is the polyester base and has no emulsion. The dull surface should face the screen.

Examined under a microscope, countless tiny *crystals of silver bromide* are seen embedded within the gelatin (Figure 17). Silver bromide is a salt of silver which, when exposed to x-radiation, will begin to turn dark. The process is analogous to silverware which tarnishes from exposure to light over long periods of time. When the film is later chemically processed, this "tarnishing" of the exposed silver bromide crystals is completed to the point that they are entirely black (Figure 17).

The production and composition of x-ray film is more thoroughly described in Chapter 15, but this will serve as an introductory overview for the beginning student.

Figure 17. Photomicrograph (2500 X) of silver emulsion. (*Left*) Before exposure, the emulsion is seen to be made up of countless tiny crystals of silver bromide isolated from one another by gelatin. (*Right*) After exposure and development, the original crystals have been broken down to form clumps of black metallic silver.

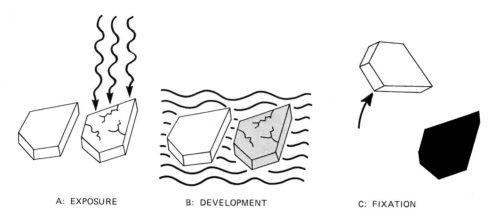

A: EXPOSURE   B: DEVELOPMENT   C: FIXATION

Figure 18. During exposure (A), x-rays cause several "fractures" or breaks in the structure of a silver bromide crystal. During processing (B), developer solution is able to penetrate deep into the "broken" crystals, converting them into black metallic silver. Unexposed crystals are intact and resist penetration by the developer solution. These intact crystals are later removed from the film by the fixer solution (C), while those converted into black silver remain on the film and form the visible image.

LATENT IMAGE FORMATION

As described in Chapter 1, x-rays are capable of ionizing matter, that is, they can cause orbital electrons to be "knocked out" of atoms. In the silver bromide crystals of an x-ray film, this removal of electrons can cause the molecules to break apart, separating the bromine from the silver. In simple terms, this damage may be thought of as cracks or "fractures" in the crystal at each point where an x-ray struck (Figure 18). Later, when the film is processed, the developing chemicals are able to recognize and "attack" those crystals already damaged by x-rays, but unable to penetrate those which are free of defects.

There are many hundreds of silver bromide molecules in one crystal, so these breaks caused by x-rays do not immediately transform the whole crystal. Rather, they break several silver atoms from the structure. These freed silver atoms tend to clump together at special locations on the crystal called "sensitization specks," forming small spots of metallic silver. These silver spots are not large enough to result in a visible, complete image. Therefore, upon exposure, a film will contain information which is not yet visible. This "invisible image" is called the *latent image.*

Although the latent image is not completely visible, the fact that a chemical change has occurred in the silver bromide crystals can be demonstrated with the following laboratory experiment:

EXPERIMENT:

You may need someone to assist by opening doors for you. In the dark room under red lighting only, remove one small x-ray film from the film bin. Hold it between your flattened hands, placing them directly opposite each other with fingers fanned. Make sure that each finger is directly opposite its counterpart on the other hand. Keeping your hands in place, exit the dark room and immediately hold the film up to an illuminator (viewbox) for a count of about ten. Quickly step back a few feet from the illuminator and have the group watch carefully as you remove both hands simultaneously. For a very brief few seconds, a lighter silhouette image of the hands will be visible.

Explanation: Those silver bromide crystals outside the hands had a latent image formed by the illuminator light. This image consisted of small spots of dark silver clumps on each crystal, making the emulsion outside the hands appear slightly darker. Upon removing your hands, the light in the room quickly causes those crystals which were previously covered to also form latent images, erasing the silhouette effect.

PROCESSING THE SILVER IMAGE

As clearly demonstrated in the foregoing experiment, the small clumps of silver which comprise the latent image are not sufficient to produce a fully visible, diagnostic image. To fully develop an image, chemical processing of the film is required.

Processing may be thought of as a chemical method of multiplying or exaggerating the effects of exposure. Those silver bromide crystals which have been "fractured" by x-rays will allow the processing chemicals to penetrate into their structure. The remaining molecules in these crystals will be broken down as the chemicals continue to separate silver atoms from bromine atoms. The free silver atoms will then adhere to the small silver spot (at the "sensitivity speck") which was originally formed from the exposure. Thus the small metallic silver spot is caused to grow many thousands of times larger, forming blackened areas on the radiograph which are visible to the naked eye.

The processing chemicals recognize and attack only those silver bromide crystals which have already been damaged by exposure to the x-ray beam, Figure 18-B.

Crystals that were not exposed are later washed away by "fixer" chemicals, Figure 18-C.

A review of Figure 14 reminds us that under dense tissues such as bone, few x-rays reach the film. In such areas, few crystals will be damaged, and therefore not many crystals will be chemically developed into clumps of black metallic silver. Rather, these crystals are washed away by fixer chemicals, resulting in light or "white" areas on the film. However, under soft tissue areas, many x-rays reach the film, causing "fractures" in the crystals. Those crystals are later recognized and attacked by developer chemicals, ultimately turning them into clumps of black silver which remain on the film after processing. This final image composed of black metallic silver is called the *visible image.*

The chemistry of latent image formation and of visible image formation is fully described in Chapters 15 and 36. The following "resume" of image production, along with Figure 18, should serve to review and clarify the basic concepts of radiographic exposure and processing.

RESUME OF IMAGE PRODUCTION

When the exposed emulsion is considered as a whole rather than as its constituent silver bromide crystals, the various stages in the production of the silver image can be diagrammatically illustrated as in Figure 19. Let us assume that an object (A)

X-RAY BEAM

Step Wedge

6

5

4

3

2

1

A

Film

B

Latent Image

6

5

4

3

2

1

Unexposed
Emulsion

C

Developed Silver Image

6

5

4

3

2

1

Undeveloped
Unexposed
Emulsion

D

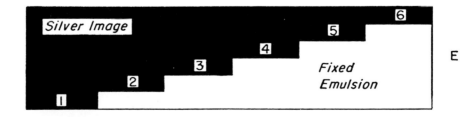

Silver Image

6

5

4

3

2

1

Fixed
Emulsion

E

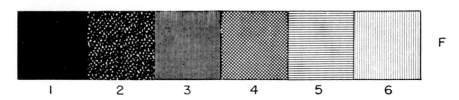

1   2   3   4   5   6

F

in the form of an aluminum step wedge is correctly exposed using an x-ray film (B) as the recording medium. When the film is represented in enlarged cross section, a latent image of the object is produced upon exposure in the silver bromide emulsion (C). The latent image is represented by the dotted area and consists of representations of the six portions of the wedge. The radiation reaching the film is of varying intensity after its passage through the various thicknesses of the wedge and the relative absorption of each thickness is represented.

The radiation passing through step number 1 of the object (A) is only partially absorbed, hence more silver bromide is exposed than that portion of the film under steps No. 4 or No. 6 wherein greater absorption takes place. Hence, upon development, the quantity of silver deposited in these areas is less than under step number 1. In other words, each step is recorded as a deposit of silver that is proportionate to the intensity of the emergent radiation reaching the film.

Upon development (D), the latent image silver bromide is reduced to metallic silver and the unexposed silver bromide (thin diagonal lines) is not affected. (Mixed with the metallic silver deposits are unexposed and undeveloped silver bromide crystals.) After the film has been treated as in fixation (E), all the unexposed and undeveloped silver bromide is dissolved from the emulsion and the metallic silver remains on the film to constitute the radiographic image of the step wedge shown in (A). When the radiographic image (F) is later viewed on an x-ray illuminator, all the various deposits of silver representing the steps of the wedge are seen in their proper silver concentration with various degrees of translucency to the transmission of light from the illuminator.

←

Figure 19. "Life cycle of a radiograph:" (A) Exposure of a step wedge and x-ray film (B) creates a latent image (C). During processing, the developer solution attacks only the exposed silver bromide crystals (D), which are changed to black metallic silver. The fixer solution then removes the unexposed and undeveloped crystals (E). The final image seen as seen on the x-ray illuminator appears as various quantities of black silver on the clear base (F).

SUMMARY

1 A *latent image* is produced on an x-ray film when incident x-ray photons *ionize* portions of a silver bromide crystal, releasing free silver atoms to collect around a *sensitivity speck*.

2. During *development*, reducing chemicals attack the exposed crystals to complete the process of breaking all of the silver atoms free from the bromine atoms to coagulate around the sensitivity speck and form a clump of *black metallic silver*.

3. Unexposed crystals, having few or no *breaks* in their lattice structure, resist development and are removed from the film during the fixing process.

REVIEW QUESTIONS

1. When x-rays were discovered, film had already been largely developed in the field of:

2. Instead of film, early radiographs were taken on:

3. What are the component layers of an x-ray film:

4. Define Latent Image:

5. What is a modern x-ray film base made of:

6. Define Chemical Development:

7. What are the crystals in the film emulsion made of prior to development?

8. What are the crystals left on the surface of the film after development made of?

9. What material is used to hold the emulsion crystals in an evenly-distributed suspension?

Chapter 3

QUALITIES OF THE RADIOGRAPHIC IMAGE

COMPONENTS OF THE IMAGE

WHAT ARE THE ESSENTIAL requirements for your eyes to be able to see? The first and most obvious answer is that they need light. But, consider what light is. Light is the flow of small bundles of energy called quanta or photons; it is a part of the same electromagnetic spectrum as x-rays are. In fact, the only real difference between x-rays and light is the length of their waves.

VISIBILITY

What you *see* is actually reflected light photons striking the nerve endings in the retina of your eyes. When twice as many photons strike your eye, the image you see appears twice as bright. It is more intense. Thus, the amount of light photons flowing toward your eyes, or the number of photons striking your retina, is referred to as the *intensity* of the light. When the light intensity is very low, you cannot recognize your surroundings, because much of the information in the actual image is not visible.

However, adequate light alone does not provide vision or create an image. Suppose that everything in your field of view was the same white light and all at the same intensity or brightness. You would be just as blind seeing blank white as you would if everything was pitch darkness. In order to see, there must be differing shades of brightness and darkness within your field of view. The greater the difference is between the shade of an object and the shade of the surrounding field of view, the easier it is to see the object. A pure black object against a white background, for example, is a most visible combination. This difference between intensities of reflected light is called *contrast*. For contrast to exist, hence for any image at all to exist, there must be two or more different intensities present. If the differences between the intensities is great, then the image is regarded as having *high contrast*. Some contrast is required for any image to exist.

However, it is possible for an image to have *too much* contrast. This situation is illustrated by the photographs in Figure 20. In photograph A, note that you cannot distinguish the edges between the girl's blouse and the background wall, the edges between the stuffed animal and the girl's blouse, or the ruffles in the blouse. These details are visible in photograph *B*. Photograph *A* possesses extremely high contrast—everything in the image tends to be reduced to either black or white, with very few intermediate shades of gray. Objects that should have been depicted as a very light gray, such as the ruffles and shadows of the blouse, are recorded instead as white, and are not discernable against a background of white. Likewise, dark gray objects are depicted as black and will not be distinguishable against a black background. This image has less visible details in it than photograph *B*. Excessive contrast has caused a loss of useful information.

On the other hand, insufficient contrast leads to an image that is not adequately visible. If there is barely any difference between two adjacent shades of gray, it will be difficult for the human eye to detect that there are indeed two shades there. If these gray shades cannot be distinguished from each other, information is again lost. Photograph *C* in Figure 20 demonstrates insufficient contrast, with an overall gray appearance. Note that the subtle dark gray shades of leaves under the bench, visible in photograph *B*, are not as visible in photograph *C*, because there is little difference between them and the dark shadow of the bench.

To summarize, note that the greatest amount of information in Figure 20 is found in photograph *B*, where the contrast level is intermediate. If contrast is too high, gray shades are exaggerated into white or black, and information is lost. If contrast is too low, different gray shades that lie next to each other become difficult to distinguish, and again, information is lost. Excessive contrast can cause as great a loss of information as a lack of contrast. The ideal amount of contrast to maximize the information in an image lies in an intermediate range and is somewhat subject to personal preference.

The word *optimum* is used to describe the ideal level of contrast that an image should have. It refers to an intermediate level which is neither too much nor too little. In radiographic imaging, the goal is not to produce *maximum* contrast, nor *minimum* contrast, but rather to produce *optimum* contrast. The same term should be used to describe the ideal intensity of light for an image: Too little light would be pitch dark,

too much would blind us. The ideal amount of light is a medium amount that we would refer to as *optimum intensity*.

One more factor affects the visibility of an object in your field of view: If it is raining heavily between yourself and the object, you may not be able to see it well. The rain represents unwanted information which obstructs the visibility of the wanted information. Undesirable information that interferes with the subject of interest is referred to as *noise*. Interference and static on your TV screen are examples of noise in an image. In radiography, fogging of the film by heat or light, static discharges and artifacts from foreign objects (several of which are illustrated in Chapters 38-39) are forms of noise. The most common form of image noise in radiography is fogging of the film by random radiation known as *scatter*.

These three functions–intensity, contrast and noise–are the *visibility functions* of an image. Maximum visibility is attained when light intensity and contrast are optimized and when noise is kept at a minimum.

RECOGNIZABILITY

In addition to the visibility functions of an image, there are *recognizability functions*. A visible image is completely worthless unless the information in it is capable of being recognized. We depend upon the geometrical integrity of the image to recognize what real object it represents. If the image is blurry, or if it's size or shape is grossly distorted, we may not be able to tell what it is, even though it is visible. Recognizability or geometrical integrity is made up of three components: sharpness of recorded detail, magnification and shape distortion.

Figure 20. Photographs demonstrating (A) high contrast with short gray scale, (B) medium contrast with longer gray scale, and (C) low contrast with excessive gray scale. Note that details visible in the stuffed animal, blouse and sidewalk disappear with excessive contrast (A). Darker gray details in the leaves, the shadow under the bench and the girl's eyebrows disappear with excessive gray scale (C). Also, note that high contrast can deceptively mimic underexposure: Photograph A appears light at a glance, yet the shadow under the bench is actually *darker* than that in B. The overall density of Photograph A is *not* light, rather, it possesses excessive contrast.

Sharpness of Recorded Detail

Sharpness of recorded detail may be described as the *abruptness* with which the edges of a particular image *stop*. To better visualize this principle, imagine yourself moving across a black-and-white photograph, perhaps in a microscopic sports car: You are passing from a white image onto a black background. If you suddenly find yourself over the black part, the edge of the white image was sharp and *stopped* abruptly. If you gradually pass from white to gray to black, then the edge of the white image is blurred and is not sharp.

Theoretically, if shadows could be cast from a *point* source of light, there would never be any blur. There would be a single, pure shadow with sharp edges. But when the source of light is an *area* such as the sun or a flashlight bulb (or an x-ray tube focal spot), there will always be partial shadows cast around the edges of the *pure* shadow. This occurs because the shadow of any given edge of the object is projected at several different angles from several different points within the area of the light source.

Figure 21 illustrates this effect. Note that when the light comes from a single point, a pure shadow with sharp edges is projected behind the object. However, single point sources of light are not found in nature. The sun, for example, has a surface *area*, and light can be emitted from many different regions across that area. This means that the shadow of a particular edge of the object will be projected by different beams of light coming from different angles. The edge of the shadow will then be projected onto the background in more than one place, resulting in an unsharp appearance called *blur*.

The *pure* shadow of an object is named

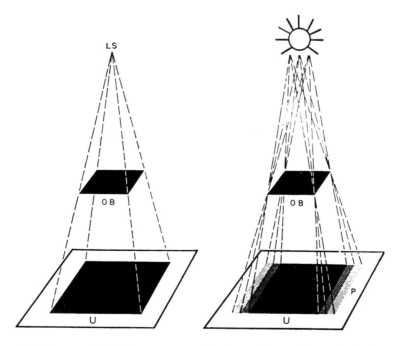

Figure 21. Diagram illustrating a pure umbra image from a theoretical point source of light (*left*) compared to the production of penumbra (p) at the edges of a shadow image by an area light source such as the sun or the x-ray tube anode (*right*).

its *umbra*. The partial shadow of the edge of an object is called its *penumbra*. Penumbra is synonymous with blur—the more penumbra that is present, the more blurry the edge appears. To demonstrate umbra and penumbra, hold your hand over an over head projector or in front of a flashlight, move it away from the light and then toward the light and observe the shadow cast. As you move your hand back and forth from the light source, you will see the blurry penumbra at the edges grow and shrink. Note that the penumbra does not only grow outward but also inward, causing the umbra portion to shrink. With enough penumbra present, you would not be able to recognize the image as the shadow of your hand.

Now consider the problems caused with recognizability when observing a very blurry image of two closely adjacent objects. As penumbra grows, the edges of the two images recorded will blur into each other and overlap. The penumbra also replaces a portion of the umbra, so that the umbra diminishes in size. When two shadows overlap in this way, they may appear as one shadow of one object, even though there are really two objects.

Since increasing penumbra invades the umbra, it is even possible for an image to deteriorate until it is all penumbra and virtually no umbra, effectively disappearing, with only a nebulous area of blurry density left in the area of the image.

Sharpness may be destroyed not only by the geometrical growth of penumbra but also by blurring due to motion. An example of motion blurring of the hand is found in Figure 33. Sharpness of recorded detail has a strong impact upon our ability to recognize images.

Magnification

Excessive magnification of the size of an image may make it difficult to recognize what real object the image represents. It is hard to tell what kind of a building you are looking at when you are standing one inch from the wall. In photography and in radiography, *magnification* may be defined as the difference between the size of a real object and the size of its image on the *picture*. Magnification is often referred to as *size distortion* and classified under the general heading of *distortion*. However, for the sake of clarity, the word *distortion* shall be used in this book only with regard to changes in the apparent shape of an image. *Magnification* shall be consistently used to describe changes in the size of the image.

Figure 22. Diagram demonstrating shape distortion. Misalignment or angling of a beam of light will project the shadow of a square object as a distorted rectangular image.

Shape Distortion

Shape distortion is defined as the difference between the shape of a real object and the shape of its image on a radiograph or photograph. In a given axis of direction, shape distortion will consist of either a foreshortening of the image or an elongation of the image. When a square object, for example, is projected onto a two dimensional film as a rectangular shadow due to angling or off-centering of the camera or x-ray tube, the true nature of the object is not recognizable and information recorded on the film may be misleading and misinterpreted (Figure 22).

Good recognizability or geometrical integrity in an image is determined, then, by maximum sharpness of detail and minimum magnification and shape distortion.

When visibility and recognizability of all of the details in an image are optimized, the greatest amount of information is provided.

QUALITIES OF THE RADIOGRAPH

The image on a radiograph must have all of the same qualities as an image you visually see–intensity, contrast, noise, sharpness of detail, magnification and distortion of shape. But, since a radiograph works differently than your eyes, some of these qualities are given different specific names. Also, each quality has its opposite, which must be named and learned about in order to critique the quality of radiographs.

DENSITY VERSUS TONE VALUE

First, the "background" intensity on a radiograph is actually a transparent *white* shade—you see the light shining through its transparent plastic base. The image on it consists of blackened deposits of metallic silver left on the film after processing. The darkest areas represent the greatest exposure (intensity) of radiation striking the film. The amount of blackening present at any given point on the film is referred to as its *density*. Thus, a very dark film is regarded as having high density, and a lighter film as having low density. The densities on a film indicate the intensity of the beam of radiation which penetrated the patient and struck the film.

During their passage through a body part, the x-rays are absorbed selectively by various tissue components. This absorption results in the production of a number of *different* silver deposits on the radi-

ograph. Obviously, the greater the number of tones present (correct tone rendition), the greater the number of structural details that can be visualized in the image.

Under standard conditions of illumination, highlights possessing little silver show little detail, and are diagnostically worthless. Also, areas of overexposure may be considered diagnostically useless since the opaqueness of the silver deposit obscures image details when the radiograph is viewed before the light from a standard x-ray illuminator (see Figure 23).

Figure 23. Series of radiographs demonstrating results of underexposure (A), correct exposure (B), and overexposure (C). Note the loss of visible details in the bones at both extremes.

The opposite of density is *tone value*. Tone value refers to the amount of light (from an illuminator, for example) that is able to pass through the film at a given point and strike your eyes. If there is less silver deposited in an area of the film, more light will shine through it, it will appear *whiter* or clearer and has a high tone value. High tone value, then, is the same thing as low density. A device called a densitometer is used to measure the densities on radiographic films. What this device actually does is to detect the amount of light passing through the film at a certain point. So it really measures tone value and then *converts* the measurement into a density reading algebraically. The density values read off of a densitometer range from 0 to 4.0, with a reading of 0 indicating that all of the light striking the film passes through it, and a reading of 4.0 indicating a pitch black density with virtually no light passing through.

Since neither blank white areas nor pitch black areas on the radiograph contain useful information, those densities that might be considered as "useful" range from a very light gray shade (slightly darker than the film base) to a very dark gray shade just short of black. *This range of useful densities extends from 0.25 to 2.5 as measured on a densitometer.*

CONTRAST VERSUS GRAY SCALE

Radiographic *contrast* is the proportional difference between two adjacent densities, measured as a ratio, not as a subtracted difference. If one density is twice as dark as the adjacent density, the contrast would be measured as 2/1 or 2. A very contrasty radiograph appears to be more *black and white*, whereas a low-contrast radiograph appears to be gray overall. Figure 24 shows how density levels can change without contrast being affected. Note that as long as all densities on the film increase or decrease by the same proportion, the ratios of difference between them remain the same and contrast is equal.

The opposite of radiographic contrast is *gray scale*. There is considerable confusion about the difference between contrast and scale, primarily because of the terminology commonly used. The term *contrast scale* is sometimes used, but combining the word *contrast* with *scale* seems contradictory and is certainly confusing. This book shall consistently utilize the terms *gray scale* or *scale* to refer to this image quality.

Radiographic gray scale is the *range* of different densities present in an image. When there are many different shades of density (many grays), the radiograph has long scale. Conversely, when few densities are present, the radiograph has short scale. To understand the relationship between contrast and gray scale, consider a 10-foot-high staircase. The staircase may be built to have 10 individual stairs, each one being one foot tall, or it may be built to have only five individual stairs. If there are

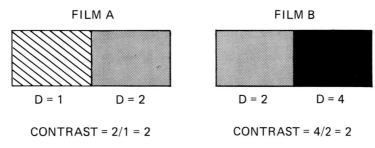

FILM A — D = 1, D = 2, CONTRAST = 2/1 = 2
FILM B — D = 2, D = 4, CONTRAST = 4/2 = 2

Figure 24. Diagram illustrating a change in density without a change in contrast. The *ratio* of difference between the two adjacent densities remains the same even though *Film B* is twice as dense overall. An image can be darker and still have high contrast.

SHORT SCALE

Figure 25. Step wedge diagram and PA chest radiograph illustrating short gray scale.

SHORT WAVELENGTH
PRIMARY
RADIATION

STEP WEDGE

REMNANT
RADIATION

AGGREGATE OF
SILVER DEPOSIT
ON X-RAY FILM

RADIOGRAPHIC
IMAGE AS SEEN
ON ILLUMINATOR

LONG SCALE

Figure 26. Step wedge diagram and PA chest radiograph illustrating long gray scale.

only five stairs, each one must be two feet tall–there is a greater difference between the stairs. A greater difference from one stair to the next results in fewer total stairs. Conversely, if there are many stairs, there must be a smaller degree of difference from one to the next. With this staircase concept in mind, examine the *aggregate silver deposits* diagrammed in Figures 25 and 26. High contrast implies short scale, because when there are great differences between densities, there can only be a few densities present (Figure 25). With low contrast, there will be long scale (Figure 26).

A good radiograph is one that possesses a correct balance of densities (gradation) over the entire gray scale. The contrast should be such that, with prevailing exposure technics, good differentiation is shown between tissue details portrayed over the whole area of diagnostic interest, without loss of detail in the lighter or darker areas of the radiographic image.

The scale of densities that determines the contrast and the visibility of details is directly influenced by the x-ray wave length which, in turn, is regulated by the factor of kilovoltage. This fact is also demonstrated by Figures 25 and 26. An aluminum step-wedge is shown being irradiated by x-rays; the exposed x-ray film in enlarged cross section is shown beneath the step-wedge; and the resulting radiographic image as it appears when viewed on the illuminator is depicted below the film cross section in both illustrations.

Short Scale

In the diagram (Figure 25) it is assumed that long wave length radiation is directed toward a step- wedge. The radiation easily penetrates step No. 1 and the remnant radiation strongly affects the silver emulsion. Upon development, a radiographic density representing step No. 1 is produced. This density appears opaque when viewed on the illuminator. Step No. 2 is also easily penetrated and although the intensity of the remnant radiation is somewhat reduced by absorption, another opaque density is produced. The radiation is greatly absorbed by step No. 3 resulting in remnant radiation of such low intensity that a translucent density with a gray tone is produced. The x-rays traversing step No. 4 are largely absorbed and the remnant radiation has just sufficient intensity to produce a density with a light gray tone. The radiation passing to steps Nos. 5 and 6 is almost totally absorbed and the film covered by this area is not exposed because there is too little remnant radiation. Differentiation between densities Nos. 1 and 2 representing the thin portion of the wedge cannot be made when the image is viewed on the illuminator. The film area that should contain details of steps Nos. 5 and 6 is devoid of silver, hence, there is no image. Steps Nos. 3 and 4 are represented by two densities of different tone value. A representative image of the entire wedge was not recorded because of an inadequacy of remnant radiation. Note that the differences between densities are wide and that the number of densities are too few to portray a complete image of the subject.

This diagram illustrates the fact that radiographic details of an object cannot be seen in the image unless there are discernible differences in tone value between densities and that there must be a silver deposit on the film if a detail within the object is to be demonstrated. The above situation is typical for *short scale* or high contrast.

When an image of a body part is rendered with densities that are either excessive or virtually nonexistent with a short range of widely different intermediate translucent densities, short scale exists. Such radiographs are pictorially pleasing to look at, for they possess instant eye appeal but they have little diagnostic worth and are economically wasteful.

When low kilovoltage is used for thin tissue parts such as the hand, elbow, etc., greater contrast occurs between the bones and the flesh. In fact, a point may be reached in which the thinner portions such as the skin and subcutaneous tissues and even some muscle detail are obliterated by opaque silver deposits; and, some bone detail may also be lost because the denser bone tissue absorbs so much radiation that little remnant radiation reaches the film. Even when exposures are increased to impractical limits by the mAs factor in order to obtain satisfactory bone detail, opaque silver deposits will still obscure details of the less dense fleshy areas.

On the other hand, when the exposure is decreased to exhibit flesh details satisfactorily, then osseous details are lost. In other words, as kilovoltage is decreased, the number of intermediate tones diminishes and the over-all amount of information diminishes in the same ratio. So only those details in the image produced by exposure factors that happen to be optimum for the area are rendered with maximum visibility and the remainder of the image becomes diagnostically useless.

There are occasions when it seems advisable to shorten the gray scale in a specific area but when this is done, there is always that danger of losing detail visibility in other adjacent areas. On the whole, the entire image exhibiting short scale is invariably incomplete, for details that represent the thinner and thicker portions of the body part are not always shown. Short scale has its place only as a special procedure and in more adequately visualizing details of *small* tissue areas and then only after preliminary survey radiographs have been made. Typical examples of short scale are shown in Figure 27.

Long Scale

Portraying the same situation as shown in Figure 25, but using *shorter wave length radiation*, the diagram, Figure 26, exhibits a

Figure 27. Typical radiographs exhibiting various degrees of short gray scale.

Figure 28. Typical radiographs exhibiting long gray scale. An abundance of details is shown because the kilovoltages used were optimum to penetrate the various tissues present.

different result. The radiation readily penetrates all portions of the wedge and the selective degree of absorption by each step has permitted remnant radiation to emerge with different intensities that are recorded as separate translucent densities. These densities of varying tone value represent the several steps in the wedge. The transition between tones is gradual and each tone is distinctive. The image is completely informative and is typical of long scale. Desirable long scale is produced when the kilovoltage is adjusted to delineate all normal structures satisfactorily. Absorption of radiation by the silver bromide crystals decreases as the kilovoltage increases and when exposures are correct there is little opportunity to produce excessive densities in the image.

In the case of human radiography, when the scale of densities representing a departure from the normal occurs, the image becomes open to pathologic or physiologic suspicion. In the final analysis, the criterion of good diagnostic contrast is whether one sees all one expects to see. Compare the radiographs shown in Figures 25 and 26 with the photographs in Figure 20.

Long scale is characterized by a large number of translucent densities of varying tone value, each of which represents some structural element of the part examined. The transition between tones is gradual. Long scale makes possible visualization of small units of image density. The short wave length radiation employed effects greater penetration of the tissues resulting in an abundance of remnant radiation of varying intensity that, in turn, produces a large number of translucent densities (Figure 26). The gray scale, however, should never be so long that differentiation between structures is difficult. If the maximum of diagnostic information is to be obtained in the survey film, a compromise must be made between the radiograph with short scale or that exhibiting the longer scale. Typical examples of long scale are shown in Figure 28.

A medium level of contrast will allow the most information to be visible on a radiograph. Too much contrast can cause the loss of information, just as too much gray scale can do the same.

Figure 29 uses magnetic resonance images of the spine to illustrate these important concepts: Images **A** and **B** both have too short of a gray scale (excessive contrast). **A** was taken with a lighter overall, density level, and **B** with a much darker setting, in order to show that *the use of a lighter or darker technique does not correct the image when gray scale is insufficient.* Images **C** and **D** were taken with long gray scale, using similar density settings. Although **C** is light and **D** is dark, *both* of these images demonstrate more details and more information than **A** or **B** The ideal image would be a relatively long gray scale image with a density level intermediate between **C** and **D**.

FOG AND OTHER NOISE

On foggy days, details of the out-of-doors are obscured. The mist in the air scatters the light more or less evenly over a landscape so that it may be difficult to differentiate one object from another. However, on a clear day the same landscape can be seen distinctly. When a primary beam of x-rays traverses an object, some of the x-rays are absorbed while others pass directly through it; a considerable percentage, however, is scattered in all directions by the atoms of the material struck—very much as light is dispersed by a mist (Figure 30). These secondary rays comprise what is known as *scatter radiation* and are radiographically effective. Scatter radiation strikes the film from random directions and produces a. fairly uniform

Figure 29. Magnetic resonance images of the lateral spine showing (A) short gray scale and light density, (B) short gray scale and dark density, (C) long gray scale and light density, and (D) long gray scale and dark density. More details are visible in the long gray scale images.

deposit of silver over an entire image. This veil of silver overlays the image density produced by the remnant radiation and is, in reality, a form of noise known as scatter *fog.* When fog is present, the effect is as if image details were being viewed through a mist. In other words, the quality of the image is degraded. Radiographic examples of scattered radiation fog are shown in Figure 31. Observe (1) the characteristic dull gray appearance of the images and (2) the absence of important details.

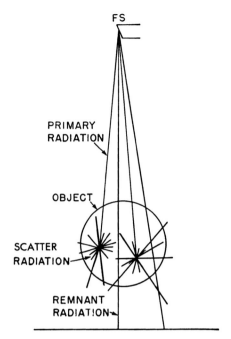

Figure 30. Diagram illustrating manner in which scatter radiation is generated when x-rays strike any form of matter. Scatter radiation is random in its direction, and destructive to the image.

Virtually the whole question of radiographic quality is related to the effect of scatter radiation fog on the visualization of detail. Its effect is greatest on those elements of an object that are farthest from the film. Visibility of these details may be greatly lessened and on occasion they may not even appear in the image. By controlling the amount of scatter radiation reaching the film during an exposure, details become more pronounced with resultant improvement in image quality. Rendition of all anatomic details, then, becomes more in accord with the actual absorption properties of the tissues irradiated. Also, reduction in fog makes possible easier visualization of details representing small differences on tissue absorption.

The scatter radiation reaching the film has more of the quality of the longer wave lengths (lesser penetration) than the remnant radiation. Its intensity is modified either (1) by the *absorbing action* of the tissues through which it must pass, or (2) by the *distance* from the film to its origin in the tissues. Scatter radiation originates from a multiplicity of sources and is, therefore, unfocused and random. Even with present-day accessories, it is not always possible to control it completely. The supplemental density superimposed by this radiation on the image is like a veil; it actually increases the over-all density of the image and limits the ability to see radiographic details clearly. In fact *a desirable range of densities (gray scale) is usually destroyed and important detail is obscured by this common form of image noise.*

Gray Scale, Fog and Density

It is essential to understand that every "gray" radiograph is not necessarily fogged. Long gray scale is often desirable in an image. Fog is never desirable. Yet, both make the image appear more "gray." Long gray scale can improve the image, or in excessive amounts it can degrade the image, but fog is *always* destructive.

When gray scale is increased, contrast is reduced. But, when fogging occurs, *both gray scale and contrast are reduced.* This is possible because fog is a *blanket* of density which covers every useful density on the radiograph. Therefore, those densities which should have been a very light gray shade are completely lost to the image as the fog darkens them, and there are less densities altogether present. This is more fully discussed in Chapter 12.

It is quite easy to confuse an overexposed *burned-out* radiograph with a fogged radiograph, so it is important to understand that a darker film is not necessarily a *fogged* one. Fogging is caused by scattered radiation. It is possible to simply overexpose a

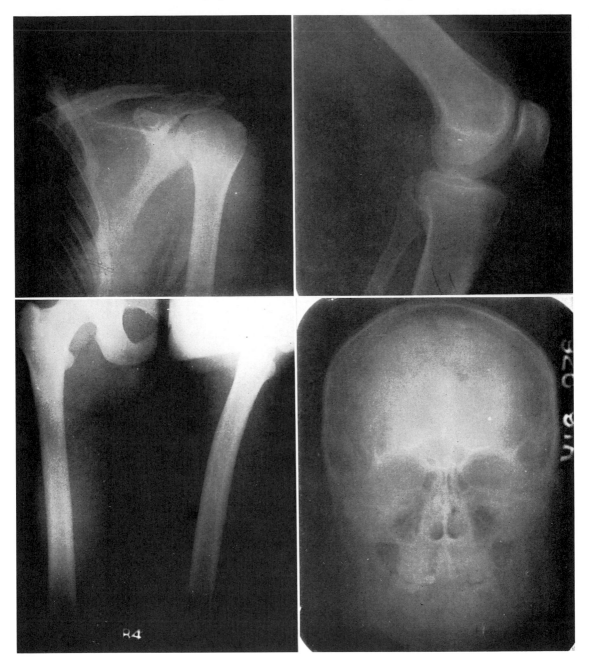

Figure 31. Radiographs exhibiting evidence of scatter radiation fog. Note the general loss of detail visualization because of degraded contrast.

film with too much radiation without scatter levels changing. Figure 32 shows the difference between an overexposed radiograph and a fogged radiograph. Note that a fogged radiograph is not necessarily very dark but can be quite light and still present a *washed*-out gray, low-contrast appearance. An excessively dark film may be simply

Figure 32. Radiographs demonstrating the difference in appearance between an overexposed image (A) and a fogged image (B). Note that a fogged image can actually be lighter in density, as within the orbits and at the top of this skull.

overexposed, or it may be both overexposed and fogged.

Artifacts

Any impertinent, useless, grossly distorted, or false information which obscures the useful details in an image may be referred to as *noise.* Scatter fog has already been described as the most common form of radiographic noise. In addition, a radiograph may be fogged from exposure to white light or excessive exposure to darkroom safelights, or it may be *chemically* fogged from excessive temperatures, excessive development times, or improper solution concentrations during processing.

Many other artifacts too numerous to list here constitute forms of image noise. A few examples are torn paper or dirt inside screen cassettes, iodine or barium spilled onto sponges or patient gowns, removable objects in or on the patient such as hairpins, dentures and jewelry, scratches and splashed chemicals on the film.

Static electricity discharges on the film can be caused from rough handling, pressure from stacking boxes of film on their sides rather than on end, automatic film conveyor systems and low humidity. These discharges cause branching or radiating black exposure marks on the finished radiograph, one of the most common and destructive types of artifacts. Another type of artifact which is often misunderstood is the *false* image. False images are images created by patient motion, tomographic movements or other geometrical anomalies that blur and superimpose true images into each other. Although these images are often referred to as distorted images, it should be clarified that they are newly *created* images which do not represent any real anatomical object at all and, therefore, are completely *false*. Further discussion, examples and illustrations of these types of artifacts are found in Chapters 34, 38 and 39.

Regardless of origins or causes, all of these artifacts obscure the visibility of the useful portions of the radiographic image and, therefore, constitute image noise.

GEOMETRICAL INTEGRITY

An image must have geometrical integrity with the object that it represents in order to be recognizable. That is, it must have close to the same size and shape as the real object, and it must not be blurred into the surrounding details, or else it might be mistaken for some other object. Hence, *geometrical integrity* refers to the recognizability of an image.

The most important component of geometrical integrity is the *sharpness* of recorded detail. As previously described, sharpness is the abruptness of image edges. Sharpness may also be described as the *lack* of penumbra or blur at image edges. In Figure 33, a radiograph demonstrating blur due to motion shows blurred edges and loss of details in the bones of the hand.

In radiography, a very common misconception occurs when the *visibility* of edges is confused with the *sharpness* of edges in an image. Compare the two chest radiographs in Figures 25 and 26 and see if you can determine which radiograph has sharper

Figure 33. Radiograph of the hand showing blurred edges of bones and loss of details within the bones due to motion.

edges between the ribs and the background lung density. The answer is that they are both equally sharp. High-contrast radiographs are not only deceptively appealing to the human eye but they also create the *false* impression that they are sharper. The longer-scale radiograph is not blurred, and the edges of the ribs have no more penumbra present than those in the short-scale radiograph. They *stop* just as abruptly. However, the rib edges in the long-scale radiograph are less *visible* than those in the short-scale version, because they possess less contrast, which is a visibility function. Edges of image details, just like all of the other parts of the image, have both visibility and recognizability components. Edges that are more visible must not be construed as necessarily being sharper. Conversely,

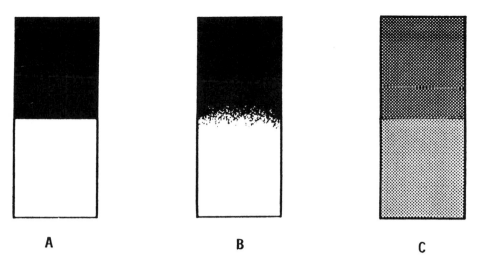

A   **B**   **C**

Figure 34. Blur versus fog. Image A shows no blur and no fog. Image B shows blurring, but with high contrast since there is no fog, while image C shows poor contrast due to fog, but with high sharpness at the edge of these densities, since there is no blur.

penumbra or blur must not be confused with fog.

Figure 34 illustrates the difference between unsharpness (blur) and poor contrast such as might be caused by fog. In this illustration, **A** shows a high contrast image with a sharp edge between the two densities. In **B**, the high contrast is still present, but the edge is blurry, gradually changing from one density to the other. In **C**, very poor contrast causes the edge between the two densities to become less *visible*, but it is still sharp, because it "stops" abruptly. Blur is not present in **C**.

Geometrical penumbra and motion are the two most important causes of blur or unsharpness. Blur may also be caused by poorly constructed film and intensifying screens, referred to as "materials unsharpness," or by absorption defects at the edges of an object. These special types of blur are discussed in later chapters. To summarize the types of unsharpness, they are (1) geometrical penumbra, (2) absorption penumbra (see chapter 24), (3) motion unsharpness and (4) materials unsharpness.

Magnification of a radiographic image can also be quantitatively measured by detecting a difference between its size and the actual object's size in *both dimensions or axes*, lengthwise *and* crosswise. If the length or width of the image is equal to the same measurement on the real object, no magnification is present. In a magnified image, both the length and the width of the image will measure larger than the object by equal proportions. For magnification to be present, the *umbral* portion of the image must increase in size. When the penumbra expands *without* the umbra increasing, the image is not magnified but only blurred.

If the length of an image should measure differently than the length of the real object it represents while its width is unchanged, the image is *shape distorted*, it is not magnified. The shape of an object might be grossly represented as the ratio between its length and its width. For example, if the length and width are equal, their ratio would be 1:1 and you might have a square or a circle shape. If the length is twice as long as the width, however, their ratio

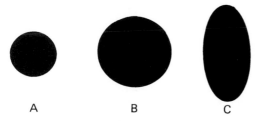

A B C

Figure 35. Diagram showing difference between magnification and shape distortion. If image measurement changes in *both* axes (length and width) equally, a magnified but still circular image results. Only when one axis changes *more* than the other does shape distortion occur, producing an oval shadow in this case.

would be 2:1 and you might have a rectangle or an ellipse shape. The shape only changes when this ratio changes.

For example, the radiographic "shadow" of a spherical object will be a circle with equal width and "length," having a *shape ratio* of 1:1, Figure 35-A. Suppose that the circular image measures *both* 20 per cent longer and 20 per cent wider than the real object. The *shape ratio* of the image is now 1.2:1.2 = 1:1 = 1. The ratio of length to width is unchanged from that of the real object, and there is *no shape distortion* present. There is, however, *magnification.* The image is larger, but still has the same circular shape, Figure 35-B.

For *shape distortion* to be present, one dimension (axis) of the image must be changed by a different proportion than the other dimension. Length must change *more* than width, or vice versa. In Figure 35-C, the *width* of the image measures the same as the original width in *A*, but the *length* of the image is increased. If the length is doubled, the new *shape ratio* (length/width) is 2:1 = 2. This is different from the original shape ratio of 1, and indicates that distortion has occurred. If the length were cut in half while the width remained at 1, the new shape ratio would be 1/2:1 = 1/2, again indicating shape distortion. Any time one

dimension or axis of the image changes differently than another, the result will be a different shape.

Suppose that *both* the length and width increase, but the *length* grows three times longer while the width only doubles. The new shape ratio is 3:2 = 1.5, and shape distortion has occurred. In this case, however, magnification has *also* occurred because *both* dimensions were increased. This image was both magnified and distorted.

Specifically, if the image measures longer in one axis than the real object, it is said to have *elongation* distortion. If it measures shorter in *one* axis, it is said to have *foreshortening* distortion. If it changes equally in *both* axes, it is *magnified.*

Blur, magnification and distortion reduce the recognizability of information, can cause misleading information or create false information, and can lead to the complete loss of some information on a radiograph.

RESOLUTION

The ability to distinguish two adjacent details as being separate and distinct from each other is called *resolution.* A well-resolved image detail will have *both* high visibility and optimum recognizability. The two most important aspects of the resolution of a particular image detail are its *contrast* compared to other details nearby, and its *sharpness* or acutance against background details.

Chapter 24 fully explains how contrast and sharpness are closely related to each other, because they both affect the resolution of the image. In other words, both sharpness and contrast are essential to the *resolution* of image details.

Nonetheless, contrast and sharpness are different image qualities, and they must not be confused, even though they are related.

Figure 36. Resolution template images showing that overall image resolution can be lost by either (A, arrow) blur resulting in ragged edges that begin to run into each other, or (B, arrow) a loss of contrast, even though the edges are "sharp." In both cases the individual lines are more difficult to distinguish.

High contrast images can still have poor resolution if edges are blurred. Sharp images can still have poor resolution if contrast is low, as illustrated in Figure 36.

Thus, the resolution of information in the image depends upon both visibility and geometrical integrity. The actual measurement of the resolution in a radiographic image can be made by exposing resolution pattern templates (Figure 132). Made of lead foil, such templates provide an image of black-and-white line pairs which gradually diminish in width. The smaller the line pairs which can be visibly distinguished on the radiograph, the greater is the resolution. In a blurred image, the penumbral shadows at the line edges will grow into each other so that the smaller lines cannot be distinguished.

The smaller the lines that can be clearly recorded on the film, the more pairs of these lines would fit into a certain area on the film. A functional unit of measurement for image sharpness can thus be derived. This unit is *line-pairs per millimeter*, abbreviated *LP/mm*. The more line-pairs per millimeter that can be resolved clearly, the greater the resolution of detail.

The overall image quality may be defined as the total amount of diagnostic information resolved in the image. Overall image quality is dependent upon the entire imaging system–the combination of a particular type of film and cassette with the x-ray machine used and all related variables.

SUMMARY

To summarize, any image must be both visible and recognizable in order to be of value in providing information. The visibility of the image is best when its intensity (density) is adequate, its contrast and gray scale are balanced, and its noise is minimal. The image is most recognizable when its geometrical integrity is maintained with the real object it represents. This occurs when sharpness of recorded detail is maximized

and when magnification and shape distortion are minimized.

HIERARCHY OF IMAGE QUALITIES

An overview of the relationship between all of the radiographic image qualities is presented in graphic form in Figure 37, and a concise table of definitions of imaging terms follows.

Figure 37. Hierarchy of radiographic image qualities.

DEFINITIONS OF IMAGE QUALITIES

1. **Density:** The degree of *blackness* in an area of the image, determined by the amount of silver deposited on the film in that area.

2. **Tone Value:** The amount of light that is able to pass through an area on the film, or its *translucency*. The opposite of density.

3. **Contrast:** The ratio of *difference* between two adjacent densities on the film.

4. **Gray Scale:** The *range* or number of different densities present on the film. The opposite of contrast.

5. **Noise:** Any unwanted, *useless information* recorded on the film which obscures the visibility of the desired image. Includes fog, static and artifacts.

6. **Fog:** A form of noise, fog is a veil of *useless density* covering portions of the desired image. It is caused by randomly scattered radiation which carries no useful signal or image.

7. **Sharpness of Recorded Detail:** The *abruptness* with which the edges of an image stop. Also, the lack of penumbra in an image.

8. **Blur:** See **Penumbra.** The lack of sharpness, or the presence of penumbra, in an image.

9. **Penumbra:** A *partial shadow* at the edges of an image, whereby its transition into the adjacent density is gradual rather than abrupt.

10. **Magnification:** The *difference* between the size of a real object (measured in all axes) and the size of its umbral image on the radiograph.

11. **Distortion of Shape:** The *difference* between the *shape* of a real object and the shape of its image on the radiograph, consisting of either *elongation* or *foreshortening* of the image in one axis.

12. **Visibility Factors:** Those factors which directly affect the ability to see an image, including density or tone value, contrast or gray scale, and noise including fog.

13. **Geometrical Integrity (Recognizability) Factors:** All those *geometric* factors in an image which directly affect the ability to discern the nature of the real object it represents. These include sharpness of detail, magnification, and shape distortion.

14. **Resolution:** The ability to distinguish adjacent details as being *separate* from each other, controlled by both visibility factors and geometrical factors.

15. **Radiographic Image Quality:** The total amount of useful diagnostic information resolved in an image, controlled by all of the visibility and geometrical factors.

DISCREPANCIES IN TERMINOLOGY

Unfortunately for the radiography student, there are pronounced discrepancies in the imaging terminology used by different educators and authors. Attempts have been made by certifying agencies to standardize terminology, and some progress has been made. But, confusion still abounds because these efforts were based upon the popularity, rather than the utility, of the terms chosen. Those with dissenting opinions have been tenacious and controversy continues.

As a reference to help the student "translate" between other textbooks and this one, the following discussion and *Table I* are included, listing some of the most common terms used for each image quality.

The terms "density" and "contrast" are widely standardized in conventional use and should pose no problem to the student. Image *gray scale* is frequently called "contrast scale." This is a very confusing practice, since gray scale is the *opposite* of contrast. It is suggested that the student focus on the words "scale" or "range" whenever they are used, and try to ignore the attachment of the word "contrast" in this context. This book will consistently use *gray scale* in reference to the range of different densities present in an image.

Image "noise" is generally understood to include any unuseful densities or artifacts which obscure the desired image. Since "fog" meets this definition, it is categorized in Figure 37 as a type of noise. Although noise and fog may be categorized in different fashions, their definitions are widely standardized.

In the 1980s, the American Registry of Radiologic Technologists chose the term "recorded detail" to be used on its certification examination in reference to the sharpness or abruptness of the edge of an

TABLE I
Terminology for Image Qualities

Image Quality	A.R.R.T. Term (1993)	Other Terms Used
Density	Density	
Contrast	Contrast	Contrast Resolution
Gray Scale	Contrast Scale Scale of Contrast	Latitude
Noise	Noise, Artifacts and Fog	
Sharpness of Recorded Detail	Recorded Detail	Detail Resolution Spatial Resolution Definition Sharpness
Magnification	Size Distortion	
Shape Distortion	Shape Distortion	
Visibility	Visibility	
Geometrical Integrity (Recognizability)	Sharpness of Detail	
Radiographic Quality or Resolution	Radiographic Quality or Resolution	Detail Clarity

image. The single word "detail" is perhaps the most abused of all imaging terms. It has been variously defined as the overall quality of an image, the total amount of information in an image, the visibility of small images, the geometrical integrity of the image including shape distortion and magnification, and the sharpness of image edges. To make matters worse, the plural term "details" is generally used to point out the many small components of an image, as in "visibility of details" and "recognizability of details." For these reasons, we shall try here to consistently use the term *sharpness of recorded detail* when discussing the abruptness of edges. The term "detail" will not be used in any other context regarding image qualities.

A complication arises from the adoption by the A.R.R.T. of the phrase "sharpness of detail" to collectively describe sharpness, magnification, and distortion. In other words, in Figure 37 "sharpness of detail" would replace that box labelled *recognizability functions.* Thus, the A.R.R.T. placed "recorded detail" as a subset of "sharpness of detail," using the word "detail" on two levels of the hierarchy of image qualities. The student should beware of mixing up such terms.

One other discrepancy bears full explanation: It is common to refer to the magnification of an image as "size distortion." This allows a category labelled "distortion" to be listed in the hierarchy of image qualities, with two divisions–size distortion and shape distortion. The student should be aware of the term "size distortion," but as with "detail," it is confusing to employ the word "distortion" with two different meanings. Therefore, "magnification," a straightforward term with which most people are familiar, will be used in this book. A careful review of Table I should help the student cope with different textbooks.

REVIEW QUESTIONS

1. Define Density:
2. Define Contrast:
3. Define Gray Scale:
4. Define Noise:
5. Define Penumbra:
6. Describe the two types of Shape Distortion:
7. Define Sharpness of Detail:
8. Define Resolution:
9. Define Radiographic Quality:
10. What are the three Visibility Functions in an image:
11. Why is *very* long gray scale not desirable in an image?
12. Why is penumbra present to some degree in all radiographic images?
13. Why is very high contrast not desirable in an image?
14. Explain how a radiograph could be fogged and yet light at the same time:
15. List the three image qualities which should always be minimized:
16. What is the useful range of image densities as measured on a densitometer?
17. List the four types of unsharpness:

Chapter 4

INTERACTIONS OF X-RAYS WITHIN THE PATIENT

THE ENDEAVOR OF EVERY radiographer is to control the six radiographic image qualities listed in the previous chapter. The *visibility* functions are completely essential to the radiographic image. All of the visibility functions are controlled by the relationship of the electrical technique variables to the patient-status variables. In other words, visibility is entirely dependent upon the interaction of the x-ray beam, which is controlled electrically, with the atoms inside the patient. Each visibility quality of the image is directly controlled by one of two types of atomic interactions. It is important that radiographers understand these interactions well enough that they can translate the results on the radiograph into the causes within the x-ray beam and the patient.

TYPES OF INTERACTIONS

Although detailed explanations of the various atomic interactions of x-rays may be found in radiographic physics texts, a simplified overview will be provided here so that reference may be made effectively throughout the chapters of this book to the ultimate causes and controls of the condition of the remnant beam which exposes the film.

PHOTOELECTRIC EFFECT

The *photoelectric* effect is crucial to the formation of the radiographic image. In the photoelectric effect, the energy of the x-ray photon is completely absorbed by an orbital electron in an atom. The orbital electron with the additional energy of the photon is ejected out of its orbit as a *photoelectron*, a high-speed electron (Figure 38). The photoelectron soon collides with another atom and does not leave the patient's body. There is no secondary radiation emitted, since all of the original photon's energy is absorbed into the photoelectron.

Because the original photon is completely absorbed, the radiographic film will be left blank white in that area. *The photoelectric effect is responsible for the production of contrast in the image.* This effect only occurs when the energy of the incoming photon is slightly greater than the binding energy which holds the orbital electron in its orbit.

COMPTON EFFECT

The *Compton* effect occurs when the energy of the incoming x-ray photon is much greater than the binding energy holding an orbital electron in orbit. The energy needed to eject the electron from its orbit is absorbed by that electron, but there is considerable energy left over after the ejection. The ejected electron is called a *recoil electron.* The remaining energy is re-emitted as a secondary *Compton photon,* which may be scattered in any direction (Figure 39). *Scatter* refers to any x-ray photon which has noticeably changed direction from the original beam. Scattered radiation may reach the film and cause a destructive fogging of the image. Compton may be considered synonymous with *scatter,* since 99 per cent of all scattered photons originate from Compton interactions. Scattered radiation reduces the contrast of the image and, therefore, works against the photoelectric interactions. Compton scattered interactions are also known by several other names, including *modified scattering and incoherent scattering.*

THOMPSON EFFECT

When the energy of the incoming photon is less than the binding energy of the

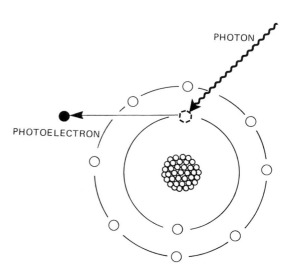

Figure 38. The photoelectric effect. The impinging x-ray photon is completely absorbed by an inner-shell orbital electron, which is then ejected from the atom as a *photoelectron.* No radiation reaches the film.

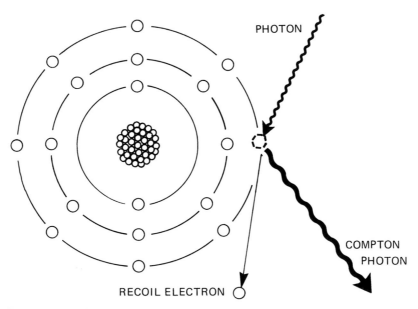

Figure 39. The Compton effect. The impinging x-ray photon is partially absorbed by an outer-shell orbital electron. The electron is then ejected from the atom as a *recoil* electron, and the remaining photon energy is emitted as a *Compton scatter photon* which may reach the film and fog it.

orbital electron, *Thompson* interaction may occur. The orbital electron absorbs the entire photon but is not ejected from its orbit. The electron is raised to an excited state of energy for a fraction of a second, after which it emits a secondary photon with the original energy. This secondary photon, although it is unchanged in energy from the original, may be emitted in any direction and is therefore considered as *scatter* (Figure 40). However, Thompson scattering accounts for only 1 per cent of all scatter produced within the patient. Further, these photons have low energy and are less likely to reach the film. Therefore, Thompson scatter is of little consequence in affecting the radiographic image. Thompson scattering is also known as *unmodified scattering, coherent scattering,* and *classical scattering.*

OTHER INTERACTIONS

Since primary photons can ionize atoms, *characteristic* interactions similar to those occurring in the anode of the x-ray tube may also occur within the patient. After any ionization (photoelectric or Compton interaction), the atom is left with an orbital vacancy and soon pulls in an electron to fill it. The loss of energy from the electron falling in is emitted as electromagnetic radiation. However, the "size" of atoms of soft tissue in the patient is extremely small compared to the "size" of the tungsten and rhenium atoms in the anode. Since the energies of characteristic photons are dependent upon atomic binding energies, the "smaller" atoms in the patient will emit only very low-energy photons, so low in energy that they will not be x-rays at all but ultraviolet or visible light, which will not make it out of the patient. Characteristic interactions in the patient cannot have any effect at all upon the radiographic film.

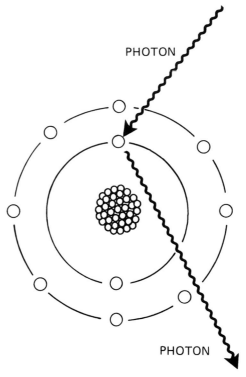

Figure 40. The Thompson effect. The impinging x-ray photon is *temporarily* absorbed by an orbital electron, then re-emitted with its original energy, but in a different direction as a *scatter photon* which may reach the film and fog it.

Scatter Versus Secondary Radiation

It is important to understand that *secondary* radiation refers to any radiation resulting from interactions within the patient, but that *scatter* refers only to that secondary radiation which has been emitted in a direction different than the original beam. Since some secondary radiation is emitted in directions equal to or very close to the original direction of the primary x-ray beam, it would not be considered as scatter. Nonetheless, *most* secondary radiation is scatter. Scattered radiation, travelling in random directions, becomes more or less evenly distributed across the film and cannot possess any subject contrast between one area and another. Therefore, it cannot carry any useful image to the film but only fogs the film overall, destroying the visibility of the information recorded by the primary and unscattered x-rays.

Even when grids (Chapter 13) are used to eliminate the severely scattered x-rays in the remnant beam, still as much as 75 per cent of the radiation exposing the film is secondary radiation which has interacted within the patient but which was not re-emitted at a sufficiently changed angle from the primary beam to be absorbed by the grid. Hence, grids eliminate only the most severely scattered x- rays but do not come close to eliminating all secondary radiation. When grids are not used on thick anatomy, over 90 per cent of the recorded image is attributable to secondary radiation.

PRODUCTION OF SUBJECT CONTRAST

As described in the previous chapter, *contrast* is essential to the visibility of a radiographic image. The primary concern when discussing the interactions between x-ray beam photons and the atoms of tissue within the patient is their effect upon image contrast. The mechanism by which *scatter* radiation produced by the Compton interaction fogs the image and reduces image contrast will be explained later in this chapter. The most significant influence upon the overall contrast of the radiographic image is the *subject contrast* produced by the interaction of the x-ray beam with the various tissues of the body.

Subject contrast is produced by the *differential absorption* between the various tissues of the body, which is already present before the x-ray beam strikes these tissues. Simply put, a tissue such as bone stands out from the "background" density of soft tissue because the bone absorbs more x-rays than soft tissue does. For the purposes of this discussion, it must be remembered that *both* the Compton interaction and the photoelectric interaction cause attenuation of the x-ray beam. (Even though the Compton interaction may be considered as only a partial absorption event so far as the energy of a single incoming photon is concerned, bear in mind that the emitted sec-ondary photon is less likely to reach the film because of its reduced energy, and if the emitted secondary photon is significantly scattered in direction and strikes the film somewhere else, the area of the film directly beneath this event remains unexposed. Therefore, the Compton interaction may be loosely considered as an "absorbing" event, even though it does not produce the "total absorption" which the photoelectric interaction does.) *All interactions, whether Compton, Thompson or photoelectric, represent some degree of absorption of the x-ray beam. All interactions attenuate the x-ray beam.*

The differential absorption of the x-ray beam by different tissues is a direct consequence of the *percentage* of the x-ray beam absorbed by all interactions, versus the penetration of the x- ray beam. Subject contrast is represented by the *ratio* between the overall absorption factors for two adjacent tissues. For example, let us examine the subject contrast of bone against soft tissue, and then determine how this would change if some disease caused the soft tissue to double in its physical density: Suppose 100 x-rays per square inch are incident upon the body. Let us assume that, of these 100 x-ray photons, the soft tissue absorbs 50 by the photoelectric interaction, and scatters 10 by the Compton interaction, thus leaving 40 x-rays that penetrated through to the film. The overall attenuation factor would be 60 per cent (photoelectrics plus Comptons), as shown in Figure 41. Meanwhile, the bone, which is much denser, absorbs 70 x-rays by photoelectric interaction and scatters 20 by Compton interaction. Of the original 100, only 10 x-rays penetrate completely through the bone, and the overall attenuation factor for the bone is 90 per cent. The bone has a much higher attenuation factor (90%) than the soft tissue (60%). The *ratio* between the attenuation factors for the bone and the soft tissue is 90/60 = 9/6 = 1.50. This is a fairly high ratio, and we expect the bone to stand out with high contrast against the soft tissue background.

Photoelectric = 50 ⎰ Attenuation
Compton = 10 ⎱ Factor = 60%
Penetrating = 40

Total = 100

Photoelectric = 70 ⎰ Attenuation
Compton = 20 ⎱ Factor = 90%
Penetrating = 10

Total = 100

SUBJECT CONTRAST = 90/60 = 1.50

Figure 41. Diagram of the production of subject contrast between bone and soft tissue. In this case, photoelectric and Compton interactions in soft tissue combine to absorb 60% of the beam. In bone, all interactions combine to absorb 90% of the beam. The subject contrast produced is the *ratio* of the two attenuation factors: 90%/60% = 1.50.

Now, suppose that the patient has a disease which causes a severe increase in the fluid content of the soft tissues (edema). We would expect this additional fluid to increase the overall physical density of the soft tissue. The molecules of fluid are more concentrated; there are simply more atoms per cubic millimeter for x-rays to "run into." Some of these events will result in photoelectric interactions and some in Compton interactions. Let us assume that in the soft tissue both interactions have increased by some 30 per cent, Figure 42.

There are now occurring 67 photoelectric interactions and 13 Compton interactions. This leaves only 20 x-rays from the original 100 which will penetrate clear through to the film. The attenuation factor of the diseased soft tissue then increases to a factor of 80 per cent instead of the original 60 per cent. How does this change the subject contrast between the soft tissue and the bone? The attenuation factor for the bone is still 90 per cent, so the *ratio* between the two tissues is 90/80 = 9/8 = 1.13. There is much less difference between the tissues.

Figure 42. Diagram of the change in subject contrast from Figure 41 if a disease increases the physical density of the soft tissue by some 30%. Both photoelectric and Compton interactions increase in number, and the attenuation factor rises to 80%, with only 2 out of 10 photons penetrating through the soft tissue. The subject contrast between the soft tissue and the adjacent bone is now reduced to 90%/80% = 1.13.

In this hypothetical case, the edema within the soft tissue ultimately caused the ratio of attenuation between bone and soft tissue to decrease from 1.50 to 1.13. There will be less difference between the two radiographic densities of these tissues produced on the film. Contrast will be reduced.

Note that to measure the contrast between the two tissues above, the ratio between their attenuation factors is used, dividing one factor into the other, rather than the subtracted difference: In his text, *The Physical Principles of Diagnostic Radiology*, Perry Sprawls clearly defines image contrast. He states, "Actually, it is the ratio of the penetration factors, rather than the difference, which determines the amount of contrast." Dr. Sprawls provides the mathematical formula for subject contrast as:

$$C_s = \left\{ 1 - \left(\frac{P_o}{P_t} \right)^x \right\} \times 100$$

where P_o and P_t are the penetration factors for the two tissues. Note that these two factors are not subtracted one from the other. One is divided one into the other to form a ratio. (The other parts of this formula are simply designed to result in an answer which is a percentage figure.)

There are three essential aspects of tissues which determine their attenuation properties and the resulting subject contrast: The thickness of each tissue, the physical density of each tissue, and the average atomic number of each tissue.

TISSUE THICKNESS

As a tissue becomes thicker, the attenuation of the x-ray beam increases exponentially. A rough rule of thumb for body tissues in general is that for every 4 to 5 centimeters of additional tissue thickness, the attenuation of the x-ray beam is doubled, and the penetration of x-rays through to the film is cut in half. The actual mathematical relationship of tissue thickness to subject contrast is a somewhat complicated logarithmic formula, and unnecessary here. Suffice it to say that the thickness of a tissue is directly related to its attenuation factor: The thicker the tissue, the greater the attenuation of the x-ray beam. In accordance with the above rule of thumb, a body part which is 4 centimeters thicker than another part composed of the same tissue will absorb about twice as much of the beam, and the image will turn out about one-half as dark in this area.

Suppose that tissue A has an attenuation factor of 40 per cent, and tissue B has a factor of 10 per cent. The subject contrast between tissue A and tissue B is $40/10 = 4.0$. Then, let tissue B increase in thickness by 4 centimeters. This would double its attenuation factor from 10 per cent to 20 per cent. The subject contrast would now be $40/20 = 2.0$. Clearly, in this case the contrast has been *reduced* from 4.0 to 2.0. On the other hand, let tissue *A* increase in thickness by 4 centimeters, thus increasing its attenuation factor from 40 per cent to 80 per cent. With tissue B at the original 10 per cent, the subject contrast would then be $80/10 = 8.0$, and contrast has *increased* from 4.0 to 8.0. Hence, changes in tissue thickness may cause the contrast to either decrease or increase, depending on which tissue changed.

TISSUE DENSITY

The physical density of a substance refers to the amount of physical mass that is concentrated into a given volume of space, such as grams per cubic centimeter. In the patient, it may be considered as the concentration of atoms or molecules of tissue. At higher tissue densities, there are more atoms or molecules in a given space. At lower densities, atoms or molecules are less concentrated and there is more space between them.

Clearly, if the number of atoms in a space is doubled, there will be twice as high a probability that an impinging x-ray photon will hit one of the atoms. If the tissue density is cut to one-half the original, it will be one-half as likely that an impinging x-ray will interact with an atom in that space. This probability applies equally to Compton interactions and photoelectric interactions. Therefore, it may be said that the occurrence of all interactions is *directly proportional* to the physical density of the tissue through which the x-rays are passing.

Radiographic contrast will occur between two tissues in the image if they are extremely different in physical density, simply because the one tissue will absorb much more radiation altogether (by both types of interactions) and leave a lighter, less exposed area on the film. For example, air in the lungs is a gas and therefore has an extremely low density compared to soft tissue, which is equivalent in density to liquid. The density ratio of soft tissue to air is roughly 1000:1. Since the soft tissue will absorb 1000 times more radiation than the air, visible image contrast results.

Three types of body tissues may be distinguished from each other on a radiograph primarily because of the effect of tissue density: soft tissues (muscles and glands), fat, and gasses such as air in the lungs. Soft tissues absorb more x-rays than fat or gas and result in the lighter shades on the film, with fat appearing slightly darker and gas appearing the darkest.

Most radiography, however, involves the visualization of bones or of contrast agents. Bones, metals and contrast agents are not significantly different from soft tissue in their physical densities. These materials appear with contrast on the radiograph because of their high atomic numbers (larger atomic "size") but not because of any significant difference in density.

TISSUE ATOMIC NUMBER

Most radiographic procedures fall in the categories of skeletal procedures and artificial contrast procedures. Soft tissues cannot be radiographically distinguished from each other without some form of intervention to artificially provide subject contrast. Contrast agents—substances usually based on the iodine atom or the barium atom—are introduced into cavities in soft tissue where possible to provide an image.

Contrast agents, bone and metallic objects are visible on radiographs primarily because of the difference between their atomic numbers, that is, how "large" their atoms are. This is why iodine (atomic number = 53) and barium (atomic number = 56) are so effective at absorbing x-rays. Barium not only has 56 positively-charged protons within its nucleus, but it also has, under normal conditions, 56 electrons in its orbital shells. Interestingly, barium and other atoms with high atomic numbers are *not* actually larger in *diameter.* The outermost shell of the barium atom is only slightly larger in diameter than the single electron shell of hydrogen (atomic number = 1). As the nucleus of an atom becomes larger and larger, the additional positive charge of the protons "pulls" all of the electron shells in closer to the nucleus. So, atoms with more shells have them "packed" in tighter and closer to the nucleus. This also means that all of the electrons within these shells are now packed more tightly within the small volume of space which the atom occupies. This concentration of the electrons within the space of the atom's diameter is referred to as *electron density.*

Hence, "larger" atoms are not spatially larger in actual size, but rather they are more *dense* with electrons. The likelihood, then, that an x-ray photon will be absorbed by one of these electrons is greatly enhanced for high atomic number elements. A particular tissue is comprised of several different types of atoms combined into molecules. Thus, the atomic number of a tissue must be expressed as an average, which takes into account the number of each different atom within these molecules. For example, the average atomic number of soft tissue, mostly composed of water, is 7.4. (Water is composed of two atoms of hydrogen, each of atomic number 1, and one atom of oxygen with atomic number 8. The average atomic number, then, must fall between 1 and 8. It averages closer to 8 because the oxygen has a much greater effect than the two small hydrogen atoms.)

To summarize, there are *two* aspects of tissue which determine its ability to attenuate an x-ray beam: The *physical density* of the tissue, which is the number of atoms per volume of space, and the *average atomic number* of the tissue, which relates to the electron density or the number of electrons per volume of space within each atom. Bone, metallic objects and contrast agents are demonstrated on radiographs primarily because of their *atomic numbers* being different from soft tissue. Gasses such as air, and fat, show up on radiographs primarily because of extreme differences in their physical *density* when compared to that of soft tissue.

X-RAY BEAM ENERGY (KVP)

Changes in the energy levels of the x-ray beam, controlled primarily by the selected kilovoltage, dramatically alter the penetration characteristics of the x-rays. As illustrated in the last chapter, a high-kVp beam penetrates more different types of tissues and records them on the image as varying shades of gray density. As the number of shades of gray within the image increases, the difference between these densities becomes less. Gray scale is increased, and correspondingly, contrast is decreased. These effects are again due to the penetration of the beam versus the overall attenuation factor, and will hold true regardless of the particular prevalence of the photoelectric effect or Compton effect in relation to each other.

However, there are implications for the relative prevalence of these two interactions as we study image contrast. Figure 43 is a graph showing the prevalence of the photoelectric interactions and the Compton interactions occurring in different tissues at increasing kVp levels. As you examine this graph, you will note that the

photoelectric curves plummet quickly toward zero at high kVps, but the number of Compton interactions occurring only decreases slightly. There are less interactions of all kinds, but since the photoelectrics are so quickly lost, *the Compton scatter interaction becomes the more prevalent of the two* at high kVp levels.

The photoelectric effect only occurs at discrete energy levels where the kilovoltage of the incoming photon is slightly higher than the binding energy of the nucleus which holds the orbital electron in its shell. This means that changes in kVp will have a considerable effect upon the occurrence of photoelectric interactions.

As the kVp is increased to exceed binding energies by large amounts, the occurrence of photoelectric interactions drops quickly to near zero. The photoelectric

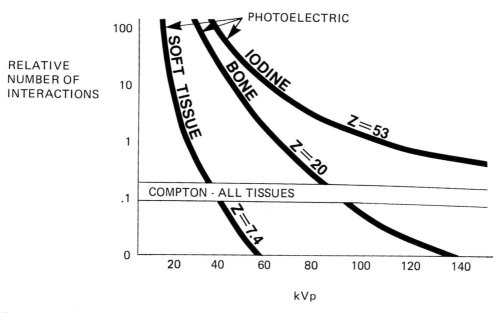

Figure 43. Graph showing the *relative* predominance of photoelectric and Compton interactions at increasing kVp levels. All interactions decrease in number at higher energies, as more of the x-ray beam penetrates through. However, photoelectrics quickly decrease to zero, especially in soft tissue, leaving Compton as the predominant interaction at high kvps. Also note that photoelectric interactions occur in much greater numbers in higher atomic number tissues such as bone, whereas Compton interactions occur at about the same rate for all tissues.

effect only occurs in the inner shells of the atom which are close enough to the nucleus to have significant binding energies. The use of atoms with larger nuclei and higher atomic numbers will raise the binding energies of these inner shells. When binding energies are increased enough to more closely match the particular kVp being used, without exceeding it, more photoelectric interactions will occur. Note that at 40 kVp, many more photoelectric interactions occur in bone tissues having an average atomic number of about 20 than do in soft tissue with an average atomic number of 7.4. For a given tissue, however, photoelectric interactions drop off rapidly as the kVp is increased. The greatest number of photoelectric interactions is achieved when kVp is low and tissue atomic number is high.

Compton interactions occur only in the outer shells of an atom. Because these shells have so little binding energy, their electrons are not selective in absorbing x-ray photons. Changes in atomic number do not affect these outer shells much. Furthermore, in the Compton interaction, only a portion of the photon energy is absorbed by the orbital electron, so that a variety of photon energy levels can result in the interaction taking place. As binding energies are not significant, the electrons are not selective, and any portion of the photon energy can be absorbed, the occurrence of Compton interactions is not affected much by changing atomic numbers of tissues, nor is it affected much by changes in kVp. Specifically, higher kVp levels will penetrate the patient more and less Compton interactions will occur, but this reduction is very slight compared to the reduction of the photoelectric effect (Figure 43). Compton interactions may be considered as almost constant, regardless of atomic number or kVp.

Now consider what happens within soft tissue when the kVp is increased from 40 to 80. In soft tissue at 40 kVp, there are roughly equal numbers of photoelectric and Compton interactions. About one-half of all interactions taking place are photoelectrics, which completely absorb the x-ray and leave the image on the film "white." At 80 kVp, there are virtually *no photoelectric interactions* occurring within soft tissue. No portion of the film under this tissue will appear "white." The image of the soft tissue at 80 kVp is being created only by penetrating rays and Compton scattered rays. The penetrating rays provide blacks and grays in the image, and the Compton scattered photons further gray the image. The only interactions occurring are "gray-producing interactions." The *bone tissue* at 80 kVp *will* have "whites" within its image, because there are still plenty of photoelectrics (about one-half of all interactions) occurring in the bone.

Let us now increase the kVp to 120 for a solid column barium study, and the graph illustrates that the same fate awaits the bone tissues: At very high kVp levels, the photoelectric interactions even within bone have almost disappeared. The bone densities in the image now consist of mostly penetrating x-rays and scattered x-rays. This is why bones appear so poorly on barium studies. The barium itself, similar to the iodine curve on the graph, still produces plenty of photoelectric interactions even at this very high kVp.

COMPTON SCATTER RADIATION

The key to understanding the effect of Compton scattered radiation upon image contrast is that *scattered radiation is random in its distribution, and therefore adds an equal density to all areas of the image.* Figure 30 in the preceding chapter shows how scattered radiation is emitted in all directions from the patient. The chance that a particular scattered ray will strike the film where a bone image should be is equal to the chance that it will strike an area where a soft tissue image should be. Thus, as shown in Figure 31 in the last chapter, the entire image is fogged with a "blanket density."

By assigning a value to this blanket fog density, it is easy to demonstrate how the scattered radiation reduces image contrast: Suppose a simple image is composed of an area of bone that measures 1.0 on the densitometer, surrounded by a soft tissue area of darker density which measures 2.0 on the densitometer. The contrast of this image is found by the ratio of the two densities, $2/1 = 2.0$. Now suppose that scattered radiation lays down a "blanket" of fog across the film, and that the fog density, if measured separately, would have a value of 0.5 on the densitometer. A fog density of 0.5 has been added to all tissue densities in the image. The density of the bone area now measures 1.5, and the soft tissue area now measures 2.5. The contrast of this fogged image is found by the ratio $2.5/1.5 = 1.67$. Contrast has been reduced, from the original 2.0 to 1.67. There is less obvious difference between the bone and the soft tissue areas, because of the addition of the fog density to both. Scatter radiation and the fog it produces are always destructive to the image.

X-RAY BEAM INTENSITY

The following chapters proceed to analyze the effect of each radiographic variable upon image contrast. It will be of immense help to understand that anything which simply alters the overall *intensity* of the x-ray beam, the *quantity* of radiation reaching the film, will *not* affect image contrast unless the change also alters one of the variables already discussed in this chapter. Two examples are changing mAs and changing source-image receptor distance (SID): If the mAs is cut to one-half the original, there will be one-half as many x-rays entering the surface of the patient, one-half as many photoelectric interactions will occur, one-half as many Compton interactions will occur, and one-half as many x-rays will penetrate through to the film. In like fashion, if the x-ray tube is moved somewhat closer to the film such that the concentration of radiation striking the patient is doubled, photoelectric interactions will double in number, Compton also, and penetration will also be doubled. As long as the *percentage of penetration* or the *ratio of attenuation* are unchanged, image contrast is not affected.

Remember from the previous chapter that an image can certainly be twice as dark or twice as light overall, yet maintain the same contrast, which is the *ratio* between its densities. This is what happens when beam intensity alone is changed. The mere quantity of radiation is not a controlling factor for image contrast, within the ranges of normal diagnostic practice.

SUMMARY

1. The *photoelectric* interaction, because of its total absorption of x-rays, produces necessary *contrast* in the image.

2. The *Compton* interaction is responsible for 99 per cent of the *fog* in the image and must be controlled.

3. *Scatter* is that secondary radiation which has significantly changed *direction* from that of the primary beam. It arises from both Compton and Thompson interactions.

4. *Subject Contrast* is produced by the differential absorption of tissues, and is measured as the *ratio* of the attenuation factors for two adjacent tissues.

5. *Subject Contrast* and is affected by tissue thickness, the physical density of tissue, the average atomic number of tissue, and the kVp of the x-ray beam. It is not directly affected by changes in beam intensity.

6. As *kilovoltage* is increased, the photoelectric interactions occurring in a given tissue fall off rapidly in number, while the Compton interactions only decrease slightly. *Contrast* in the image is lost because of the loss of the *photoelectric* absorption.

7. When *atomic number* is increased by the use of positive contrast media, the number of *photoelectric* interactions rises sharply, while Compton interactions remain at about the same level, thus restoring high image *contrast*.

8. Against a background of soft tissue, *subject contrast* is produced for metals, contrast agents and bone tissue primarily because of their *atomic number*. Gasses such as air in the lungs, and fat tissue are made visible primarily because of extreme differences in their *physical density* when compared to soft tissue.

9. Since *scattered radiation* from the Compton interaction is randomly distributed, it adds a fog density equally to all areas of the image. This added density diminishes the ratio between these densities and thus reduces contrast.

REVIEW QUESTIONS

1. What are two other names for the Compton interaction:

2. Draw a sketch of the Compton interaction, and label all parts:

3. A photon is completely absorbed by an inner-shell orbital electron in the patient, and the electron ejects from its orbit. Name this interaction:

4. Define scatter radiation:

5. What effect does increasing the x-ray beam energy (kVp) have on the *total* number of all interactions in the patient?

6. What effect does increasing the x-ray beam energy (kVp) have on the *proportion* of Compton scatter interactions compared to photoelectric interactions?

7. A photon with *much* more energy than the electron binding energies of the tissue through which it passes is most likely to undergo what type of interaction?

8. A photon with just *slightly* more energy than the electron binding energies of the tissue through which it passes is most likely to undergo what type of interaction ?

9. Roughly how much of the radiation striking the film is secondary?

10. Bone has a density only slightly greater than soft tissue. Why, then, does bone show up with high contrast against soft tissues on radiographs?

11. If barium causes just as many compton scatter interactions as normal fluids in the stomach, why does it show up so white on radiographs?

12. List the end product(s) of the Compton interaction:

Part II

VISIBILITY FACTORS

Chapter 5

MILLIAMPERE-SECONDS

MILLIAMPERAGE, ABBREVIATED *mA*, is a measure of the quantity of electrical current flowing through a circuit. It is a rate representing the number of electrons passing through a point in the circuit per second. The milliamperage control on an x-ray machine is actually the *rheostat* in the filament circuit and controls the *intensity* of the electron flow rate. Higher milliamperage settings send more electrons through the filament per second, heating it to a greater temperature each time the *rotor* switch is depressed. Because of the high temperature of the filament, more electrons are *boiled off* and made available to accelerate across the tube and strike the anode.

The number of x-rays produced in the beam is directly proportional to the number of electrons striking the anode. Therefore, the intensity of the x-ray beam is directly proportional to the milliamperage set.

Exposure time, abbreviated *s* (for *seconds*), is simply the amount of time over which the beam is on and the exposure is occurring. Since mA is a rate, the mA multiplied by the exposure time *s* will indicate the total intensity of the entire exposure. In a similar way, the rate miles per hour (MPH) multiplied by the hours of travel will indicate the total miles travelled. Milliampere-seconds (abbreviated *mAs*) is a measure of the total quantity of electricity which flowed through the circuit during the exposure and, therefore, indicates *the total quantity of x-rays used in the exposure.*

EFFECT ON X-RAY BEAM SPECTRUM

As described in Chapter 1, an x-ray beam is heterogeneous, having many different energy levels in it, and the spectrum of the beam may be graphed by plotting the number of x-rays produced at each energy level. Figure 44 shows how a change in milliamperage or exposure time affects the x-ray beam spectrum, changing the intensity at each energy level by an equal proportion, but not affecting peak, minimum or average energies. The solid curve represents the original x-ray beam, and the dashed curve depicts the new beam if the mAs is doubled.

If the mA is doubled, twice as many x-rays will be produced from the x-ray tube during the time the exposure occurs. If the mA is unchanged, but exposure time is twice as long, once again there will be twice as many x-rays in the total exposure. In either case, the height of the x-ray beam spectrum curve as shown in Figure 44 will double. The total area under the dashed line represents the total number of x-rays produced, and this area has doubled from the original beam.

Note in Figure 44 that the number of x-rays having just 10 kilovolts of energy has doubled. The number of x-rays at the average energy, 30 kV, has also doubled. There are also twice as many x-rays produced having 70 kV of energy. When total *mAs* is doubled, the number of x-rays produced *at all energies* will be doubled. This means that the minimum, peak, and average energies of the x-ray beam will be unchanged. For example, in Figure 44 the *average energy* of the original beam (solid line) is 30 kV. When the intensity of the new beam is doubled (dashed line), the average energy is still 30 kV. The *quantity* of the x-ray beam has increased, but the *quality* or penetrating ability has not.

Figure 44. Graph demonstrating the effect of doubling the mAs on the x-ray beam spectrum. The number of photons produced at *every* keV level is doubled. Therefore, the minimum, average and peak energies remain the same.

RECIPROCITY LAW

The milliampere-seconds factor, indicated by the symbol mAs, directly influences radiographic density when all other factors are constant. It is the product of the *milliamperage* (mA) and the duration of the exposure time in *seconds* (s). Either factor of mA or s may be changed at will to conform to required radiographic exposures as long as their product—mAs—remains the same. For example, approximately the same radiographic density will be obtained whether 50 mA is used for 1/10 second or 10 mA for 5/10 second—both conditions entail the use of 5 mAs.

An important concept advanced by Bunsen and Roscoe in 1875 states that the reaction of a photographic emulsion to light is equal to the product of the intensity of the light and the duration of exposure. This is known as the reciprocity law. The phenomenon occurs in radiography only when intensifying screens are used, because exposure of the film under these circumstances is chiefly caused by the fluo-

rescent light emitted by the screens and very little by x-rays.

Failure of this law may be observed when extremely short exposures (less than 5/100 second) with high mA or extremely long exposures and low mA are used even though the total quantity of x-radiation exposing the film remains the same. Fortunately, it is not necessary to be concerned about this effect in routine work, for today it is seldom encountered because it has been largely compensated by the characteristics of the x-ray film emulsion. Therefore, the mAs value may be considered reliable for use as an exposure factor in general radiography.

In radiography, the reciprocity law states that the density produced on the film will be directly proportional to the exposure received by the film. The intensity of the total exposure is controlled by total mAs. Therefore, *radiographic density will be directly proportional to the mAs used.*

ARITHMETICAL RELATIONS

RELATION BETWEEN MILLIAMPERAGE AND TIME

RULE. The mA required for a given radiographic density is inversely proportional to the time of exposure when remaining factors are constant. This rule may be expressed by the following formula:

$$\frac{\text{(A) Original mA}}{\text{(B) New mA}} = \frac{\text{(F) New Time}}{\text{(E) Original Time}}$$

Example 1. Assume that 10 mA (A) and an exposure time (E) of 0.5 sec. was employed in making a radiograph. It is desired to decrease the exposure time (F) to 0.05 sec. What milliamperage (B) would be needed to assure comparable radiographic densities?

Solution. A, E, and F are known and B is unknown.

$$B = \frac{AE}{F}$$

$$B = \frac{10 \times 0.5}{0.05} = \frac{5}{.05} \quad 100\text{mA Answer.}$$

Example 2. Assume that 10 mA (A) and an exposure time (E) of 0.5 sec. was employed in making a radiograph. It is desired to increase the milliamperage (B) to 100. What time of exposure (F) would be needed to obtain comparable radiographic densities?

Solution. A, E, B are known and F is unknown.

$$F = \frac{AE}{B}$$

$$F = \frac{10 \times .5}{100} = \frac{5}{100} \quad 1/20 \text{ sec. Answer.}$$

DECIMAL EQUIVALENTS OF FRACTIONAL EXPOSURES

In computing mAs values, it is often convenient to use the decimal equivalent of the exposure time fraction. Table II lists decimal equivalents of commonly employed exposure fractions. It will be recalled that in any fraction, the number above the line is called the *numerator* and the number below the line, the *denominator*. For example, in the fraction $3/20$ the number 3, above the line, is the numerator and the number 20, below the line, is the denominator. Table II is arranged so that the numerators of fractions are listed horizontally, at the top of the table; and the denominators are listed vertically, in the columns to the left and the right. The body of the table contains the decimal equivalents of various combinations of numerators and denominators.

Example. To determine the decimal equivalent of the fraction $3/10$, find the numerator 3 in the horizontal row at the top of the table. Then, find the denominator 10 in the left-hand *vertical* column; now, follow the horizontal row of decimals on line 10 until it meets the vertical column containing the numerator 3. At the intersection of these columns, the decimal equivalent of the fraction $3/10$ is indicated as 0.3. The mA may be multipled by this decimal to obtain the mAs value.

TABLES OF mAs VALUES

Table III makes possible rapid determination of mAs values when the time of exposure and the milliamperage are known. To use the table, find the exposure to be employed in the left-hand vertical column; then, in the horizontal row at the top of the table, find the mA value to be used. The required mAs value is found at the point where these two columns meet in the body of the table.

Example 1. An exposure of $1/30$ second was employed in a given projection at 100 mA. What is the mAs value?

TABLE II

Table for Determination of Decimal Equivalents of Fractional Exposure Times

| | *Decimal Equivalents of Fractional Exposures* | | | | | | | | | | | | |
| | *Numerators* | | | | | | | | | | | | |
	1	2	3	4	5	6	7	8	9	10	11	12	
2	0.5	1.	1.5	2.	2.5	3	3.5	4.	4.5	5.	5.5	6.	2
3	.333	.666	1.	1.33	1.666	2.	2.33	2.66	3.	3.33	3.66	4.	3
4	.25	.5	.75	1.	1.25	1.5	1.75	2.	2.25	2.5	2.75	3.	4
5	.2	.4	.6	.8	1.	1.2	1.4	1.6	1.8	2.	2.2	2.4	5
6	.167	.333	.5	.667	.835	1.	1.167	1.333	1.5	1.667	1.833	2	6
7	.143	.286	.429	.572	.715	.858	1.	1.143	1.286	1.429	1.57	1.7	7
8	.125	.25	.375	.5	.625	.75	.875	1.	1.125	1.25	1.375	1.5	8
9	.111	.222	.333	.444	.555	.666	.777	.888	1.	1.111	1.222	1.333	9
10	.1	.2	.3	.4	.5	.6	.7	.8	.9	1.	1.1	1.2	10
11	.09	.18	.27	.363	.455	.545	.636	.727	.818	.090	1.	1.09	11
12	.083	.167	.25	.333	.415	.5	.583	.667	.75	.833	.917	1.	12
15	.067	.134	.2	.267	.333	.4	.467	.533	.6	.667	.733	.8	15
20	.05	.1	.15	.2	.25	.3	.35	.4	.45	.5	.55	.6	20
24	.042	.083	.125	.167	.208	.25	.292	.333	.375	.416	.458	.5	24
30	.033	.067	.1	.133	.167	.2	.233	.267	.3	.333	.367	.4	30
40	.025	.05	.075	.1	.125	.15	.175	.2	.225	.25	.275	.3	40
60	.017	.033	.05	.067	.083	.1	.117	.133	.15	.167	.183	.2	60
120	.008	.017	.025	.033	.042	.05	.058	.067	.075	.083	.092	.1	120

Solution. Find $5/30$ second in the left-hand vertical column of Table III, then, locate 100 in the horizontal row at the top of the table. Follow the horizontal line at the $1/30$ level to the right until it meets the vertical column headed by 100 mA. The mAs value common to both columns is found at this point, and the answer is 3.33.

Example 2. An exposure of 0.07 seconds was given in a specific projection at 50 mA. What mAs was employed?

Solution. Locate 0.07 seconds in the left-hand vertical column of Table III; then, locate the value 50 in the horizontal row at the top of the table. Follow the horizontal line at the 0.07 level to the right until it meets the vertical column headed by 50 mA. The mAs value common to both columns is found at this point and the answer is 3.5.

WORKING WITH DECIMAL TIMERS

Radiographers must often adjust techniques using decimal timers or fractional timers. Such mAs conversions are normal-

TABLE III
Milliampere-Seconds (mAs)

Time Decimals	Time Fractions	Milliamperes 25	50	100	200	300	400	500	600
0.0083	1/120	0.21	0.42	0.83	1.67	2.5	3.33	4.17	5.
0.007	—	0.18	0.35	0.7	1.4	2.1	2.8	3.5	4.2
0.01	1/100	0.25	0.5	1.	2.	3.	4.	5.	6.
0.0125	1/80	0.31	0.63	1.25	2.5	3.63	5.	6.25	7.5
0.0167	1/60	0.42	0.83	1.67	3.33	5.	6.25	8.33	10.
0.02	1/50	0.5	1.	2.	4.	6.	8.	10.	12.
0.025	1//40	0.62	1.25	2.5	5.	7.5	10.	12.5	15.
0.033	1/30	0.83	1.67	3.33	6.67	10.	13.33	16.67	20.
0.035	—	0.88	1.75	3.5	7.	10.5	14.	17.5	21.
0.05	1/20	1.25	2.5	5.	10.	15.	20.	25.	30.
0.067	1/15	1.67	3.33	6.66	13.33	20.	26.67	33.33	40.
0.07	—	1.75	3.5	7.	14.	21.	28.	35.	42.
0.083	1/12	2.08	4.16	8.33	16.67	25.	33.33	41.67	50.
0.1	1/10	2.5	5.	10.	20.	30.	40.	50.	60.
0.125	1/8	3.13	6.25	12.5	25.	37.5	50.	62.5	75.
0.133	2/15	3.33	6.67	13.33	26.67	40.	53.33	66.67	80.
0.15	3/20	3.75	7.5	15.	30.	45.	60.	75.	90.
0.167	1/6	4.17	8.33	16.7	33.33	50.	66.67	83.33	100.
0.2	1/5	5.	10.	20.	40.	60.	80.	100.	120.
0.25	1/4	6.25	12.5	25.	50.	75.	100.	125.	150.
0.3	3/10	7.5	15.	30.	60.	90.	120.	150.	180.
0.35	—	8.75	17.5	35.	70.	105.	140.	175.	210.
0.4	2/5	10.	20.	40.	80.	120.	160.	200.	240.
0.5	1/2	12.5	25.	50.	100.	150.	200.	250.	300.
0.7	—	17.5	35.	70.	140.	210.	280.	350.	420.
0.75	3/4	18.75	37.5	75.	150.	225.	300.	375.	450.

ly done mentally, rather than with pencil and paper. On x-ray machines, the most used mA stations are in multiples of 100. On the exposure timers, the most used decimal times consist of two digits after the decimal, that is, they are "hundredths" (e.g., 0.35, 0.02). This provides an easy starting point for practicing decimal conversions. To figure the total mAs, get into the habit of moving the decimal point on the exposure time two places to the right, in your mind. Then ignore the two zeros on the mA station while multiplying. You are simply canceling the hundreds with hundredths.

For example, find the total mAs for

300 mA at 0.05 seconds.

Moving the time decimal two places to the right, you have 5. Ignoring the two zeros on the mA, you have 3. This is simply 3 times 5, or 15 mAs.

Think of 300 mA at 0.08 seconds as simply 3 times 8, or 24 mAs. And, 100 mA at 0.025 seconds is 1 times 2.5, or 2.5 mAs.

If there are three digits after the decimal, as in 0.008 seconds, you will use the same method but will still be dealing with a decimal in multiplying. For example, 200 mA at 0.008 seconds should be thought of as 2 times 0.8 for a total of 1.6 mAs. If there is only one digit behind the decimal point, such as 0.4 seconds, again move the decimal two places over. This time it will add a zero to your time number, so you will consider 0.4 as 40. Hence, 200 mA at 0.4 seconds will be thought of as 2 times 40, for a total of 80 mAs. Think of 100 mA at .2 seconds as 1 times 20. And, 500 at .8 is 5 times 80 or 400 mAs.

Do the following exercise, calculating total mAs values *mentally*. When completed, check your answers from the Appendix.

EXERCISE #1

$$mA \quad x \quad time \quad = \quad mAs$$

1. 100 @ .05 =
2. 100 @ .8 =
3. 100 @ .125 =
4. 200 @ .02 =
5. 200 @ .125 =
6. 200 @ .3 =
7. 200 @ .035 =
8. 300 @ .7 =
9. 300 @ .04 =
10. 300 @ .025 =
11. 300 @ .006 =
12. 400 @ .04 =
13. 400 @ .016 =
14. 400 @ .33 =
15. 400 @ .007 =
16. 500 @ .03 =
17. 500 @ .7 =
18. 500 @ .125 =
19. 600 @ .25 =
20. 600 @ .008 =

WORKING WITH MILLISECOND TIMERS

Modern radiographic equipment with a high-capacity generator may use a millisecond timer. As with decimals and fractions, the mathematics involved is simple, yet a little practice is very helpful in developing the required skill. To convert a millisecond exposure time into a decimal time, simply move the decimal three places to the *left* and delete any zeros at the end of the number. For example, the decimal time for 700 milliseconds is 0.700 = 0.7 seconds, and 350 milliseconds is 0.350 = 0.35 seconds.

If the millisecond time has only one or two digits, zeros must be added in front of it (to the left of it) as the decimal point is shifted to the left. For example, the decimal time for 50 milliseconds is 0.05 seconds—one zero must be added before the "5" as the decimal points shifts to the left. The decimal time for 25 milliseconds is 0.025 seconds. What is the decimal time for 4 milliseconds? Shifting the decimal point three places to the left and adding two zeros in front of the "4", the answer is 0.004 seconds.

When converting decimal times into milliseconds, the decimal is moved three places to the *right*, adding zeros as required. Thus, 0.8 seconds is 0800. = 800 milliseconds. Two zeros were added as the decimal shifted to the right. What is 0.15 seconds in milliseconds? Moving the decimal to the right three places requires adding one zero. The answer is 0150. = 150 milliseconds. A decimal time of 0.135 seconds is 135 milliseconds.

Complete the following brief exercise *mentally*, without paper or calculator. Then check your answers in the Appendix.

EXERCISE #2

Decimal = *Milliseconds*

1. 0.75 =
2. 0.3 =
3. 0.125 =
4. 0.04 =
5. 0.083 =
6. 0.0333 =
7. 0.005 =
8. 0.0012 =

Milliseconds = *Decimal*

9. 200 =
10. 167 =
11. 250 =
12. 35 =
13. 70 =
14. 15 =
15. 8 =
16. 1200 =

When calculating mAs conversions with millisecond times, you may move the decimal point on the *mA* to the left three places and multiply, but it is often easier to move the decimal for the *exposure time* three places to the left and multiply the mA by this number. In other words, it is usually easier to convert the millisecond time into a decimal time, as we have just practiced in EXERCISE #2–then multiply the mA value by the decimal time. Now try the following mAs calculations, finding the total mAs mentally. These problems are identical to Exercise #1, but these use millisecond times instead of decimal times. Check your answers from the Appendix.

EXERCISE #3

mA x *time* = *mAs*

1. 50 @ 50 ms =
2. 50 @ 300 ms =
3. 100 @ 500 ms =
4. 100 @ 35 ms =
5. 100 @ 8 ms =
6. 200 @ 200 ms =
7. 200 @ 125 ms =

mA x *time* = *mAs*

8. 200 @ 35 ms =
9. 300 @ 33 ms =
10. 300 @ 6 ms =
11. 300 @ 25 ms =
12. 400 @ 250 ms =
13. 400 @ 80 ms =
14. 500 @ 5 ms =
15. 600 @ 150 ms =
16. 600 @ 12 ms =

WORKING WITH FRACTIONAL TIMERS

Exposure timers reading in fractions are somewhat more difficult than decimals to work mentally, yet they tend to follow patterns, and with just a few memorized pairs of numbers you can do most of them. At each mA station, certain pairs of numbers always go together. For example, at the 100 mA station, fives and twos always go together:

100 mA at $1/2$ second is 50 mAs
100 mA at $1/5$ second is 20 mAs
100 mA at $1/50$ second is 2 mAs
100 mA at $1/20$ second is 5 mAs

and so on. Zeros may be added, or decimal points moved, but a time fraction using a 5 will always result in a total mAs involving a 2, and vice versa.

The 100 mA Station

At the 100 mA station, the following pairs of numbers always go together–commit them to memory before you go on. The best way to memorize them is to get a study partner to drill you as if it were an oral test.

3 and 33
4 and 25
5 and 2
6 and 16
7 and 15
8 and 12

These numbers are rounded up or down to make it easier to memorize them. For example, **100 mA at $1/6$ second** is actually **16.67 mAs**, and would normally round up to **17**. However, it is easier to remember **16** because the mind associates the sixes in $1/6$ and 16 together. The results are close enough for any radiographic technique. Likewise, $1/8$ of 100 is actually 12.5, and $1/12$ of 100 is actually 8.33. In these units on fractions, all answers will be rounded out. The goal is for you to *mentally* derive a good estimated technique, not an exact answer. Memorizing the pairs of numbers will not tell you where to put any decimal points—you will have to learn that by practice. Try Exercise #4 and check your answers in the Appendix.

EXERCISE #4

		ma	x	time	=	mAs
1.	100 @			$1/2$	=	
2.	100 @			$1/20$	=	
3.	100 @			$1/50$	=	
4.	100 @			$1/8$	=	
5.	100 @			$1/12$	=	
6.	100 @			$1/120$	=	
7.	100 @			$1/15$	=	
8.	100 @			$1/40$	=	
9.	100 @			$1/30$	=	
10.	100 @			$1/6$	=	

The 200 mA and 50 mA Stations:

Having memorized the number pairs for the 100 mA station, you can figure the total mAs for the most time settings at the 200 and 50 mA station simply by doubling or halving the answer you would get at 100 mA. For example, once it becomes second-nature to you that 100 mA at $1/60$ second is 1.7 mAs, whenever you see 200 mA at $1/60$ second you can simply double 1.7 in your mind for a total of 3.4 mAs. If 100 mA at $1/30$ second is 3.3 mAs, 50 mA at $1/30$ second will be approximately 1.6 or 1.7 mAs.

Practice these conversions for typical fractions in Exercise #5 and review you answers from the Appendix.

EXERCISE #5

		mA	x	time	=	mAs
1.	200 @			$1/8$	=	
2.	50 @			$1/20$	=	
3.	200 @			$1/5$	=	
4.	200 @			$1/120$	=	
5.	50 @			$1/120$	=	
6.	200 @			$1/40$	=	
7.	50 @			$1/30$	=	
8.	200 @			$1/60$	=	
9.	200 @			$2/3$	=	
10.	200 @			$1/7$	=	

The 300 mA Station

The 300 mA station is an odd number and produces its own unique number pairs when a fractional timer is used. For example, at the 300 mA station **fives** and **sixes** always go together; $1/5$ **second** yields **60 mAs** total, while $1/6$ **second** produces **50 mAs**. The following pairs of numbers always go together when using 300 mA. Commit these to memory, drilling with a study partner if you can:

> 5 and 6
> 15 and 20
> 12 and 25

Other combinations can be made, but these three pairs are used very commonly. For other times, such as $1/8$ second or $1/7$ second, it is easier to simply use the paired number you memorized for the 100 mA station, and then triple that number. For example:

300 mA at $1/8$ second: Remember that at the 100 mA station **eights** always pair with **twelves**. So think of this as:

= 3 sets of 12

= appx 36 mAs

Proceed to Exercise #6. Then check your answers in the Appendix.

EXERCISE #6

	mA	x	time	=	mAs
1.	300 @		$1/5$	=	
2.	300 @		$1/60$	=	
3.	300 @		$1/20$	=	
4.	300 @		$1/15$	=	
5.	300 @		$1/12$	=	
6.	300 @		$1/120$	=	
7.	300 @		$1/25$	=	
8.	300 @		$1/40$	=	
9.	300 @		$1/80$	=	
10.	300 @		$1/7$	=	

Other mA Stations

Technique conversions can be made at other mA stations by building on the previous exercises. For the 600 mA station, the total mAs values learned at the 300 mA station can simply be doubled. The same thing can be done with the 400 mA station, doubling the results from the 200 mA station. Furthermore, any of these can be solved by going back to the number pairs you memorized for the 100 mA station. Proceed to Exercise #7 and review your answers from the Appendix.

EXERCISE #7

	mA	x	time	=	mAs
1.	400 @		$1/20$	=	
2.	600 @		$1/5$	=	
3.	500@		$1/4$	=	
4.	600@		$1/40$	=	
5.	600 @		$1/30$	=	
6.	400 @		$1/60$	=	
7.	400 @		$1/8$	=	
8.	600 @		$1/120$	=	
9.	400@		$1/12$	=	
10.	500 @		$1/15$	=	

Complex Fractions

Complex fractions involve numerators other than "1" on the top, such as $2/5$ or $7/20$. You must convert them in two steps, dividing the bottom denominator into the mA station first, and then thinking of the top number as "sets."

For example, to solve:

200 mA at $2/5$ second

First, ignore the top numerator in the fraction, considering it as a "one"–in other words, find $1/5$ of 200. When you have this number, multiply it by the top of the fraction thinking in "sets," as follows:

$1/5$ Of 200 = 40

2 SETS of 40 = 80 mAs

200 mA at $7/20$ second should be thought of as **7 sets of 10**, and **300 mA at $3/15$ second** would be **3 sets of 20**. Using this approach, solve all of the problems in Exercise 8 mentally, then check your answers in the Appendix.

EXERCISE #8

	mA	x	time	=	mAs
1.	100 @		$2/5$	=	
2.	100 @		$2/15$	=	
3.	100 @		$3/20$	=	
4.	200 @		$3/5$	=	
5.	200 @		$3/15$	=	
6.	200 @		$7/20$	=	
7.	400 @		$2/5$	=	
8.	300 @		$4/5$	=	
9.	300 @		$3/20$	=	
10.	400 @		$3/20$	=	

CONVERTING FRACTIONAL AND DECIMAL TIMES

A radiographer who is used to working with decimal timers should be able to quickly adapt to an x-ray machine employing a fractional timer. The reverse is also true, and both types of machines are commonly found. It turns out that the math for doing this is very similar to the mathematics used for mAs conversions.

For example, to convert the fraction $1/6$ into a decimal number, 6 is simply divided into 1.00 for an answer of 0.16. Note how similar this operation is to taking $1/6$ second at 100 mA to obtain 16 mAs. The only difference is the placement of the decimal point.

Changing Fractions into Decimals

To change a fraction into a decimal, simply divide the numerator (top) by the denominator (bottom). But, first place a decimal point to the right of the numerator and add as many zeros as needed to complete the division. For example, to find the decimal equivalent for $3/20$:

$$\frac{3.0}{20}$$ Temporarily remove the decimal:

$$\frac{30}{20}$$ Remove the extra zeros

$$\frac{3}{2} = 1.5$$ Now, "replacing" the decimal place to the left in the answer

$$\frac{3.0}{20} = 0.15$$

You may find it even easier to pretend that the numerator is an mA station, in multiples of 100. To illustrate:

$$\frac{3.0}{20}$$ Think of the numerator, 3.0, as the 300 mA station

$$\frac{300}{20}$$ Recall from the previous section that at 300 mA, the number pair 15 and 20 always go together:

$$\frac{300}{20} = 15$$ Now, since you added two zeros the numerator above, you must move the decimal two places to the left in your answer:

$$\frac{3.00}{20} = 0.15$$

In the following exercise, convert each fraction listed into its decimal equivalent. For unusual fractions, simply divide the numerator by the denominator. Review your answers in the Appendix.

EXERCISE #9

	Fraction		Decimal
1.	$2/3$	=	
2.	$1/5$	=	
3.	$1/6$	=	
4.	$1/7$	=	
5.	$1/8$	=	
6.	$1/12$	=	
7.	$1/15$	=	
8.	$1/20$	=	
9.	$1/30$	=	
10.	$1/40$	=	
11.	$1/60$	=	
12.	$1/80$	=	
13.	$1/120$	=	
14.	$2/15$	=	
15.	$3/20$	=	
16.	$2/5$	=	
17.	$3/5$	=	
18.	$4/5$	=	
19.	$3/15$	=	
20.	$7/20$	=	

To convert a decimal number into a fraction requires three steps: First, the numerator (top of the fraction) is found by simply writing out all of the non-zero figures to the right of the decimal point. Then to find the denominator (bottom of the fraction), write 1 for the decimal point, and a zero for each decimal place after it. For example, find the fractional equivalent for 0.0125:

0.0125 For the numerator, write out nonzero figures to the right of the decimal point:

125 is the numerator.

For the denominator, write a 1 in place of the decimal point. There are four figures or decimal places to the right of the decimal point (.0125), so you will write four zeros after the one:

10,000 is the denominator.

The fraction is: $\dfrac{125}{10,000}$

Finally, reduce the fraction if possible to its lowest common denominator. In the example above, 125 and 10,000 do not have a lower common denominator, and the fraction cannot be reduced. Following is an example of a decimal number which can be reduced after converting it into a fraction:

0.6   For the numerator, write the non-zero figure to the right of the decimal point:

6 is the numerator.

For the denominator, write a 1 for the decimal point and a zero for each place after it:

10 is the denominator.

The fraction is:

$\frac{6}{10}$ Six and ten share a common denominator– they are both divisible by 2. Reduce the fraction by dividing both numbers by 2:

$\frac{6/2}{10/2} =$

$\frac{3}{5}$ This fraction cannot be further reduced, and is the answer.

In the following exercise, convert the decimal numbers listed into equivalent fractions, then check and review your answers in the Appendix.

EXERCISE #10

	Decimal	Fraction
1.	0.05	=
2.	0.0333	=
3.	0.2	=
4.	0.75	=
5.	0.025	=
6.	0.6667	=
7.	0.143	=
8.	0.002	=
9.	0.08	=
10.	0.167	=
11.	0.125	=
12.	0.6	=
13.	0.0625	=
14.	0.00833	=

FINDING MA AND TIME COMBINATIONS FOR A DESIRED MAS

Probably the most common mathematics problem a radiographer faces every day is that of having a desired total mAs in mind, and trying to mentally determine an mA-time combination that will yield that total. In this case, you must decide what mA station your desired total mAs will divide into easily. With a little practice, the correct time fraction will then come to mind.

One unique thing about fractions (which you will not find in working with decimals) is that some of the answers can only be found in "complex fractions" as we have defined them. To solve these, you must again learn to think in "sets," such as using two sets of 20 mAs to obtain 40 mAs.

For example, how would you obtain **80 mAs** using the **200 mA** station? Since 80 does not divide *evenly* into 200, no usable fraction with a "1" on top as the numerator can be found, (that is, to simply divide it out, you will get 2.5 as the denominator, resulting in a fraction of $1/2.5$–this is a complex fraction that will not be found on the timer knob). However, if you learn to recognize that **80 is two sets of 40**, you can find a usable time:

First, **divide 40 mAs into 200 mA = 5.**

5 is the denominator of your fraction.

In other words, the fraction used to obtain 40 mAs is $1/5$

Now, simply go back and take *two sets* of $1/5$, by changing the numerator to 2.

The answer is $2/5$ second.

80 mAs = 200 mA at $2/5$ second

(80 mAs = two sets of 40 mAs)

The following exercise will "warm you up" to finding these sets of numbers. For each total mAs listed, express it as so many sets of a smaller number which will easily divide into one of the typical mA stations. There are ONE or TWO answers to each problem, but no more, because, for that smaller number, you must choose a number which does not require further reduction. For example:

120 mAs can be expressed as _____ sets of _____?

If you use **6 sets of 20**, this ratio can then be reduced to **3 sets** (of 40). It is not a good answer.

One good answer is **3 sets of 40**, since this number of sets cannot be further reduced.

Another good answer is **2 sets of 60**, since, again, this number of sets cannot be further reduced. (One set of 120 is absurd, because there is no 120 mA station available.)

Note that sets of 40 will be evenly divisible into the **200 mA station**, while sets of 60 will be divisible into the **300 mA station**.

It sounds complicated at first, but try the exercise, and you will find it is not as hard as you might have expected. Check your answers in the Appendix.

EXERCISE #11

1. 80 mAs can be expressed as _____ sets of _____.
2. 45 mAs can be expressed as _____ sets of _____.
3. 66 mAs can be expressed as _____ sets of _____.
4. 75 mAs can be expressed as _____ sets of _____.
5. 180 mAs can be expressed as _____ sets of _____.
6. 120 mAs can be expressed as _____ sets of _____.
   OR as _____ sets of _____.
7. 160 mAs can be expressed as _____ sets of _____.
   OR as _____ sets of _____.
8. 240 mAs can be expressed as _____ sets of _____.
   OR as _____ sets of _____.
9. 90 mAs can be expressed as _____ sets of _____.
10. 320 mAs can be expressed as _____ sets of _____.

In the following two exercises, the total mAs desired is given along with the mA station to be used. You must mentally decide which time to use. Use only those times which are available on most x-ray machines. On the first exercise the answers must be expressed as fractions, on the second one they must be decimals. Do the exercises *mentally*, then check your answers in the Appendix.

EXERCISE #12

ANSWERS MUST BE IN FRACTIONS

Total mAs = mA x seconds

1. 2.5 mAs = 100 mA x _____
2. 7 mAs = 100 mA x _____
3. 3.3 mAs = 100 mA x _____
4. 1.7 mAs = 100 mA x _____
5. 1.25 mAs = 100 mA x _____
6. 0.8 mAs = 100 mA x _____
7. 40 mAs = 100 mA x _____
8. 2.5 mAS = 50 mA x _____
9. 40 mAs = 200 mA x _____
10. 120 mAs = 200 mA x _____
11. 5 mAs = 200 mA x _____
12. 14 mAs = 200 mA x _____
13. 6 mAs = 300 mA x _____
14. 20 mAs = 300 mA x _____
15. 2.5 mAs = 300 mA x _____
16. 45 mAs = 300 mA x _____
17. 180 mAs = 300 mA x _____
18. 240 mAs = 300 mA x _____
19. 80 mAs = 400 mA x _____
20. 240 mAs = 400 mA x _____

EXERCISE #13

ANSWERS MUST BE IN DECIMALS

Total mAs = mA x seconds

1. 2.5 mAs = 100 mA x _____
2. 7 mAs = 100 mA x _____
3. 16 mAs = 100 mA x _____
4. 3.3 mAs = 100 mA x _____
5. 1.7 mAs=100 mA x _____
6. 40 mAs = 100 mA x _____
7. 2.5 mAs = 50 mA x _____
8. 1.25 mAs = 50 mA x _____
9. 25 mAs = 200 mA x _____
10. 120 mAs = 200 mA x _____
11. 5 mAs = 200 mA x _____
12. 2.5 mAs = 200 mA x _____
13. 14 mAs = 200 mA x _____
14. 50 mAs = 300 mA x _____
15. 6 mAs = 300 mA x _____
16. 21 mAs = 300 mA x _____
17. 180 mAs = 300 mA x _____
18. 75 mAs = 300 mA x _____
19. 80 mAs = 400 mA x _____
20. 240 mAs = 400 mA x _____

CONTROL OF DENSITY

Milliampere-seconds is the primary electrical control over image density, because it affects *only* image density. This relationship is a direct proportion. Whether the rate of x-ray intensity is doubled by mA or the exposure time is doubled, density will double. Since total image density is a direct function of total mAs, it may be said that mA and exposure time are inversely related to each other for a given image density level. That is, if the mA were doubled, the exposure time should be cut to one-half to maintain the original density.

EXPERIMENT:
TIME-DENSITY RELATION

Purpose. To demonstrate the relation between exposure time and radiographic density when all other factors are constant.

Theory. When all other factors but time are constant, the quantity of x-rays emitted by the x-ray tube increases in direct proportion to the time of exposure. Thus, the quantity of x-rays applied in 1 second is approximately doubled when the exposure is 2 seconds, etc. Since radiographic density is influenced by this action, increasing the time increases the density and vice versa.

Procedure

1. The time-density relation can also be demonstrated by making two series of posteroanterior radiographs of the hand (Figure 45), employing 35 and 50 kVp. Series A is made with 35 kVp and all other factors are constant except exposure time, which is increased in accordance with the rule of thumb for changing density. Series B is made with 50 kVp and all other factors are constant except exposure time, which is increased in the same manner as in Series

A. The following materials and factors are employed.

Materials Factors	Film:	Screen-type, 8 x 10-inch
	kVp:	35 (Series A)
	kVp:	50 (Series B)
	mA:	100
	SID:	36 inches

Variable Factors	Exposure No.	Time	mAs
	1	$1/10$ sec.	10
	2	$2/10$ sec.	20
	3	$4/10$ sec.	40
	4	$8/10$ sec.	80

Comment. With all factors constant except time, the two series of radiographs demonstrate the progressive increase in density that results when the exposure time is increased.

a. Series A. In this series (Figure 45 *Top*) the densities do not adequately increase as the time of exposure increases, because the penetration of the radiation is relatively small, i.e., 35 kVp. Prolonged and impractical exposures would, therefore, be necessary to produce radiographic densities that might be satisfactory.

b. Series B. When an optimum kilovoltage of 50 is employed for this projection of the hand (Figure 45, *Bottom*) a greater intensity of radiation is provided and any desired density may be obtained simply by increasing or decreasing the time of exposure. The most satisfactory density is provided by 40 mAs.

EXPERIMENT:
mA-DENSITY RELATION

Purpose. To demonstrate the relation between milliamperage and radiographic density when all other factors are constant.

Theory. When all other factors except milliamperage are constant, radiographic density increases in direct proportion to the milliamperage and vice versa.

Figure 45. Demonstration of the effect of exposure time on radiographic density when an absorber (hand) is used, (*Top*) using 35 kVp, and (*Bottom*) using 50 kVp. The respective total mAs values are noted on each radiograph.

Procedure

1. The mA-density relation may be demonstrated by three posteroanterior radiographs of the hand wherein the following materials and exposure factors were employed. All factors but mA are constant:

Materials Factors	Film:	Screen-type, 8 x 10-inch	
	kVp:	50	
	Time:	$^1/_2$ sec.	
	SID:	36 inches	
Variable Factors	Exposure No.	mA	mAs
	1	10	5
	2	50	25
	3	100	50

Comment. The radiographs of the hand (Figure 46) demonstrate that as the milliamperage increases, the radiographic density increases. The radiographic effect is similar to the influence of time on density. Compare exposures No. 1 and No. 3 and note that the latter has greater density because ten times the milliamperage of No. 1 was employed.

EXPERIMENT: mA-TIME RELATION

Purpose. To demonstrate the interrelation of milliamperage and exposure time with respect to radiographic density when all other factors are constant.

Theory. The milliamperage required for a given radiographic density is inversely

Figure 46. Demonstration of influence of mA on radiographic density with absorber (hand). The respective exposures are (1) 100, (2) 200 and (3) 300 mA.

proportional to the exposure time when all other factors are constant.

Procedure

1. The mAs density relation is demonstrated by three posteroanterior radiographs of the hand, the following materials and exposure factors being employed.

Materials	Film:	Screen-type, 8 x 10-inch	
Factors	kVp:	50	
	SID:	36 inches	
	mAs:	50	
Variable	Exposure No.	mA	Time
Factors	1	10	5 sec.
	2	50	1 sec.
	3	100	$^1/_2$ sec.

Comment. The radiographs (Figure 47) demonstrate that as the milliamperage is increased and all other factors but time are constant, the latter may be reduced to equalize radiographic densities. Since milliamperage and time directly influence density, in actual practice the mA is usually established as a constant and the exposure time as a variable. The greater ease with which small changes in time can be made with modern timers suggests this procedure.

Figure 47. Demonstration of the compensatory (inverse) relationship between mA and exposure time on radiographic density. Time was adjusted downward in inverse proportion to the mA increases which are indicated on each radiograph, to maintain equal total mAs.

VISIBLE DENSITY CHANGE

Generally, the most common cause of repeated exposures is improper density—the radiograph turns out too light or too dark. A repeated exposure doubles the radiation dose to the patient in order to obtain a particular view. It seems unconscionable that a third exposure might be necessitated, thus tripling the patient dose, because the radiographer did not accurately assess the needed technique correction the first time. Every radiographer should have developed the fundamental skill to confidently determine how much a technique must be increased or decreased by observing the original radiograph. An exercise to help develop this skill is found in Chapter 24.

By far, the most common error in making such technique adjustments for improperly exposed radiographs is to *not make a big enough change.* For example, to compensate for a light radiograph, it is somewhat common to "go up one step in time." In most cases, this is a foolhardy notion, since the resulting radiograph may not appear obviously darker than the original, and another repeat could easily result. This is demonstrated in Figure 48 using manual techniques. Note that in this case a 25 per cent increase in exposure did *not* result in an obviously darker radiograph. The 47 per cent increase in mAs did result in a darker film.

This is not to say that a 25 per cent increase in mAs is *never* visible, but for most daily procedures it is not worth risking this type of increase and the additional repeat it may lead to. What is needed is a good rule of thumb for minimum technique corrections, to ensure that the change will be substantial enough to make a difference. A traditional rule of thumb was to always adjust technique (mAs) by at least one-third. The advent .of rare earth screens has indeed lowered this amount slightly, but not as

dramatically as some authors have suggested: Educators should beware that if this type of experiment is performed in the lab using a step-wedge penetrometer, results as low as 17 per cent may be obtained. Such results must not be translated into clinical practice for two very important reasons: First, the step-wedge is made of homogeneous material whereas the human body is composed of heterogeneous tissues forming thousands of trabecular densities, so that greater changes are required before they become obvious in the image. Second, the step-wedge is small in thickness and produces very little scatter radiation, whereas the human body produces large amounts of scatter. This also obscures density changes so that they are less obvious. The rule of thumb we seek must address practical clinical results on real patients.

In practice, a 25 per cent increase may

Figure 48. Demonstration of minimum mAs adjustment to cause a visible change in image density for knee radiographs. Radiograph B shows a 25% increase in mAs from the previous Radiograph A: Note that the density of B is *not visibly darker than A.* Radiograph C shows a 47% increase in mAs, which does result in an obviously darker image. Factors = 58kVp, A = 6.8 mAs, B = 8.5 mAs, C = 10 mAs.

not be visible, while a 25 per cent *decrease* usually is. The 25 per cent decrease results in an exposure that is $3/4$ of the original mAs. The new exposure ratio is $3/4$. The opposite of this change, that is, a corresponding *increase* in technique, is actually **4/3** ($3/4$ inverted). That is, if technique must be reduced to $3/4$ to be visibly lighter, it would be expected that an increase to $4/3$ would be needed to be visibly darker. Expressed as a percentage, $4/3$ of the original technique is a 33 per cent increase. Thus, a workable rule of thumb using modern screens is: ***Always decrease technique by at least a quarter, always increase technique by at least a third.***

Suppose that the radiologist asks for a repeated exposure in order to darken the image, and the technologist makes this correction by increasing "one step in time." There are two inherent problems with this approach: First, it is not specific. What exact percentage of change is achieved at the next "step" on the exposure timer depends upon the range of times involved and the particular format in which the manufacturer of the equipment designed the timer. The "next step in time" on one machine might be a 25 per cent increase, while that on another brand of equipment might be as different as 50 per cent. Second, many steps on a typical timer fall well below the one-third increase required for a visibly darker density on the finished radiograph. As an example, if 300 mA at $1/5$ second, or 60 mAs, were used on a light radiograph, the next step in time would likely be $1/4$ second. At 300 mA, $1/4$ second would yield 75 mAs total, or an increase of 15 mAs from the original mAs. Fifteen added to sixty represents an increase of 25 per cent or $1/4$, below the one-third

increase required to really see any difference. This radiograph would not be visibly distinguishable as being any darker than the first.

The rule of thumb for minimum technique corrections is affected by the response, reciprocal or otherwise, of the image receptor system, but is not brought about by it. The need for such a rule is simply based upon the limitations of the human eye in distinguishing subtle density differences. It is important to note that the discussion thus far has dealt only with *minimum* visible changes, not with *recommended* changes. The older rule of thumb, "reduce technique by at least $1/3$ or increase it by at least $1/2$," is still quite functional as a *recommendation*. In fact, when using automatic exposure control or "phototiming," the most common selections for increasing technique are +25%, +50% and 75%. Given these choices, as shown in Figure 191 in Chapter 28, it is almost always wiser to select the +50% in order to darken up an image, thus increasing technique by $1/2$.

Another general rule of thumb has proven valuable when correcting for *serious* underexposures and overexposures: It is useful for the radiographer to think of substantial technique corrections in factors of 2. Most serious underexposures can be corrected by doubling the initial mAs. In the case of serious overexposures, cutting the mAs to one-half the initial value will usually suffice. There are certainly situations that require more dramatic alterations, and the density correction exercise in Chapter 24 addresses these. But, this "factor of 2" concept is workable in perhaps 80 per cent of the circumstances when a radiograph turns out much too light or very dark.

UNDEREXPOSURE AND QUANTUM MOTTLE

During a light rain shower, you can see the individual raindrops on a sidewalk. If you count the raindrops in each square foot, you you can see that they are not evenly distributed, but that more fall in some areas than in others. When a heavy rainfall comes, the same uneven distribution of raindrops is still there. But, you can no longer tell, because the sidewalk is now saturated with rain and there are no dry spots between the drops.

The x-ray beam is a *shower* of x-rays which have a random distribution just like a rain shower. When very low mAs values are used, there are few photons striking the film and you can see the uneven distribution of densities resulting. The radiograph appears *grainy*–that is, very small blotches of density are seen across the film. These blotches are referred to as *quantum mottle,* a mottling of the film caused by the quanta or photons in the beam. Mottling indicates that insufficient mAs values were used. To correct it, the intensity of the beam must be increased by increasing mAs.

EFFECT ON CONTRAST

Radiographic contrast is determined by the ratio of penetrating x-rays between different types of tissues within the patient as explained in Chapter 4. As shown in Figure 44, changes in mAs control the total number of photons produced but do *not* change the proportion of photons at one energy level to another energy level. For example, the number of photons having 35 keV may be doubled, but the number of photons having 70 keV will also be doubled so that their proportion to each other remains the same. Milliampere-seconds cannot have any effect upon the types of interactions taking place, only upon their total numbers.

For example, doubling the mAs will have the following effects: Twice as many x-ray photons will enter the surface of the patient. In soft tissue, twice as many photoelectric interactions will occur and twice as many Compton scatter interactions will occur, so that the overall absorption of x-rays has doubled. *However, there will also be twice as many photons penetrating completely though the soft tissue without interacting.*

Everything doubles, including the number of penetrating rays. Therefore, the *ratio* of penetration or absorption in the soft tissue is unchanged–this tissue still has the same subject contrast characteristics. The same is true for bone tissue: Twice as many x-rays are absorbed, but twice as many penetrate through as well, so that the penetration or absorption *ratio* is unchanged and the bone still possesses its characteristic subject contrast.

As illustrated in Chapter 4, image contrast will not change as long as the absorption ratios between the tissues is unchanged. Let us assume that, originally, the absorption ratio for the soft tissue was 90 per cent, and that the ratio for the bone was 70 per cent. Doubling the quantity of x-rays entering the patient does not change these ratios. Thus, the contrast between the bone and the soft tissue will still be 9/7. Contrast is unchanged.

Figure 24 in the last chapter shows that a radiograph can be twice as dark overall, and yet still possess the same contrast. Figure 45, just a few pages back, demonstrates the same concept if you observe the two middle radiographs on the bottom row, using 20 mAs and 40 mAs respectively. The soft tissue may appear twice as dark, but as long as the bone *also* appears twice as dark, the ratio of density difference *between* the bone and the soft tissue will still be equal. (Note that in evaluating image contrast, the *background* density must be ignored–comparisons should only be made between between the different tissue areas *within the anatomy*, in this case, the soft tissue density versus the bone density.) For practical purposes, *mAs should not be considered as a variable affecting contrast.*

Now, if *extreme* changes in mAs are made, an exception occurs which also can be seen in Figure 45 by observing the two extreme ends of this series of radiographs:

On the one hand, if there is just insufficient exposure to the film to produce any reasonable density, all tissues, both bone and soft tissue, will appear nearly blank white, and the contrast between them is lost. On the other hand, if extreme amounts of mAs are used so that the film is grossly overexposed, the soft tissue areas will have reached the maximum density the film can produce–"pitch black," while the bone areas will continue to darken, and contrast will diminish. These are both exceptional cases: Note that in Figure 45 the difference in mAs to illustrate these effects was *8 fold*, while in daily practice, changing technique by 8 times would be unheard of. *The mAs should never be considered as a controlling factor over image contrast* when used in diagnostic ranges.

EXPOSURE TIME AND MOTION

Long exposure times are not the direct cause of motion. But in chest radiography, for example, heart motion is unavoidable, and can only be eliminated radiographically by the use of very short exposure times. In addition, the longer the time, the greater the chance for peristaltic motion, breathing motion or movement of the patient to occur. Therefore, exposure time should be considered as a *contributing cause* of motion during radiographic procedures. Generally, the shorter the exposure time, the sharper the recorded detail.

EFFECTS ON OTHER QUALITIES

Milliamperage and exposure time have no direct effect upon magnification or distortion–because mA and time are essentially electrical factors and have nothing to do with geometry.

SUMMARY

1. Milliamperage is an electrical factor controlling the *rate* of x-ray emission from the x-ray tube.
2. Milliampere-seconds (*mAs*) multiplies this rate by the exposure time and represents the *total exposure* intensity.
3. Milliampere-seconds is the primary control for image *density*. This is for two reasons: First, density is directly proportional to mAs, and second, mAs has no direct affect upon the other image qualities in the practical ranges.
4. For a given mAs value, mA and exposure time are inversely related to each other. A higher mA and a shorter time can be used, as long as the total mAs is equal, to achieve a certain image density.
5. When correcting mAs for and improperly exposed radiograph, *decrease by at least $1/4$ or increase by at least $1/3$ to produce a visible change in the density.* For serious corrections, generally change mAs by a factor of 2.
6. Insufficient mAs can lead to visible quantum mottle in the image.

REVIEW QUESTIONS

1. What electrical factor controls the rate of the x-rays coming from the tube?
2. In controlling image density, why is it important to talk of total mAs rather than just mA or time separately?
3. Give two reasons why mAs should be considered as the primary control for image density:
4. In maintaining a given density, mA and time are _____ related to each other.
5. The reciprocity law states that the resulting density on a radiograph should be directly proportional to:
6. 1.6 mAs may be obtained by using 100 mA at _____ second.
7. The fraction $1/8$ second is equal to which decimal number:
8. 80 milliseconds is _____ second in decimal time.
9. 240 mAs may be obtained by using 300 mA at _____ second.
10. In normal ranges, changing the mAs does not affect image contrast because the number of incoming photons does not alter the _____-contrast of the tissues.
11. What would be a good practical reason for using a low mA and a long exposure time to achieve a given total mAs?
12. When repeating a radiograph that was too dark, always decrease mAs by at least _____ to ensure a visible difference.
13. When repeating a radiograph that was too light, always increase mAs by at least _____ to ensure a visible difference.
14. When repeating a radiograph that was much too dark or much too light, always change mAs by at least a factor of _____.
15. What can cause the uneven distribution of x-rays within the beam to show up as a "grainy" appearance on the radiograph?

Chapter 6

KILOVOLTAGE PEAK

KILOVOLTAGE ABBREVIATED keV or kV, is a measure of the electrical force or *pressure* behind a current of electricity, which causes it to flow. In the x-ray machine, the kilovoltage control is actually the *autotransformer* in the high-voltage circuit. Whenever a potential difference exists between two points in a conductor, one end having a relative negative charge and the other end a relative positive charge, a current of electrons will flow through the conductor. The greater the difference is in electrical charge or potential, the more *pressure* is exerted on the current to flow, and the more kilovoltage is measured. While mAs actually measures the quantity of electrons flowing through a wire, kV measures the quality, or the *energy* level, of the electrons flowing through it.

Due to the rotation of the magnetic fields in a generator that produces electricity, the actual kilovoltage of a current varies in strength up and down in a sinewave pattern, rising to a peak and then falling back to zero repeatedly. Since the kilovoltage is constantly changing, we must measure it in terms of either an average value or as a peak value attained during the cycle (Figure 49), hence the use of the term *kilovolt-peak*, or *kVp*.

EFFECT ON X-RAY BEAM SPECTRUM

The kVp control meters on typical x-ray equipment read in peak kilovoltage, but it is important to remember that this reading indicates the energy of only a very small portion of the current. Most of the current is much less than the peak kilovoltage. Since the x-rays produced cannot possibly have any more energy than the electrons

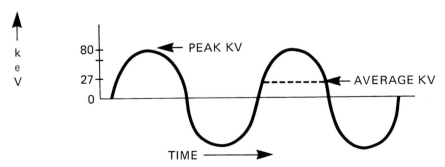

Figure 49. Graph of sine wave showing the changing kilovoltage during normal electrical cycles. Kilovoltage must be measured as a peak value or as an average value. For single-phase equipment, the *average* kilovoltage is about one-third of the *peak* kilovoltage.

that produced them, this also means that only a few x-rays will actually have the peak kilovoltage of energy, with the average having much less, about 1/3 of the peak.

The characteristic curve of the spectrum of energies in an x-ray beam plots the kV energy level against the number of x-rays produced at each kV, i.e. the intensity at each kV level, as shown in Figure 50.

Note that the greatest number of x-rays for an 80 kVp beam occurs at about 27 kVp. When kVp is increased, as shown by the dotted curve, peak energy of the x-ray beam increases to the right, average energy increases, and the total number of x-rays produced (indicated by the total area under the curve) is also slightly increased.

Figure 50.   Graph of x-ray beam spectrum changes resulting from an increase in kVp. The peak and average energies of the beam increase, while the minimum energy remains the same. Also, the total number of x-rays emitted from the x-ray tube increases by 25% to 40%.

When the kilovoltage applied across the x-ray tube is increased, the electrons emitted from the filament accelerate to a greater speed before reaching the anode. Since they have a higher energy, they are capable of losing more energy when they interact with the atoms in the anode. X-rays with higher energy levels can be produced. Not

all of the additional x-rays produced will have higher energies than those already in the beam, but many will, and the average energy of the beam will increase (Figure 50).

At the same time, electrons traveling at higher speeds are likely to undergo *more* interactions, producing more x-rays. Reviewing the *bremsstrahlung* interaction in Chapter One, one can surmise that, since an electron is only *partially* slowed down from this interaction, the electron may undergo *several* bremsstrahlung interactions before losing all of its speed. This means that one electron can produce several x-rays, one from each interaction. At higher kilovoltage, the electrons enter the anode material at higher speeds, and can undergo yet more interactions before losing all of their energy. More x-rays will be produced, shown in Figure 50 as a *higher* spectral curve. Therefore, the *quantity* as well as the *quality* of the x-rays produced increases at higher kilovoltage levels.

Even though more x-rays are produced at all energy levels, those with low energies will be absorbed by filtration. The *minimum* energy of the beam is denoted in Figure 50 as the point to the left at which the curve is cut toward zero. This portion of the spectrum curve is unchanged. The minimum energy of the x-ray beam is controlled by filtration, not by kVp.

An x-ray beam with higher energy will be capable of *penetrating* through more different types of tissue.   As discussed in Chapter Four, such a change in penetration will affect the gray scale, and consequently change the image contrast, on the finished radiograph. Higher kVp levels also result in more x-rays being initially produced, and with higher penetration power, these are more likely to reach the film, darkening the density.   Therefore, changes in kVp have profound effects on *both* image *contrast* and image *density*.

CONTROL OF CONTRAST

Subject contrast, the difference in intensity between one portion of the remnant x-ray beam and another, is completely essential for a radiographic image to be produced. Three situations, all of which can be related to kVp, can prevent this production of subject contrast in the image. In the first case, insufficient penetration of the x-ray beam through the tissues leads to a failure to record each different tissue as a density on the radiograph. Two underpenetrated areas will both be recorded as blank white, so that there can be no distinction between them. In the second case, alteration of the directions of the remnant x-rays by scattering interactions within the patient leads to a crossing over of exposure intensities, so that there is less distinction between them. In the third case, extreme overexposure of the film leads to all areas reaching a level of pitch-black density, so that there can be little or no distinction between them.

PENETRATION AND GRAY SCALE

The most important function of kVp is to, provide penetration of the x-ray beams through the patient's tissues. At higher levels of kVp, the penetrating ability of the x-rays is increased. Therefore, *more* different types of body tissues may be penetrated and recorded on the radiograph as a representative density. As greater numbers of different tissues are recorded on the radiograph, more different gray shades will be present in the image. Gray scale increases. Penetration is a primary controlling factor over image gray scale.

Let us examine this relationship more closely by considering low, medium, and high kVp levels one at a time: If kVp is so low that there is insufficient penetration, virtually all tissues are recorded as a light or "white" density on the image, and by definition, there is little contrast. As kVp is gradually increased, tissues with lower atomic numbers are recorded as gray shades, while bones, barium, iodine and other tissues with higher atomic numbers are still "white." Differential absorption, due to "subject contrast or tissue contrast" is now established. Gray scale can now be measured in the image, but the scale is too short, with only a few different shades of light gray and white present. Continuing to still higher energies, bones and similar tissues become penetrated and are recorded as light grays, while other tissues are seen as medium grays and dark grays. Eventually, if the kVp is high enough, even barium and iodine will be penetrated enough to be recorded as a light gray rather than a blank white (which possesses no radiographic information).

By increasing the kVp, more and more different types of tissue are recorded on the film, more different shades of gray are produced, and gray scale is gradually lengthened.

As discussed in Chapter Three, gray scale is the opposite of image contrast, and when there are many more different shades of gray present in the image, the result is that there is less of a difference from one gray shade to the next. Hence, contrast is reduced.

This implies that even when scatter fogging of the radiograph is eliminated as a consideration, changes in kVp will still have a considerable effect upon image contrast by virtue of their control over beam penetration. *Higher kVp levels will increase the gray scale, reducing contrast.*

Demonstration No. 1

The influence of kilovoltage on gray scale can be demonstrated by a series of radiographs of a dry skull (Figure 51). The absence of soft tissues in the specimen eliminates in large measure the influence of scatter radiation on the image. The images, therefore, may be considered substantially free of scatter radiation fog. The radiographs were exposed in 10 kVp increments from 50 to 100 kVp. The density effect of each kilovoltage was offset by compensating mAs. As a guide in mAs compensation, a step-wedge was recorded in each radiograph—the density of its third step being used as a "control." This density was maintained constant for all kilovoltages. The procedure made it possible to demonstrate the gray scale characteristics of each skull image produced by each advance in kilovoltage.

In the 50-kVp film, very high image densities are exhibited and there are also areas in which no details appear because of a lack of sufficient silver deposit. Penetrating radiation was needed to traverse the) thicker and denser structures, such as the jaws, pars petrosae, and superior portions of the vault. As the kilovoltage is advanced, some details in these latter structures begin to appear. At 90 and 100 kVp, all structures are thoroughly penetrated and all radiographic details are visible. In comparing the 50-kVp and 100-kVp radiographs, a difference in "brightness" of the images is manifest. The lower kilovoltage film attracts the eye at once because of its brilliance. The eye ignores the fact that a large number of details representative of

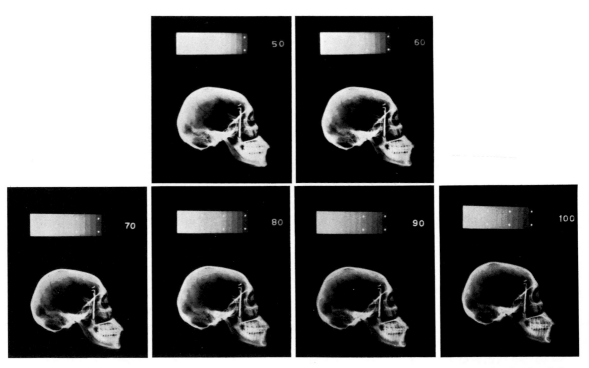

Figure 51. Radiographs of a dry skull demonstrate that the increased *penetration* obtained at higher kilovoltages leads to lengthened image gray scale. Note that with no soft tissue present, scatter is negligible. Therefore, this effect is entirely due to increased penetration of various tissues. The kVp used is shown on each image.

the anatomy are absent. The few details that are adequately recorded are composed of rather heavy silver deposits and a *rapid* fall-off in image density occurs in areas representing the thicker or denser anatomical structures. Also, the distribution is unequal. At 100 kVp, there is a uniform distribution of translucent densities over the entire image. This radiograph has a lower level of "brightness," but the image contains an abundance of details which are so necessary for diagnostic purposes. Whenever great "brightness" or brilliance of an image immediately attracts the eye, short scale exists as shown in the 50-kVp film. Whenever a lower level of brightness exists and the image contains an abundance of details, long scale exists as shown in the 100-kVp film. The former is to be avoided and the latter to be attained.

Comment. From this demonstration it may be seen that, when secondary radiation is efficiently controlled, kilovoltage becomes the factor of radiographic scale. Note that the scale lengthens as the kVp rises. Also, the radiographs exhibiting the greatest number of details are made with low mAs and higher kVp values.

Demonstration No. 2

Purpose. To demonstrate the influence of kilovoltage on radiographic gray scale.

Theory. As kilovoltage increases and the mAs is adjusted to secure approximate equalization of translucent densities of a given body part, radiographic scale increases.

Procedure

1. A series of four posteroanterior chest radiographs of average thickness (22-23 cm.) was made employing the following materials and exposure factors:

Materials	Film:	Screen-type, 14 x 17-inch	
	Screen:	Average speed	
Variable	Exposure No.	kVp	mAs*
Factors	1	50	20
	2	60	8.33
	3	80	3.33
	4	100	1.66

Comment. In this experiment (Figure 52) a circular area about 2 inches in diameter over the inferior portion of the right upper lobe of the lung was selected as a density guide since it possesses average pulmonary tissue density. As the kilovoltage was increased, the mAs was adjusted so that translucent densities in this area of each radiograph showed essentially the same details. With each successive rise in kilovoltage, details of heavier and more dense tissue structures gradually made their appearance in the entire images, indicating gradual penetration by the more abundant shorter wave length x-rays.

The 80 kVp radiograph demonstrates all essential thoracic detail. No added diagnostic features become visible when 100 kVp is employed. However, unmistakable evidence of an unduly long scale is shown in this radiograph. Note that many details are absent in the 50-kVp radiograph that are visible in the 80-kVp radiograph, particularly those portions of the image that represent thick structures. In other words, as the kilovoltage increases, more densities become visible—the gray scale becomes longer—up to a certain point (80 kVp). Above this level, the scale is much too long. The experiment demonstrates that kilovoltage controls the scale of radiographic densities by means of which image details become visible.

*To offset the influence of increasing kilovoltages on density, the mAs values were selected to produce translucent densities.

Figure 52. Radiographs of the chest demonstrating the effect of increasing kilovoltage upon image contrast and gray scale. Radiograph No. 1 was taken at 50 kVp, No. 2 at 60 kVp, No. 3 at 80 kVp, and No. 4 at 100 kVp.

INFLUENCE OF SCATTER FOG

As explained in Chapter 4, higher-energy x-ray beams result in a drastic loss of photoelectric interactions, leaving high *proportions* of Compton interactions, which result in scattered x-rays. Although Thompson interactions also emit x-rays in random directions, Compton interactions account for over 99 per cent of all scattered x-rays reaching the x-ray film. Any radiation emitted as the result of interactions within atoms in the patient's body are considered as *secondary* radiation. Not all secondary radiation is significantly scattered. A small amount may be emitted in very nearly the direction of the original x-ray which caused the interaction and, therefore, will still be carrying an image.

An image cannot exist without *subject contrast,* the difference in radiation intensity between two areas in the remnant beam, exiting the patient. The area under a bone, for example, would have much less intensity left than the area under soft tissues, since the bone attenuates more of the original beam. It may, therefore, be said that the remnant beam *carries* an image or a signal. The subject contrast carried by the remnant beam is directly responsible for the image contrast on the finished radiograph. Most of the secondary radiation resulting from Compton interactions is scattered in random directions. Subject contrast can only exist in the remnant beam while the x-rays are travelling in roughly parallel, straight lines. When scattered rays cross over the remnant beam from one area to another, it no longer carries an image but only causes an overall, general increase in the density on the film (Figure 53). Scattered radiation cannot carry the contrast differences required for an image to exist.

Fog as Noise

Since scatter radiation cannot carry any useful signal, it contributes nothing of value to the radiographic image. It can only be destructive, veiling over the useful image with a nebulous layer of density called *fog.* This fog obscures image details, reducing their visibility.

Any useless information recorded on the radiograph which obscures the desired image becomes a form of *noise.* A certain degree of noise is present in any image. The visibility of the image is enhanced by keeping this noise level low in proportion

Figure 53. Diagram showing how subject contrast is lost in the remnant beam by scattered x-rays randomly crossing over image boundaries and fogging the film.

to the useful signal. It should be recalled that in radiography, the useful signal is produced primarily by the occurrence of photoelectric interactions within the patient, which result in subject contrast in the remnant x-ray beam. At high levels of kVp, these photoelectric interactions are rapidly lost, while much of the scatter interactions remain. This remaining noise then comprises a larger *proportion* of the total information reaching the x-ray film. The fogging effect of the scatter radiation becomes visible in the image.

In addition to these differences in the proportions of interactions, two other effects of higher beam energy levels upon scatter radiation must be remembered: First, at higher kVp levels the scattered radiation produced will also have higher energies, making it more likely to penetrate out of the body and reach the film. Second, the higher the energy of the scatter radiation, the more it tends to be emitted in a forward direction, rather than backward or to the side, so more of it strikes the film. Together, these two effects more than compensate for the slight reduction in Compton interactions graphed in Figure 43 so that *the net amount of scatter radiation reaching the x-ray film is gradually increased at higher energy levels.*

High kVp techniques, then, result in low contrast images for three reasons:

1. Increased penetration of the primary beam through various tissues lengthens the image gray scale.

2. Photoelectric interactions are rapidly lost, leaving a high Compton/photoelectric ratio—On the radiograph, "white" densities are lost and fog becomes more visible in the image.

3. Scatter radiation produced by the Compton interaction is both more energetic and scattered in a more for- **ward direction, and the increased amount of scatter *reaching the film* produces more fog in the image.**

Fog darkens the relatively light areas of the image, while those areas which are already pitch black cannot become visibly any darker. The diffuse exposure of the various areas of the film to fog results in less difference between their densities. Contrast is reduced.

Increased scatter radiation reaching the film constitutes a second mechanism by which image contrast is reduced when increasing kVp.

Figure 54. Photograph of paraffin emitter and associated objects used to illustrate the influence of kilovoltage on the production of scatter radiation in Figure 55.

Demonstration

The influence of kilovoltage on the proportion of scatter radiation and its fogging effect on the image is illustrated by a series of radiographs shown in Figure 55. The arrangement of a paraffin block to be used as the emitter of scatter radiation, a dried femur, and a slab of 1/8-inch lead and a lead sheet barrier in relation to an x-ray film is shown in Figure 54. The dried

Figure 55. Radiographs of paraffin emitter and associated objects. Kilovoltages are noted on each radiograph. Note the presence of scatter fog (from the paraffin) in areas and 3 at high kVp levels.

femur and lead produce such small quantities of scatter radiation within the 40 to 100 kVp range that neither can be considered an effective emitter. A sheet of $1/8$-inch lead when wrapped around the emitter on three sides served as a barrier to the scatter radiation that would reach the film on one side upon exposure. Radiographs A-D, Figure 55, were made with the bone and lead sheet placed on *top* of the emitter, thereby creating a 2.5-inch OID for these objects. The lead strip and the femur were permitted to project over the lead barrier on both sides of the paraffin block as shown in Figure 54. The radiographs were made with a constant mAs factor of 40. The kVp employed for radiograph A was 40; B, 60; C, 80; and D, 100.

Comment. The radiographs A-D demonstrate that as kilovoltage increases and all other factors are constant: (1) radiographic density and fog increase in the presence of an emitter of scatter radiation and (2) full penetration is effected at 60 kVp. In each radiograph, there are six image areas (1, 2, 3, 4, 5, 6) that should be observed as the kilovoltage is increased and all other factors remain constant.

1. Area 1 is that portion of the image of the femur that is covered by the image of the paraffin emitter. It is affected by the increasing density effect of the kilovoltage and the scatter radiation emitted by the paraffin block. As the kilovoltage increases, the density of this area increases. The ease with which details are visualized becomes less and less until they are virtually obliterated by the excessive density in the 100-kVp film (D).

2. Area 2 is that portion of the image of the femur that projects over and *beyond* the lead barrier. Since the lead barrier prevents scatter radiation from affecting this portion of the image of the femur, the increased density is solely due to the increased kilovoltage. This area becomes overexposed in the 100-kVp radiograph (D).

3. Area 3 is that portion of the image of the lead strip covered by the image of the paraffin emitter. Because the object-film-distance of the lead strip is 2.5 inches, scatter radiation undercuts the lead and this image area becomes fogged. In the 40-kVp radiograph (A) there is only small evidence of fog in this area. As the kilovoltage increases, as shown in radiographs B, C, and D, the fog becomes greater. Because the lead strip is not penetrated by the primary radiation, the silver deposit in this image area may be entirely attributed to exposure by scatter radiation.

4. Area 4 is that portion of the image of the lead strip that extends beyond the lead barrier. No appreciable change in density of this image area occurs because no primary radiation penetrates the lead and no scatter radiation reaches this image area from the emitter.

5. Area 5 is that portion of the image of the femur projecting over the *unshielded* side of the emitter. Details in the femur image nearest the emitter are fogged, but the fogging effect diminishes as the bone becomes more remote to the emitter. Here, the inverse square law has an opportunity to become effective in reducing the fogging action of the scatter radiation.

6. Area 6 is that portion of the image representing the lead strip that projects over and beyond the unshielded side of the emitter. The diminution in fogging by undercutting as the strip becomes more remote is shown. The condition is similar to that shown for area 5 except for the fact that details are not present in the image area.

OVEREXPOSURE BY KILOVOLTAGE

The real function of beam penetration, controlled by kVp, is to leave a sufficient intensity of x- rays in the remnant beam to expose the film and thus produce an image. It is possible to extend the penetration capacity of the beam to such an extreme level that a great majority of the x-rays penetrate through every type of tissue in the patient. For example, the use of 120 kVp for any procedure other than chest radiography or barium studies will result in an overexposed film. At this kVp level, even the bones are unable to attenuate more than a few of the x-rays. With increased numbers of x-rays penetrating through the patient, the actual intensity of the remnant beam increases. With excessive amounts of x-rays exposing the film, light areas will turn darker gray, while pitch-black areas will remain pitch black (having used up all of the silver crystals available in the film emulsion). Radiographic contrast will be lost, as the image will have no more light areas present (Figure 56).

Figure 56. Non-grid radiographs of the shoulder showing effect of kVp overexposure. Kilovoltage used is noted on each radiograph. Note the fog on the 78 kVp image.

CONTROL OF DENSITY

The single most essential quality of the x-ray beam is its *penetration*, the ability to pass through an object and reach the x-ray film to expose it. Without penetration, there can be no production of x- ray images, no densities on the film. Penetration is the opposite of attenuation (see Chapter One). Seventy-five to eighty per cent of the typical diagnostic x-ray beam is attenuated within the patient, so that the average remnant beam has about 20 per cent of the intensity of the original beam. It may then be said that the penetration of the typical x-ray; beam is about 20 per cent or $^1/5$ Penetration is a characteristic of the energy level or quality of the x-ray ream and is therefore controlled by kVp. The higher the kVp, the higher the penetration of the beam.

Greater penetration through the object

Figure 57. Illustrations of the relationship between beam penetration and radiographic density. (A) and (B) effects of long wave length (low energy) radiation, (C) and (D) effects of short wave length (high energy) radiation. Radiographs of the hand (E) through (H) that simulate the theoretical conditions shown above.

results in higher intensity levels of the radiation reaching the film, which increases film exposure and image density. Although kVp is a controlling factor for image contrast, it will also affect image density each time it is altered, a consideration which must be kept in mind constantly as the radiographer manipulates electrical technique factors.

Since x-ray energies are inversely related to their wave lengths, it may be said that x-ray wave length controls penetration, affecting film exposure and image density.

Long Wave Length Exposure

Reference to Figure 57 will serve to explain theoretically the penetration and absorption of x-rays. In diagram (A), a small unit of an x-ray beam of long wave length (low kVp) is projected toward an object. The predominantly long wave length x-rays are shown to partially penetrate the object but none emerges to expose the film because they have been absorbed by the object. Actually, a limited number of the shorter wave lengths in this primary beam do penetrate the object and expose the film slightly as shown in (E). For practical radiographic use, however, their number is so small that they cannot be depended upon to produce a satisfactory image with a practical exposure time. When the *number* of long wave length x-rays is increased (B), they are also absorbed and fail to reach the film. The radiograph of the hand (F), was made employing the same wave length as in A but the exposure was very long and impractical. A satisfactory image was not obtained. Because the wave length was very long and insufficiently penetrating for the thicker portions of the hand, no appreciable gain in the amount of silver

deposit occurred except in the image details representing the very thin tissues (fingers).

Short Wave Length Exposure

When the wave length is shortened by increasing kVp, (C), and a small unit of this x-ray beam is directed toward the object, penetration of the object easily takes place. The emergent x-rays (remnant radiation) sensitize a small unit of silver bromide emulsion in the x-ray film that upon development changes to a deposit of black metallic silver–a radiographic density. This is comparable to the image shown in (G), wherein weak radiographic densities in the image representing the *thicker* portions of the hand indicate that the radiation is sufficiently penetrating but it is inadequate in quantity. The radiation may now be considered *qualitatively* correct and penetration of the hand attained. However, the *number* of short wave length x-rays is still too small to expose the film sufficiently and produce a satisfactory image. With the same kilovoltage and an increase in exposure a satisfactory image is obtained (D) and (H).

Demonstration No. 1

Purpose. To demonstrate that radiographic densities increase as the kilovoltage increases when an absorber (hand) containing structures of varying absorption properties is employed.

Procedure

1. A series of four posteroanterior radiographs of the hand was made employing the following materials and factors:

Materials	Film:	Screen-type, 8 x 10-inch
	Exposure holder:	8 x 10-inch
Factors	SID:	36 inches
	mA:	100
	Time:	0.2 sec.
	mA:	20
Variable	Exposure No.	kVp
Factors	1	40
	2	50
	3	60
	4	70

Comment. In this series of radiographs (Figure 58) the over-all density of the radiographs increases with the kVp. The over-all density of the No. 3 radiograph made with 60 kVp is greater than that of No. 1 made with 40 kVp. Successive increases in kilovoltage cause corresponding increases in density due to greater tissue penetration, since less radiation is absorbed by the tissues and more reaches the film because of the shorter wave lengths. However, it should be noted that in each radiograph less radiation emerged from those portions of the hand representing the bones than from those representing the flesh—less silver deposit is rendered in the bone images than that representing the adjacent soft tissues because bone absorbs a greater amount of radiation than does soft tissue.

Figure 58. Demonstration of kVp-density relation. Kilovoltages are noted on each radiograph. Note the dramatic change in density caused by a 10 kVp adjustment.

Demonstration No. 2

In medical radiography it can also be shown in a series of posteroanterior chest radiographs, Figure 59, that as the kilovoltage advances, radiographic density and gray scale increase. This series of radiographs was exposed with a range of 60 to 100 kVp in increments of 10 kVp. The mAs and all other factors were constant.

Since the lungs are full of air, very little scatter fog is produced. The increasing gray scale can be attributed primarily to enhanced penetration. However, at 100 kVp, overexposure occurs, and scatter fogging becomes apparent. The ideal kVp in this particular case would be 90 kVp.

SUFFICIENT PENETRATION

X-ray film requires a certain minimum exposure in order for the silver crystals to be developed into black metallic silver deposits and produce density. It actually takes several x-ray photons, not just one, to sensitize a silver crystal enough to be developed successfully into black metallic silver during processing. Suppose that the kVp you have set results in 10 per cent penetration through the patient. Suppose further that the particular x-ray film you are using requires at least 200 photons striking each square millimeter of emulsion in order to develop an image. If a setting of 100 mAs were to result in 10 photons striking each

Figure 59. Series of chest radiographs demonstrating that as the kilovoltage advances and all other factors are constant, density increases dramatically. Kilovoltages used are noted.

square millimeter, then an increase to 200 mAs would produce 20 photons striking each square millimeter; at 500 mAs there would be 50; and at 1000 mAs (about the limit of most x-ray equipment), there would still only be about 100 photons striking each square millimeter. When penetration is insufficient, it cannot be realistically compensated for by more intensity. For practical purposes, no amount of output of the x-ray tube will ever compensate for inadequate energy in the beam. From a technique standpoint, *no amount of mAs will ever compensate for insufficient kVp.*

Excessive mAs values are dangerous to the patient and are not justified in medical radiography. All medical radiography can be adequately performed within a range of 50 to 120 kVp. It is well to remember that when a kilovoltage is to be assigned to a given projection, one must think of it in relation to *tissue penetration*, and whether the radiation will penetrate the part and provide remnant radiation of a quality and quantity that will produce a satisfactory

image. The following example will illustrate the futility of employing an inadequate kilovoltage.

Demonstration No. 1

A series of direct-exposure posteroanterior radiographs of the hand on screentype film (Figure 60), was made to determine a mAs value that would produce a translucent image of all structures in the hand. For the initial radiograph 45 mAs was used at an SID of 36 inches. The kilovoltage applied was 30. For each succeeding exposure, the mAs was doubled in an attempt to produce an image with the required concentration and distribution of silver deposit. A final mAs value of 1440 was employed, but the image was still unsatisfactory. The lack of penetrating radiation in sufficient quantity made the objective entirely hopeless. By exposing the hand with 50 kVp, 50 mAs, and an SID of 36 inches, a diagnostic image (G) was obtained. Obviously a mAs of 1440 at 30 kVp was a most impractical exposure since the diagnostic objective was not attained. Opaque densities obscured detail in the phalanges and insufficient silver in the carpal area prevented details being seen in that region. However, the 50-kVp radiograph provided an image in which *all* densities were translucent and details in the entire image were clearly recorded when a comparatively short exposure was employed.

Demonstration No. 2

A second example of this principle is demonstrated in Figure 61, where only 50 kVp was employed on a chest radiograph. It should be recalled that chest radiography is primarily for examination of the heart, not only the lungs. Therefore, adequate penetration is determined by attempting to see some details of the spine through the heart tissue. In this example, 50 kVp was insufficient to penetrate the heart tissue, even after the mAs was doubled twice. Note that although the lung areas are shown somewhat well upon doubling the mAs and were completely overexposed upon re-doubling the mAs, the heart area is still underpenetrated and inadequate for diagnosis.

Figure 60. Series of direct exposure radiographs of the hand taken at 30 kVp (A through F) to demonstrate that no amount of mAs can practically compensate for insufficient kilovoltage. Note that even at (F) with 1440 mAs, the bones are still not adequately demonstrated. In (G) the kVp is increased to 50, and an adequate view is finally obtained. MAS values used: A: 45, B: 90, C: 180, D: 360 mAs, E: 720 mAs, F: 1440 mAs, (G) was taken at 50 kVp and 50 mAs.

OPTIMUM kVp

A certain optimum kVp is required to expose the x-ray film properly. As discussed in the first chapter, whether a given photon with a certain energy level will be attenuated or not by an atom depends largely upon the atomic number of the atom, i.e. how many electrons it has. The penetration level required for an x-ray beam to make it through a particular body part is determined by the *proportions* of the various atomic numbers of the tissues making up that body part. When exposing a lateral lumbar spine, roughly 90 per cent of the tissue being penetrated is soft tissue, with an atomic number averaging about that of water, and only 10 per cent is bone. But when exposing a lateral L5-S1 joint, the overlaying iliac bones of the pelvis are added to the sacrum and spine so that roughly 20 per cent of the tissue being pen-

Figure 61. Screen exposures of the chest taken at an insufficient 50 kVp. Respective mAs values are shown on each radiograph. Note that after two doublings of the mAs, the heart and mediastinum are still not penetrated.

etrated is bone and only 80 per cent soft tissue. With a higher *ratio* of bone, which has a much higher atomic number than soft tissue, increased penetration is needed. Similarly, filling the stomach with barium causes as much as 25-50 per cent of the tissue to be penetrated to have the atomic number of barium. The average atomic number of the abdomen in that area is increased. In these procedures, the tissue of interest (the bone or barium) must be penetrated so that the radiologist can see *through* it to the other side of the organ. If it is not penetrated, the film will be blank white where the barium or bone is, and the only information the radiologist can read is the information at the *edges* of the organ, only about 10 per cent of the information he needs to see. It is like looking at a silhouette of the organ, where you cannot discern anything within the shadow, but only the edges. Figure 62 demonstrates this condition. Adequate kVp is essential to the visibility of information on the radiograph.

However, once sufficient penetration of the body part has been achieved, further increases in kVp result only in more scatter fogging of the film, with no further gain in the other image qualities. So rather than talk about *maximum* or *minimum* kVp levels, we discuss only *optimum kVp*. Optimum kVp is the minimum level of

kVp available which still provides adequate penetration of the body part. Optimum kVp does *not* vary from machine to machine, between different phases of machines, different receptor systems or dif-

Figure 62. Radiograph of barium-filled stomach taken with 80 kVp. Note that with inadequate penetration through the barium, the only details visible in the stomach are those at the very edge of the barium bolus. Such a silhouette image is of little diagnostic value.

ferent sizes of patients. It is based solely upon the relative proportions of the types of tissues in a body part. The recommend- ed optimum kVps listed in Table IV should be memorized and can be applied general- ly to most situations.

THE 15 PER CENT RULE

The relationship between kVp levels and image density is not a linear, propor- tionate one. In some ranges the effects will differ from other ranges of kVp. This means that there can be no exact rule made regarding the effect of kVp upon density which can be applied in all instances. Nonetheless, objective experience with this factor has demonstrated that a very rough rule of thumb, called the *15 per cent rule,* may be reasonably applied to most situa- tions using average ranges of kVp. The 15 per cent rule states that: *A 15 per cent change in kVp will result in a change in density by a factor of 2.* If kVp is increased by 15 per cent, the radiographic density will roughly double. If it is decreased by 15 per cent, the density will be cut roughly in half. Students should memorize and practice applying this rule in all of the various ranges of kVp, because it will be used in daily practice.

The 15 per cent rule works for *two* rea- sons: As described at the beginning of this chapter, an increase in kVp results in *both* an increase in radiation output and an increase in beam energy. Many physics texts use the "kVp-squared rule" to predict the *output* change caused by adjusting kVp. *This rule does not apply to image density,* because it does not also take into account the energy changes in the x-ray beam. By this rule alone, if the kVp were increased by 15 per cent, radiation output would go up by 35-45 per cent. (For example, changing from 50 to 60 kVp would yield $60^2/50^2 = 3600/2500 = 1.44$ times more radiation, or 44 per cent more radiation

TABLE IV

Optimum kVp for Different Procedures

Procedure	Optimum kVp
Hand/Wrist	54
Elbow/ Foot	60
Ankle	64
Knee	70
Femur/Shoulder/Sinus/Ribs	76
Cervical/Thoracic Spine (all views)	76
General Torso Anatomy (Pelvis, Abdomen, Lumbar Spine)	80
All Iodine Procedures (IVP, cystogram, etc.)	80
Non-Grid Chest	80
Air Contrast/Barium Studies	90
Esophagram	90
Solid-Column Barium Studies	110
Grid Chest	110-120

*NOTE: Unlisted procedures may be extrapolated with fair accuracy by splitting the difference between the two adjacent anatomical parts listed. For exam- ple, the humerus would be half-way between the elbow and the shoulder, yielding about 66kVp. Tangential or partial types of skull procedures, such as the mandible, would be about equal to the cervi- cal spine at 70 kVp. Most techniques ever needed can be derived from this basic list.

emitted from the x-ray tube.) But the effects of *increased penetration* must also be added to this output in order to predict the end result for image density. With a high- er average energy in the x-ray beam, a much greater percentage of the x-rays inci- dent upon the body make it through to the film. When this effect is added to the increased original output, the *total* amount of *remnant* radiation reaching the film is increased by nearly 2 times or 100 per cent. The image will be twice as dark.

There is a "physics" formula which approximates the 15 per cent rule for density. It is:

$$\frac{(kVp_2)^4}{(kVp_1)^4} = \frac{D_2}{D_1}$$

Rephrased in common English, this formula states that the density will change according to the fourth power of the change in kVp. In effect, this is the 15 per cent rule stated algebraically, and it results in similar answers. In daily practice, however, radiographers must have a rule of thumb which can be quickly calculated mentally. The 15 per cent rule is perfectly adaptable to this need, and is the most usable rule for radiographers in predicting the effects of kVp upon image density.

Students and technologists often hear the phrase, "go up or down 10 kVp." While this approach is functional in many situations, it is not nearly as accurate as the proper calculation of a 15 per cent change applied to the initial kVp range. The saying originates, in fact, from taking 15 per cent of the average kVp for all diagnostic procedures–about 70 kVp, 15 per cent of which is 10.5. To find 15 per cent of a given kVp quickly "in your head," just take 10 per cent of it and then add one-half that much again. Examine the three pairs of techniques in Table V. Using the 15 per cent rule, you should be able to determine that each pair consists of two roughly equivalent techniques in terms of radiographic density.

It is also important to remember, in solving density problems, that you must apply the 15 per cent rule in *steps*. For example, suppose that you want to cut your mAs to 1/4 of the original and maintain the density

by adjusting kVp. First, you must think in terms of doubling or halving the mAs in steps. So, 1/4 of your original mAs represents two steps of cutting it in half. Therefore, to compensate you must change kVp in such a way as to effectively double the density two times, or in two steps, for a total change of four times. Now, rather than simply take 30 per cent of the original kVp and add it, which will result in an inaccurate answer, you must add 15 per cent once and then calculate 15 per cent of *that result* and add it again in a second step. For example, if you began with 80 kVp, you would first add 15 per cent of 80 = 12 to get 92 kVp and then calculate 15 per cent of 92 = 14 and add that to arrive at 106 kVp. The 15 per cent rule is very helpful if you always think in terms of steps of doubling or halving the density.

A caveat is in order, however, in applying the 15 per cent rule in successive steps: It must be remembered that several decreasing steps of 15 per cent in kVp would soon lead to inadequate penetration of the anatomy under study, and, conversely, that several increasing steps would excessively fog the radiograph. As a general recommendation, the 15 per cent rule should never be applied in more than two successive steps.

Demonstration

The posteroanterior screen radiographs of the chest (Figure 63 A-F) demonstrate a typical example of the 15 per cent rule. Radiographs A-C were made with 80 kVp, 92 kVp, and 106 kVp, respectively, with slight reductions in mAs. Radiograph D was made with 80 kVp and 6.66 mAs; E, with 92 kVp and 3.3 mAs; and F, with 106 kVp and 1.7 mAs; all at a 72-inch SID. When all the mAs values were halved as the kVp increased in 15 per cent steps, as shown in radiographs D to F, the overex-

Figure 63. Series of screen radiographs of the PA chest showing examples of the effects of overexposure (A-C) and correct exposure (D-F) when using the 15 per cent rule.

posures were corrected and the overall density was reduced to an acceptable level. By using this rule-of-thumb method of halving the mAs or of doubling the mAs when 15 per cent changes in kVp are made, an image more in keeping with the desired result can be obtained.

APPLYING THE 15 PER CENT RULE

The ability to make 15 per cent kVp adjustments mentally should be second-nature to the radiographer. It is not very difficult to develop this ability, but it does require some practice. To find 15 per cent of the original kVp mentally, think of the operation as taking 10 per cent first, and then adding half as much again. For example, to find 15 per cent of 60 kVp

60 x 10% = 6	Take 10 per cent of the kVp
6/2 = 3	Figure one-half of 6
6 + 3 = 9	Add these two numbers
60 x 15% = 9	

15 per cent of 80 kVp would be 8 + 4 = 12.
15 per cent of 120 kVp would be 12 + 6 = 18.

This number is added to the original kVp to double film density, or subtracted to obtain one-half of the original density. In the above example using 60 kVp, what new total kVp would compensate for cutting the mAs to one-half? The answer is 69 kVp. What would the new kVp be if, due to overpenetration, this radiograph turned out twice too dark, and you wished to cut the density in half? The answer is 51 kVp. You should also become comfortable with applying the fifteen per cent rule in steps and in portions.

Applying the Rule in Steps

Sometimes the desired adjustment in image density is much greater than a doubling or halving. Suppose you need to repeat an extremely light radiograph due to underpenetration, and the density needs to be increased four-fold. Always translate the desired changes into terms of doublings (factors of two), and you can apply the rule. To produce a radiograph four times darker, think of this change as two doublings. To obtain two doublings, you will need to increase 15 per cent kVp *in two steps.* (It is not as accurate to simply make a 30 per cent change, and the greater the change, the less accurate this approach is.)

One practical example of a kVp adjustment using two steps of 15 per cent is found in deriving a barium technique (Upper G.I. or Solid Column Barium Enema) from a routine abdomen technique. If the technique for an AP projection of the abdomen were 20 mAs and 80 kVp, the following calculations would allow adequate penetration of the same abdomen when the gastrointestinal tract is filled with barium:

20 mAs @ 80 kVp	Routine AP Abdomen
10 mAs @ 92 kVp	First step increase of 15% (12 kVp), accompanied by one-half the mAs to maintain density
5 mAs @ 106 kVp	Second step increase (14 kVp) is 15% of 92, with another halving of the mAs

For a solid-column barium procedure (not air contrast) approximately 5 mAs at about 110 kVp would provide good penetration through the barium, while keeping overall image density at an optimum level. (For an air contrast technique, simply reduce 10-15 kVp with the mAs still at about 5.)

Applying the Rule in Portions

Suppose that you wish to increase density by 50 per cent, or 1 and $1/2$ times the original. You will recall the recommendation to think of technique changes in terms of doublings or halvings. In this context, such a 50 per cent increase should be thought of as *half-way to doubling.* (Similarly a 25 per cent reduction in overall technique would be thought of as a half-way to cutting it in half.) Since a 15 per cent increase in kVp will double the density, one-half of 15

per cent should bring the density halfway to a doubling. In other words, to increase the density 50 per cent, increase the kVp by one-half of 15 per cent.

For example, suppose a radiograph taken at 80 kVp comes out a bit light. Doubling the density would be too much. You decide to increase density by about $1/2$ or 50 per cent:

80 x 15% = 12	Find 15% of the kVp
12 x $1/2$ = 6	Find $1/2$ of that amount
80 + 6 = 86	Add this number to the original kVp
	For a radiograph 50 per cent darker, increase kVp to 86.

Complete the following exercise, using the 15 per cent rule. Some problems will require you to apply the rule in sequential steps, some in portions of $1/2$ of 15 per cent. Then check your answers in the Appendix. Be sure to do all of them *mentally* to benefit from the exercise.

EXERCISE #14

1. What is 5 per cent of 80?
2. What is 5 per cent of 50?
3. What is 15 per cent of 70?
4. What is 15 per cent of 60?
5. What is 15 per cent of 110?
6. What is *one-half* of 15 per cent of 80?
7. What is *one-half* of 15 per cent of 90?
8. What is *one-half* of 15 per cent of 120?
9. Starting at 120 kVp, what new kVp would result in a density one-half as dark as the original?
10. Starting at 40 kVp, what new kVp would result in a density twice as dark as the original ?
11. Starting at 60 kVp, what new kVp would/result in a density 50 per cent darker (half-way to double) the original?
12. Starting at 80 kVp, what new kVp would result in a density $1/4$ as great as the original?

TABLE V
Equivalent Total Techniques

The 15 per cent rule applied, each of the pairs of techniques below consists of two equivalent techniques in terms of the density that will be produced on the finished film.

A	B	C
60 mAs at 40 kVp	25 mAs at 92 kVp	15 mAs at 110 kVp
30 mAs at 46 kVp	50 mAs at 80 kVp	7 mAs at 126 kVp

Fill in the kVp in the following problems which would maintain equal density with the original technique, listed first.

13. 400 mA $1/20$ sec. 90 kVp
    300 mA $1/60$ sec. _____ kVp
14. 50 mA $1/60$ sec. 50 kVp
    400 mA $1/120$ sec. _____ kVp
15. 300 mA $1/30$ sec. 120 kVp
    400 mA $1/10$ sec. _____ kVp
16. 300 mA $1/20$ sec. 70 kVp
    150 mA $3/20$ sec. _____ kVp

ARITHMETICAL TABLE

The 15 per cent rule for kVp is useful not only for practical adjustments on a daily basis but for the development of accurate technique charts as well. Table VI was developed using the 15 per cent rule to derive mAs conversions to compensate for changes in kVp across the diagnostic ranges.

By the use of mAs multiplying factors, approximate mAs values may be obtained for changes in the kVp range of 50 to 100 in increments of five.

Some mAs values derived from this table may require the use of a time value that is not within the practical scope of the timer. It is then necessary to employ the *nearest* practical value. The resulting density difference is usually so small that it often is not recognizable. In most instances the derived mAs values are approximations and, if necessary, only slight alterations need be made for a given projection and body tissue. X-ray generators may differ in the manner in which their x-ray outputs vary with kVp and due to calibration differences. Tables cannot, therefore, be expected to apply accurately to *all* generators but they can provide a close guide to an anticipated value.

It is quite important to remember that when kilovoltage is employed to change radiographic density, radiographic contrast and the quantity of scatter radiation generated also change.

Example. Assume that 55 kVp was used in making a posteroanterior view of the chest employing 10 mAs at a 72-inch SID. Average speed intensifying screens were used. It is desired to penetrate the chest more thoroughly and to lengthen the scale of densities so that more structural details will be clearly shown in the image. A kVp of 80 was selected to accomplish the desired result. What mAs value should be employed at the new kVp?

Solution. Consult Table VI. In the left-hand column, locate the original kVp value of 55. Pass the finger horizontally across the chart until it reaches the column of multiplying factors indicated by the new kVp of 80 at the bottom of Table VI. Multiply this factor of 0.28 by the original mAs of 10. The answer is 2.8 mAs.

Demonstration

A series of posteroanterior screen radiographs of the chest (Figure 64) was made

TABLE VI
mAs Multiplying Factors for Use When Kilovoltage Is Changed
(Screen Exposures Only)

Old kVp	New Kilovoltage mAs Multiplying Factor													Old kVp
40	1.	.4	.23	.15	.11	.08	.064	.05	.04	.032	.025	.02	.017	40
45	2.5	1.	.52	.3	.22	.16	.12	.1	.076	.06	.05	.04	.032	45
50	4.	1.7	1.	.68	.5	.35	.27	.21	.16	.13	.1	.08	.066	50
55	8.	2.5	1.5	1.	.74	.56	.43	.35	.28	.22	.18	.15	.12	55
60	10.	4.	2.3	1.5	1.	.78	.6	.46	.37	.3	.25	.2	.17	60
65	12.	5.	3.	2.	1.4	1.	.8	.62	.5	.4	.32	.26	.21	65
70	16.	7.	4.2	2.6	2.	1.4	1.	.8	.6	.5	.39	.31	.25	70
75	20.	9.	5.4	3.5	2.5	1.8	1.3	1.	.76	.6	.47	.38	.3	75
80	24.	11.	6.6	4.5	3.2	2.3	1.7	1.3	1.	.8	.6	.47	.37	80
85	28.	13.	8.	5.4	4.	2.9	2.2	1.7	1.3	1.	.8	.64	.5	85
90	34.	15.	9.	6.2	4.5	3.4	2.6	2.	1.6	1.25	1.	.8	.64	90
95	48.	18.	11.	7.8	5.6	4.2	3.2	2.5	2.	1.6	1.3	1.	.8	95
100	60.	22.	13.	9.	6.8	5.	3.8	3.	2.4	1.9	1.5	1.2	1.	100
	40	45	50	55	60	65	70	75	80	85	90	95	100	

with a range of 40 to 100 kVp. The mAs was adjusted to compensate for the increasing kVp-density effect with the assistance of Table VI, the translucent over-all density of the upper right pulmonary area was used as a guide in adjusting mAs values. The over-all density values in all radiographs of this area are relatively equal.

kVp VERSUS mAs FOR DENSITY CONTROL

In the previous chapter you learned that excessive amounts of mAs will overexpose the x-ray film, and that overexposure is not the same thing as fogging the film with scatter radiation. When excessive levels of kVp are used, fog becomes visible. The film may also be overexposed, because the increase in penetration of the beam through the patient makes the remnant beam more intense, just as if mAs had been increased. Therefore, excessive kVp levels both overexpose and fog the radiograph, while excessive mAs levels only overexpose it.

It is generally *not* recommended that kVp be used as a control for radiographic density. Since mAs is directly proportional to density, it is predictable and easy to work with. Furthermore, mAs has no effect upon other image qualities such as contrast. Kilovoltage cannot be changed without affecting both density and contrast. The

Figure 64. Series of screen radiographs of the chest in which the mAs was decreased, using the 15 per cent rule, in compensation for increasing kVp. The kilovoltages are shown under the radiographs. Note that the gray scale becomes longer with higher kVp, but the overall density is maintained. MAS factors used: A: 70, B: 40, C: 20, D: 10, E: 8.3, F: 6.3, G: 5, H: 4.12, I: 3.3, J: 2.15, K: 2, L: 1.6, M: 1.6.

Figure 65. Screen exposures of the chest to demonstrate the negligible density effect with small changes in kilovoltage. The respective kVp used for each radiograph is noted.

proper use of kVp is in controlling penetration and radiographic contrast. When the proper level of contrast is achieved, then mAs should be used to adjust density for different sizes of patients.

A practical example is the barium enema examination: If you closely examine any technique chart, using the 15 per cent rule to adjust, you will find that the barium enema mAs is roughly 1/4 of the mAs for an abdomen radiograph, while the kVp for the barium enema is roughly two steps of 15 per cent increased from the abdomen kVp. First, the kVp had to be increased, because with the use of barium a new level of penetration is required and a new optimum kVp results. But, since the increased kVp will affect density as well as penetration and contrast, mAs must be reduced, using the 15 per cent rule to bring the density of the radiograph back down to a diagnostic level.

Different optimum kVp must be used for procedures involving different anatomy. But, *within a given procedure, it is critical that the radiologist be provided with the same type of contrast from one view to the next.* Changes in contrast and gray scale between a PA skull and a lateral skull in the same series can hinder the radiologist's ability to diagnose the patient's condition, because some detail which is visible on the one radiograph may not be visible on the other. *Within a given procedural series, kVp must be kept fairly stable while mAs is adjusted for the different views. This will ensure a set of films which have proper density and consistent contrast.*

VISIBLE DENSITY CHANGE

As discussed in Chapter Five, the human eye cannot discern any change in radiographic density of less than 30 per cent. There are occasions when the radiographer may wish to make a density change of this magnitude, 30-40 per cent, but the next available exposure time on the timer knob is 50, 75 or even 100 per cent. In such a situation, the use of kVp to make a small density change may be justified. But the radiographer should understand this use of kVp: guesswork has no place in a scientific discipline which affects the health of human beings. There is no call for changing "a couple of kV" when the density effect is not well understood.

Based upon the 15 per cent rule for kVp-density relations, recall that a 15 per cent kVp increase would double the image density, or increase it by 100 per cent. If a 15 per cent kVp increase represents a 100 per cent density increase, then it may be extrapolated that approximately one-third of that amount, or a 5 per cent kVp increase, would roughly represent a 30 per cent density increase. Therefore, as a rule of thumb, it should be memorized that a minimum of a 5 per cent change in kVp is required to cause any visible change in density on the finished radiograph. A quick calculation of 5 per cent of the various ranges of kVp used in diagnostic radiography will reveal that the common practice of changing 2 kVp to control density is a superstitious one. Since modern equipment normally only allows *even* changes in kVp, it is seen that in the lower ranges of kVp (50 to 80 kVp), at least a 4-kVp change must be made to really see a darker film and that a 6-kVp change is required in the ranges above 80 kVp.

Demonstration

The above facts may be illustrated by a series of posteroanterior views of the chest, Figure 65. Exposures were made employing a range of 76 to 84 kVp in 2-kVp steps; all other factors were constant: 2.5 mAs; 72-inch SID. Comparison of the densities in the 76- and 78-kVp images shows little difference. The same holds true in the 80- and 82-kVp radiographs. A definite difference exists, however, between the 76and 80-kVp and the 80- and 84-kVp images. A positive difference exists between the densities seen in the 76and 84-kVp radiographs. Hence, there is no advantage to be derived by changing kVp in increments less than 4 in this range.

EFFECTS ON OTHER QUALITIES

Note that kVp affects *all* of the visibility functions in an image—an increase in kVp causes density to increase, noise to increase (in the form of fog), and contrast to diminish. Kilovoltage does *not* affect any of the geometrical recognizability functions in the image.

kVp is an electrical factor, just as is mA, and has nothing to do with geometry. This means that it cannot possibly have any effect upon the recognizability functions of an image, which are all based on the geometry of the x-ray beam. Sharpness of recorded detail, magnification and shape distortion are not affected by kVp.

EXPOSURE LATITUDE

KILOVOLTAGE AND EXPOSURE LATITUDE

When a body part is radiographed, the absorption properties of the tissues are largely unpredictable. Naturally, the question arises as to how great an error can be made in the exposure factors without degrading radiographic quality. The term "correct exposure" does not necessarily mean that there is only one exposure factor that will produce the best diagnostic image. Depending upon the kilovoltage used, it may actually mean that many different exposures can be employed to yield radiographs that are diagnostically acceptable to the radiologist. This phenomenon is linked in what is known as *exposure latitude*— an important element in any standardized exposure system.

Figure 66. Series of lateral views of the knee to demonstrate exposure latitude. The range between 37.5 and 100 mAs (Nos. 3-6) may be considered the exposure latitude in this case.

Figure 67. Radiographs of the elbow demonstrating exposure latitude. The range between 90 and 135 mAs may be considered the exposure latitude in this case.

Exposure Latitude

Exposure latitude may be defined as the range between the minimum and maximum exposure that will produce a scale of translucent densities acceptable for diagnostic purposes. In other words, it is the *margin for error* in setting a proper technique. As previously demonstrated, the scale of image densities is determined by the kilovoltage employed. Hence, exposure latitude varies with the kilovoltage applied.

Wide Exposure Latitude

When high kilovoltage values are used, the exposure latitude is wide because long scale is produced in the image which can compensate at times for wide errors in mAs. The large number of densities of small tonal differences produced by the more penetrating radiation serves to retain image details even to the extremes of tissue thickness; that is, details in the *thin and thick* portions of the part may be shown.

Example. A demonstration of wide exposure latitude using 80 kVp and a Potter-Bucky diaphragm (8:1) is shown in Figure 66. A series of lateral exposures of a 10-centimeter knee were made employing mAs values of: (1) 12.5; (2) 25; (3) 37.5; (4) 50; (5) 75; (6) 100; and, (7) 125. SID: 36 inches. Radiographs Nos. 1 and 2 may be considered as underexposed; No. 7 as overexposed. Radiographs Nos. 3 to 6 may be considered to possess diagnostic densities and the latitude is 37.5 to 100 mAs. Between these values lies the range of diagnostic exposures, 62.5 mAs in width.

Narrow Exposure Latitude

Exposure latitude is usually narrow when short scale prevails, as produced by the lower kilovoltages. The small number of usable densities present requires that the exposure be more nearly correct to obtain densities that are representative of the thinnest or the thickest portions of the part. The gray scale however, is seldom such that all desired tissues are shown in the same image, particularly of a subject that contains a number of structural details of widely different tissue densities or thicknesses. Also, the mAs values required are usually so great as to be impractical in application.

Example. In a series of anteroposterior radiographs of the elbow (Figure 67) 60

was considered to be the optimum kilovoltage; the SID was 30 inches; the mAs was varied in steps of 15 mAs from 30 to 165. The exposure latitude in this series may be considered to be between 90 and 135 mAs, a range of 45 mAs in width. The selection of this range was based upon the fact that visualization of all required details was attained in the images although they possessed varying degrees of density. Selection of the optimum density may easily be made by choosing three adjacent radiographs in the series that approach nearest to the required density–90, 105 and 120 mAs. A desirable density may be considered as produced by about 105 mAs.

In review, the 80 kVp used for the knee radiographs in Figure 66 yielded an exposure latitude ranging across 62.5 mAs, while the 60 kVp used for the elbow in Figure 67 yielded a latitude range of only 45 mAs. When the kVp is so low that adequate penetration is not achieved, as illustrated in Figure 60 A-F, no amount of mAs will produce an acceptable density level and it may be said that the exposure latitude approaches zero. The longer gray scales achieved at high kVp levels allow a greater margin of error or exposure latitude. When the gray scale is short (for instance, at the lower kVp levels), exposure latitude is also very narrow and there is little margin for error.

CONTRAST VERSUS EXPOSURE LATITUDE

The close relationship between contrast and exposure latitude may be observed by a study of Figure 68. This relationship obviously is dependent upon the factor of kilovoltage.

Example. In Figure 68, radiographs (A-E) were made with 50 kVp at 72" SID. mAs: (A) 7.5; (B) 10; (C) 13.3; (D) 20; (E) 30. Radiographs (F-J) were made with 80

Figure 68. Two series of screen radiographs of a 23-cm chest that serve as a study in radiographic density, contrast and exposure latitude. The high contrast series A to E, taken at 50 kVp, demonstrates narrow exposure latitude. The low contrast series F to J, taken at 80 kVp, demonstrates wide exposure latitude.

kVp at 72". mAs: (F) 2.5; (G) 3.3; (H) 4.16; (I) 5; (J) 6.6.

Radiographs A-E

Note that, as the mAs increased, the overall density of the image increased; (D) and (E) contain opaque silver deposits and details are obscured. When the density level became satisfactory and the silver deposits were translucent as shown in (B) or (C), there was an absence of silver to depict details in the denser tissue areas despite the fact that mAs values of 10 or 13.3 were employed. The dosage values were too high. The contrast differences were so great that one could safely assume that many of the finer details were being lost due to lack of tissue penetration in (A) and to silver opacities in (D) and (E). This is a condition typical of high contrast. The exposure latitude was constricted between (B) and (C) which is too narrow a range for good chest radiography.

Radiographs F-J

As the mAs increased, the overall density increased: all silver deposits were translucent even in (J), which exhibits some overexposure. In (F), minimal silver deposits demonstrate details that are absent in (A). All essential details are recorded with varying levels of overall density in (F) to (I), which is typical of low contrast images. The density of (J) is a bit excessive and some details are obscured because of overexposure. The exposure latitude is wide, as represented by radiographs (F) to (I). All mAs values are small and the dosage minimal. Radiograph (G) may be considered as having received the correct exposure. Some scatter radiation fog is present but its level is within diagnostic acceptability.

Comment. The examples cited above demonstrate that when contrast prevails, the resulting narrow exposure latitude prevents the rendition of a large number of densities for diagnostic use.

A radiographer operating with an optimum kilovoltage technic is more likely to produce greater uniformity of radiographic results than one who uses a relatively low, variable kilovoltage technic. In fact, the latitude available at the higher kilovoltages is the very factor that permits consistency in radiographic results obtained with a fixed kilovoltage technic.

Rule

The following general rule may be considered basic: *The longer the scale, or lower the contrast, the greater is the exposure latitude.*

USE OF HIGHER KILOVOLTAGES

The use of the higher kilovoltages provides greater exposure efficiency in radiography for the following reasons:

1. Anatomical details in all tissue thicknesses are rendered as translucent densities. The relative absorption properties between bone and flesh are reduced making possible visualization of more structural details. At lower kilovoltages, bone detail often tends to obscure details of soft tissues that lie behind the bone. Complete penetration of bone by higher kilovoltages reveals soft tissue details that are often not visible at lower kilovoltages. The greater penetration effected by higher kilovoltage radiation makes possible the rendition of a greater number of anatomical details than when lower kilovoltages are employed.

2. Greater image sharpness *may* be obtained because shorter exposures may be employed with smaller focal spots.

3. The radiation dose to patients is reduced as the kilovoltage level increases because the body absorbs less radiation

than at the lower kilovoltages. More radiation can, therefore, reach the film to expose it, and exposures can be reduced.

4. Heat production in the x-ray tube is reduced because smaller energy loads (mAs) can be employed, thereby increasing x-ray tube life. As the kilovoltage increases, tube efficiency increases. There is more x-radiation per watt of electric power consumed when using the higher kilovoltages than there is when using the lower kilovoltages. A correct exposure may therefore be produced with less heat generated in the tube.

5. Greater exposure latitude may be secured. As the kilovoltage increases, exposure latitude increases because of the reduced absorption of body tissues created

by virtue of complete penetration. Details become visible in tissues of wide density and thickness. The absorption is greater when the lower kilovoltages are employed; consequently, exposure latitude is decreased and longer exposures are required.

6. The higher kilovoltages make possible the use of many radiographic technics that, heretofore, have been deemed too difficult to perform.

7. When the source of electric power is variable or is in a state of constant flux, the higher kilovoltages make possible more satisfactory bed-side radiography.

8. As a matter of economics, the use of higher kilovoltages causes x-ray tubes to last longer.

SUMMARY

1. Increasing kilovoltage increases beam *penetration* through the patient. This is essential to image production.
2. No amount of mAs can ever compensate for a kVp level that is *inadequate* to penetrate the anatomy.
3. Kilovoltage is the primary electrical control for image *gray scale*. Higher kVp levels penetrate more types of anatomy to expose the film, so that there are more gray shades and less unexposed blank areas.
4. Kilovoltage is the primary electrical control for image *contrast*. Higher kVp levels reduce image contrast for three reasons: (1) Gray scale is increased through enhanced tissue penetration, (gray scale opposes contrast), (2) Photoelectric interactions are lost, so that scattering interactions comprise a greater proportion of all interactions, and (3) The scatter radiation produced is more energetic and emitted in a more forward direction, causing increased

fog in the image. With lengthened gray scale, less photoelectric interactions, and increased fog, contrast will decrease.
5. The *scatter fogs* the image with a useless veil of density. Thus, increasing kVp increases the proportion of *noise* in the image.
6. Increasing kilovoltage increases image *density* dramatically. However, because kVp also affects contrast, it should not generally be used to control density. Density changes caused by kVp must be compensated for by adjusting mAs.
7. A *15 per cent* change in kVp roughly changes image density by a factor of 2, doubling it or cutting it to one-half the original.
8. A 5 per cent change in kVp (4-6 kVp in most ranges) is required to cause a *visible density change* in the image.
9. *Optimum kVp* is the minimum level required to sufficiently penetrate a body part, based upon the relative pro-

portions of bone or air to soft tissue in that part.

10. Increasing kVp increases the *exposure latitude*, so that there is a greater margin for error in selecting mAs values.

11. Kilovoltage has no effect upon sharpness of detail, magnification or distortion because it has no relationship to geometry.

REVIEW QUESTIONS

1. What, in one word, is the single most important function of kVp?
2. Explain the *three* reasons why higher kVp levels reduce contrast:
3. Define OPTIMUM kVp:
4. A chest radiograph demonstrates that the spine is not at all visible through the heart. Why would increasing the mAs to darken up the film NOT solve this problem?
5. Why is kVp not generally recommended as a density control?
6. Radiographs with long gray scale also allow more exposure latitude. What does this mean in setting techniques?
7. A technique of 100 mA, 1/2 second, and 90 kVp results in a radiograph of the abdomen which is fogged and also has motion on it. List a new technique which will solve *both* of these problems, without changing the overall density of the original:

_____ _____ _____
    mA   time   kVp

8. What is the minimum visible density change rule-of-thumb for kVp?
9. A good abdomen technique machine is 40 mAs at 80 kVp. Adding barium in the colon for a barium enema requires the same *total* technique, but much more penetration. If the mAs is adjusted from 40 to 5 mAs for the BE, what must your new kVp be: (must be within 2 kVp):
10. If scatter radiation has changed direction, why doesn't it reduce the sharpness of recorded detail in the image?

11. A graph of the x-ray beam spectrum change caused by a decrease in kVp from 100 to 70 would show an (increase or decrease) in the number of x-rays at each of the following energies:
    15 keV:
    55 keV:
    70 keV:
12. If you reduced kVp by *three steps* of 15 per cent each, even though you doubled *the mAs* three times, your radiograph may still turn out light because of:
13. Even if higher kVp levels did not increase fog on the radiograph, they would still result in less contrast and longer gray scale because:
14. The *average* energy of an 80 kVp x-ray beam is:
15. Why can't increasing mAs compensate for a below-optimum kVp?
16. Sketch a graph below showing the change in the shape and position of the x-ray beam spectrum caused by

increase in kVp from 60 to 100:
17. Higher kVp levels reduce image contrast because gray scale is _____, photoelectric interactions are _____, and fog is _____ (increased or decreased).

Chapter 7

MACHINE PHASE AND RECTIFICATION

In attempting to increase the efficiency of electrical generators, a design was developed that spins three coils of wire, rather than a single coil, within the field of a magnet. This new type of generator resulted in overlapping pulses of electricity being produced (Figure 69). Previously, x-ray machines using a single-coil generator would produce individual bursts of x-rays, one for each pulse of electricity. By *overlapping* electrical pulses, the new generator prevented the voltage from ever dropping to zero. X-ray machines using this new device emitted x-rays *continuously* instead of in pulses. The *rate* of emission from the x-ray tube was thus enhanced.

Radiographic machines using the overlapping pulses of a three-coil generator came to be known as *three-phase* machines, and those with a single coil as *single-phase*

machines. In a single-phase machine, one electrical cycle consists of *two* pulses of electricity. A three-phase machine triples this number to *six* pulses in a cycle. It was later found that, by using additional coils of wire in the *transformer* of an x-ray machine, the number of overlapping pulses of electricity could be doubled again, for a total of twelve pulses per cycle. In this way, x-ray output was increased slightly over the three-phase, six-pulse machine.

The Greek letter *phi* (Φ) is used to abbreviate the phase and is often followed by a superscript number indicating the number of pulses of electricity passing through the x-ray tube during each electrical cycle. The abbreviation $1\Phi^2$ indicates the usual two pulses of electricity produced for each cycle of a single-phase machine. Three phase machines are abbreviated $3\Phi^6$ or $3\Phi^{12}$ to

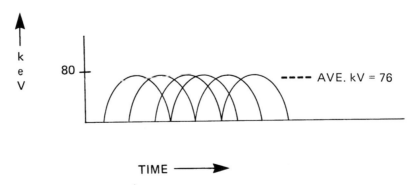

Figure 69. Diagram illustrating the overlapping of electrical pulses used in three-phase equipment to obtain continuous current and, consequently, continuous x-ray output. Also, note the ripple effect showing how three-phase equipment attains a much higher *average* keV than single-phase equipment operating at the same kVp.

122

Figure 70. Graph illustrating the electrical pulse wave form for high-frequency generators and "constant potential" generators. Output is constant and the average keV is nearly 100 per cent of the kVp set at the console.

indicate whether they are six-pulse or twelve-pulse machines.

In terms of radiographic technique, all three-phase machines are generally considered to be about twice as "hot" as single-phase machines. That is, if the same technique is used, any three-phase machine will produce a radiograph roughly twice as dark as a single-phase machine. Although a $3\Phi^{12}$ machine is slightly more efficient (about 10 per cent) than a $3\Phi^6$ machine, the difference is not enough to be of concern in setting techniques. (Recall that a 30 per cent difference would be required to be visible.) The $3\Phi^{12}$ machine still produces radiographs approximately twice as dark as a single-phase unit. Whether $3\Phi^6$ or $3\Phi^{12}$, approximately one-half of the mAs is required when compared to a single-phase machine to obtain equivalent densities.

HIGH-FREQUENCY GENERATORS

An increasingly popular type of generator is variously referred to as the *high-frequency, medium-frequency*, or *near-constant potential* generator (HFG, MFG, or CPG respectively). The popularity of this type of generator is understandable, since it can be plugged into any standard electrical outlet, is very small in size, and has about the same efficiency as a $3\Phi^{12}$ generator.

Details of its circuitry are beyond the scope of this text. Basically, a series of AC

and DC electricity converters and a "DC chopper" are used to produce an extremely high-frequency electrical current to the x-ray tube. Whereas the frequency of a single-phase unit is 60 cycles (120 pulses of electricity) per second, that of $3\Phi^6$ equipment is 360 cycles and that of $3\Phi^{12}$ equipment is 720 cycles, these new generators produce from 60,000 cycles (medium frequency) to 100,000 cycles per second (high frequency). This means that the x-ray tube is receiving up to 200,000 overlapping pulses of electricity each second, and that the voltage fluctuation is much less than one per cent, Figure 70. Just as a 3Φ machine is more efficient than a single-phase machine, a high-frequency unit is also more efficient for two reasons: First, it produces more x-rays per second (more mR/mAs), than a single-phase unit. Second, its average energy never falls more than a fraction of a per cent below the set kVp as shown in Figure 70.

The end result of this new technology is that image density is roughly doubled when compared to single-phase equipment operated at the same mAs values. Therefore, *high-frequency generators require about one-half the mAs used by single phase equipment to obtain similar image density. Techniques for high- frequency generators are roughly equivalent to those for three-phase equipment.*

EFFECT ON THE X-RAY BEAM SPECTRUM

Three-phase and high-frequency equipment are much more efficient (about twice as much) as single-phase equipment in producing a density on the radiograph. This is so for two reasons:

X-RAY QUANTITY

By overlapping electrical pulses, two additional pulses of x-rays are begun before 'the first pulse returns to zero (Figure 69). In addition, note that the *valleys* between the pulses of the original current (where it returns to zero) are now filled with the overlapping pulses of current, so that current is continuous across the x-ray tube and never falls to zero. In this manner, the total quantity of current flowing across the x-ray tube per second is increased substantially. In the case of this three- phase, six-pulse machine, the rate of x-ray output from the tube (the effective mA) is increased over the single- phase machine. The high-frequency machine overlaps thousands of pulses for the same effect, Figure 70.

X-RAY QUALITY

Overlapping the pulses results in a voltage wave form which never falls to zero but *ripples* not far below the peak voltage level (Figures 69 and 70). Compare the average energy in Figure 69 to that in Figure 49,

which represents a single-phase machine. This *ripple effect* raises the *average* energy of the x-ray beam even though the peak voltage remains the same. With a higher average voltage, the x-ray beam will be more penetrating. The intensity of the remnant beam is thus increased yet more due to a higher percentage of beam penetration through the patient.

The effects of three-phase or high-frequency current on x-ray beam quantity and quality are apparent in the beam spectrum graphed in Figure 71.

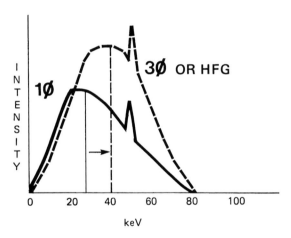

Figure 71. Graph of the x-ray beam spectra for single-phase and three-phase equipment. The three- phase machine shows a shift in average energy to higher levels (to the right) as well as an increased quantity of x-rays emitted per second (the height of the curve).

EFFECT ON DENSITY

When the increase in beam quality is added to the increase in beam quantity, the result is a radiographic density roughly double that of a single-phase machine using the same electrical technique factors

(Figure 72). This higher efficiency allows shorter exposure times, about one half those of the single phase, to be employed for like procedures. For this reason, all pediatric procedures and other procedures

Figure 72. Radiographs of the lateral skull demonstrating the maintenance of density by cutting mAs values to one-half the original when changing from a single-phase machine to a three-phase machine. Factors: (A) 20 mAs, 76 kVp, single-phase; (B) 10 mAs, 76 kVp, three-phase.

where there is a high probability of motion problems should be done in a three-phase or high-frequency room.

When changing from a single-phase room to a three-phase room, techniques for the same anatomy should be adjusted by simply cutting the mAs value to about one-half. Conversely, techniques may be doubled from three-phase to derive techniques for the same anatomy in a single-phase room. The same rules apply when changing between single-phase and high-frequency generators.

EFFECT ON CONTRAST

Because of the increased *average* kilovoltage level for the three-phase machine, penetration is increased. As described in the previous chapter, a higher penetration level means that more of the various anatomical tissues will be radiolucent to the beam and recorded as gray shades on the radiograph, and gray scale will increase. Accordingly, contrast will usually be slightly lower for a three-phase or high-frequency machine than for a single-phase machine. Although this contrast loss may be measurable using a densitometer, it is not often significant enough to detect visually. Therefore, contrast change is not a practical consideration in choosing machine phase.

EFFECT ON OTHER QUALITIES

As discussed above, three-phase or high-frequency equipment allows the use of much shorter exposure times. This reduces the *probability* of motion on the part of the patient and may therefore indirectly contribute to obtaining good sharpness of recorded detail. Nonetheless, it should be remembered that this is only an indirect relationship. It is the motion, not the exposure time, which is directly responsible for the resultant sharpness of detail. Shorter exposure times do not *guarantee* that motion will not occur any more than long exposure times guarantee that it will occur.

Sharpness of detail, magnification and shape distortion are all strictly geometrical factors. Machine phase is an electrical factor and has no relationship with geometry. It should not be considered to have any direct relationship with these recognizability functions in the image.

RECTIFICATION AND X-RAY GENERATORS

Not all x-ray equipment uses the fully rectified, pulsed electricity we have been discussing. Other variations include half-rectified units, capacitor discharge units and constant-potential generator units. These are most frequently encountered in mobile radiography, discussed in Chapter 32.

Some older mobile units may still be in use which are *half-rectified*. This means that only every other pulse of electricity is allowed to reach the x-ray tube. Whereas a fully-rectified single-phase machine produces *two* bursts of x-rays with each cycle of electricity, a half-rectified machine will produce only *one* burst of x-rays. Its output is *one-half* that of a single-phase unit, *one-fourth* that of a three-phase machine. To compensate technique when using half-rectified equipment, all mAs values must be doubled from single-phase techniques in order to produce adequate radiographic density.

Capacitor-discharge units do not use pulses of electricity at all. Rather, they store up a preset electrical charge on a capacitor (somewhat like a battery) as described in Chapter 32. This charge is predetermined by the technique (mAs) set. When the charging button is depressed, this amount of electrical charge is allowed to run from the incoming electrical line onto the capacitor. Then, when the exposure button is activated, the stored charge rushes to and across the x-ray tube, creating a single burst of x-rays. For technique purposes, the output of a capacitor discharge unit is considered to be roughly equivalent to that of a single- phase unit. The mAs values used would be double those for three-phase equipment or for battery operated units.

BATTERY-OPERATED MOBILE UNITS

Most modern "portable" or mobile x-ray units use a bank of batteries as the power source. Such a machine is charged up between uses by plugging it into a wall outlet. Electrical charge from the incoming line is stored in the batteries and later used for both driving the mobile unit and making exposures. It is essential to keep these machines properly charged between uses, or the full mAs and kVp values set by the technologist may not be attained during exposure, resulting in light radiographs.

The batteries supply a direct current. This electrical current is changed into alternating current to allow for manipulation and control at the console, and then it is changed back into direct current on its way to the x-ray tube. Direct current does not come in pulses, but is normally a steady flow of electricity. It has no voltage fluctuation like single-phase and three-phase generators produce (Figures 49 and 69). In a battery-powered unit, because the current was transformed into AC and then back into DC, a very slight voltage fluctuation results. But, this fluctuation is much less than a three-phase machine produces, and so slight that the final current is considered to be "straight" DC current rather than pulsed DC (Figure 70).

The importance of this waveform is that the average kilovoltage is essentially equal to the peak kilovoltage. It will be recalled that, with single-phase generation, the average kV produced is about one-third of the peak kV set (Figure 49). With three-phase equipment, the average kV falls between 93 per cent and 98 per cent of the peak kV, depending on whether it is a six-pulse or a twelve-pulse machine. With battery-powered mobile units, however, the average kV is virtually 100 per cent of the peak kV set at the console (Figure 70).

This explains why lower kVp settings are often used on modern mobile equipment than on stationary units in the x-ray department. For example, 80 kVp is typical for *nongrid* chest radiography in the department, such as an AP chest projection taken in a wheelchair. "Portable" chest x-rays taken with a battery-powered unit and *nongrid*, are often done at 72-74 kVp.

Lower mAs values may be used on these modern mobile machines for the same reasons. Battery-powered units are more efficient than three-phase or single-phase machines, both in terms of mAs and kVp. A rough rule of thumb is that *battery powered units require about six kVp less than three-phase, six-pulse machines.*

SUMMARY

1. Three-phase x-ray machines are twice as effective in producing radiographic *density* as single- phase machines. This is due to (1) more x-ray output per mA and (2) increased average beam energy, resulting in higher penetration.

2. When changing from a single-phase room to a three-phase room, all *techniques* may be adjusted by cutting mAs to one-half, and vice versa.

3. Three-phase machines cause a slight decrease in image *contrast* because of their increased average beam energy. Visually, however, this change is negligible.

4. Phase has no direct relation to the recognizability functions of sharpness of detail, magnification or distortion. However, the probability of motion with pediatric or problem patients can be reduced by using three-phase equipment, because shorter exposure times can be used.

5. Machines that are not fully *rectified* provide only one-half the x-ray output per mA of a single-phase, fully rectified unit. Compared to single-phase, techniques must be doubled on these machines. Compared to three-phase, they must be quadrupled.

6. *Capacitor discharge* mobile units are roughly equivalent to single-phase equipment, requiring twice the mAs that a three-phase or battery-powered machine uses.

7. *Battery-operated* mobile units are *slightly more* efficient than three-phase equipment, requiring 6 kVp less than 3Φ to produce equivalent image density.

8. *High-frequency generators* require about the same techniques as three-phase equipment to produce equal image density, and one-half the techniques used by single-phase equipment.

REVIEW QUESTIONS

1. Compared to a single-phase machine, a three-phase machine will produce an x-ray beam spectrum showing the same minimum energy, and the same peak energy but increased _____ energy.

2. What factor would you change and by how much, for a given procedure, when changing from a three-phase room to a single-phase room?

3. Explain the *two* reasons why the total density effect of the different phases of machines is different:

4. Why does a half-rectified portable x-ray unit produce lighter radiographs than, a fully rectified unit using identical techniques?

5. When changing from a three-phase machine to a capacitor discharge mobile unit, adjust mAs values to _____.

6. When changing from a single-phase unit to a high-frequency generator unit, adjust mAs values to _____.

7. For $3\Phi^6$, $3\Phi^{12}$, and high-frequency units, mAs values are roughly _____.

8. A battery-powered constant potential mobile unit will require _____ (more, less or equal) technique than a $3\Phi^6$ unit.

Chapter 8

BEAM FILTRATION

PROTECTIVE FILTRATION

WHEN ANY MATERIAL such as a sheet of aluminum is placed in the x-ray beam at the portal of the x-ray tube, the quantity and quality of the emergent radiation is altered. The effect of aluminum filtration is to screen out the long wave length non-penetrating, low-energy radiation that is not needed for routine radiography and which may be hazardous to a patient. The quantity of x-rays in the beam is reduced and the quality of the x-ray beam is increased, because removing the low-energy photons will cause an increase in the average energy of the photons in the beam. This is frequently referred to as "hardening the beam." Figure 73 shows the resulting effect upon the x-ray beam spectrum, with an increase in the average kV.

Total filtration is composed of *inherent* filtration and *added* filtration. Inherent filtration is that filtration normally occurring within the glass of the x-ray tube, the oil in the tube housing, and other devices such as beryllium windows or mirrors and windows within the collimator through which the beam must pass. Added filtration is the additional thin slabs of aluminum which may be permanently installed within the collimator and/or placed in the beam through a slot in the side of many modern collimators (Figure 74). In modern equipment, inherent filtration normally falls between 1 and 1.5 mm equivalency of aluminum. Thus, the needed additional aluminum slabs should usually be between 1 and 1.5 mm. It is not unheard-of for a radiographer to remove aluminum slabs from the slot in the collimator for a mammographic procedure or some other reason and then forget to replace them afterward. There should always be slabs of aluminum in this slot unless a radiation physicist has verified that an adequate HVL is achieved without the slabs.

If filtration is not used, the low-energy x-rays, which are not penetrating, will nearly all be absorbed within the patient. They never reach the film and, therefore, have no appreciable effect upon the radiograph, but only increase the dose to the patient (especially the skin dose). Protective filtration reduces this unnecessary hazard to the patient. Under no circumstances should radiography be performed without proper aluminum filtration in the beam.

EFFECTS ON IMAGE QUALITIES

If the filtration were increased much beyond about 3.5 millimeters of aluminum, it would begin to visibly affect the radiographic density. Such excessive filtration begins to absorb x-ray energies that are useful, in that many of them penetrate through the patient and reach the film. In addition to a visible loss of density, there would also occur a very slight increase in gray scale, or loss of contrast, due to the fact that elimination of the lower energies in the beam spectrum leads to an increase in the *average* beam energy (Figure 73). However, while this effect upon contrast might be measurable using a densitometer, it is not normally visible.

Excessive protective filtration in the beam defeats the purpose of exposing the radiograph. When density losses become

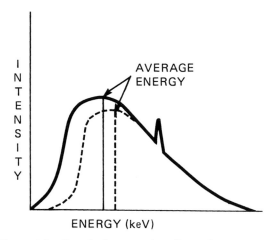

Figure 73. Graph showing the effect of increasing filtration on the x-ray beam spectrum. Minimum and average energy increase (shift to the right), but maximum energy does not. Overall intensity (the height of the curves) is reduced.

visible, they necessitate an increase in the original mAs to compensate. Such an increase in mAs simply re-introduces additional patient skin dose, which the filtration was added to eliminate.

Therefore, an *optimum* level of protective filtration has been established to achieve a maximum level of protection for the patient *without* affecting the radiographic density. Governmental regulations require that all radiographic equipment capable of operating above 70 kVp must employ the equivalent of 2.5 millimeters of aluminum total filtration. This amount eliminates the lowest-energy, most damaging x-rays in the beam—those which would *not* make it through the patient to the film anyway and therefore have no radiographic value.

For practical purposes, protective filtration should not be considered as a significant factor in *any* of the radiographic qualities, including density and contrast. For example, no increase in image density would be discernible when working with a real patient if the filtration was reduced from 2.5 millimeters of aluminum to 1.5 millimeters. This is because the additional low-energy x- rays released in the primary

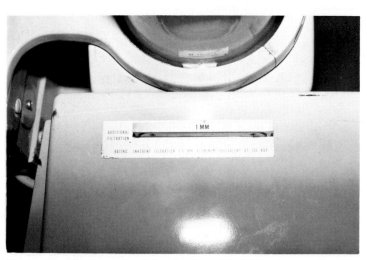

Figure 74. Photograph of the slot for added filtration on the side of a mobile unit collimator.

beam will virtually all be absorbed in the patient and never reach the film. Protective filtration becomes a factor affecting image qualities only in excessive amounts.

To summarize the effects of protective filtration upon the image qualities, remember that although it alters the primary beam prior to reaching the patient, the remnant beam which penetrates through the patient to the film is not appreciably affected. In daily practice, protective filtration has no appreciable effect upon radiographic contrast or density. It also has no effect upon sharpness, magnification or distortion since it is not a geometrical factor.

COMPENSATING FILTRATION

There are occasions when it is difficult to balance densities in radiography of large and irregular anatomical areas by making use of kilovoltage or the "heel" effect. However, by selective absorption of various portions of the x-ray beam *before* it traverses the subject, balanced densities may be secured.

Absorption of the beam can be effected by placing a *compensating filter* such as graduated aluminum in the filter channel. The material is so shaped that the beam must pass through the larger amounts of absorbing material when directed toward the thinner anatomical portions. The material should be thin or omitted for that portion of the beam passing toward the heavier parts.

Two of the most common types of compensating filters are the *wedge* filter (Figure 75) and the *trough* filter (Figure 76). The wedge filter is particularly recommended for lengthwise use on AP thoracic spines and AP feet, as well as crosswise use on lateral pelvimetry or fetogram views. The trough filter is used to obtain balanced density in both the mediastinum and the lung fields on one AP view. Other types of compensating filters can be custom made for specific needs.

In most applications of compensating fil-

Figure 75. Photograph of a wedge filter which may be inserted in the collimator rails for anatomy of graduating thickness, such as AP views of the T-spine, foot or femur.

Figure 76. Photograph of a trough filter, used for the AP T-spine.

ters, techniques will need to be increased by 8 to 10 kVp. This is due to the fact that most techniques for uneven anatomy are selected to record the thinner portions of the anatomy. In these thinner areas, the thicker end of the filter cancels out the effect of the kVp increase, while the thinner end of the filter allows the increased technique through to darken the density in the thicker anatomical parts. The result is proper density in all anatomical areas.

Special compensating filters can be custom made for particular applications such as spinal orthopedics.

In radiography of the entire spine on a 14-x-36-inch film, a normal image would exhibit high density in those portions representing the thinner tissue areas. The upper segment of the vertebral column would be overexposed because the exposure would necessarily be adjusted to suit the heavier or lumbosacral portion of the spine. This condition would still arise on occasion because the anode portion of the beam would ordinarily be directed toward the thinner area–the cervical vertebrae. Despite this arrangement, however, overexposure of the cervical area often would occur. By constructing a suitable compensating filter of barium-impregnated clay, anteroposterior and lateral views of the entire vertebral column that exhibit balanced radiographic densities may be secured (Figure 77).

Radiography of chests wherein extensive consolidations or thoracoplasties are present, shielding the normal pulmonary area with a compensating filter, permits using an exposure that is more appropriate for the diseased area or the one wherein surgery was employed without overexposing the contralateral side.

Compensating filters are also used to advantage in placental studies and orthopedic radiography. Herein, however, employment of the higher kilovoltages and the heel effect are of great assistance.

A compensating filter can even be made to produce radiographs of the total body as shown in Figures 1 and 78, wherein all densities are equalized to produce balanced images. Such a practice is *not* recommended in modern diagnosis, but these historical radiographs show how effective compensating filters can be.

Compensating filters are used to control image density, but their effect upon image contrast is negligible. Although the thicker portions of a filter may slightly increase the gray scale in those areas on the radiograph, the change is not normally visible. Compensating filters also have no effect upon sharpness, magnification, nor distortion because filters are not geometrical in nature.

Figure 77. AP and lateral radiographs of the entire spine exposed with compensating filtration. Note the balanced densities along the spine.

X-RAY BEAM QUALITY AND HVL

The quality of the x-ray beam may be thought of as its *average energy*, or its overall ability for *penetration*. The average energy of the beam depends primarily upon two factors: the set kVp and the amount of total filtration in the beam. Increasing either one of these will pull up the average energy of the beam, make it more penetrating and of higher quality.

Since filtration also plays a part, it is not accurate to refer to the quality of the beam solely in terms of the kVp. A special unit, the *half-value layer*, directly measures beam quality by determining its actual penetration ability. The half-value layer, or *HVL*, is the amount of absorber required to reduce the intensity of the x-ray beam to one half the original intensity. Requirements for HVL and its determination are fully discussed in Chapter 30.

Any increase in inherent or added filtration, or any increase in kVp, will result in a higher HVL. That is, it will take more absorber to attenuate one-half of the x-ray beam. The higher the HVL, the more penetrating the beam is.

Figure 78. Entire body radiograph of a living girl made with a compensating filter. The stomach and intestinal tract was filled with barium sulfate for their delineation.

SUMMARY

1. Normal amounts of protective filtration are used only to reduce patient radiation *dose* and in practice have no effect upon any aspect of the radiographic image. Excessive amounts of filtration, beyond recommended levels, would result in a loss of density, with no other significant image change.

2. Compensating filters are designed to reduce *density* in areas of thinner anatomy on the radiograph and have no significant effect on other image qualities.

3. Most compensating filters require an increase in *technique* of 8 to 10 kVp.

4. Overall beam quality is measured in HVL units.

REVIEW QUESTIONS

1. In an 80 kVp x-ray beam, a decrease in filtration would (increase, decrease, or not affect) the number of photons at these energies:
   a. 15 kVp:
   b. 50 kVp:
   c. 80 kVp:
2. List all of the image qualities which are noticeably affected when adding a compensating filter such as the wedge filter:
3. How much should you increase kVp when adding a thick wedge filter?
4. What is the minimum amount of protective filtration required on all x-ray machines capable of operating above 70 kVp? Be sure your answer is complete:
5. Give an example of a procedure on which you would use a wedge filter *and* explain why you would use it on *this* procedure:
6. Which image qualities would be noticeably changed when removing 0.5 mm of protective filtration from a beam which originally had 2.5 mm in it?
7. Define half-value layer.

Chapter 9

FIELD SIZE LIMITATION

The purposes of beam size limitation are twofold: (1) to reduce exposure to the patient and (2) to increase image contrast. The minimizing of patient exposure should be of paramount concern to every radiographer, and limiting the size of the x-ray beam is one of the most effective ways to minimize exposure. By controlling field size, organs with critical sensitivity to radiation such as the gonads, thyroid gland and lenses of the eyes can be kept outside of the primary beam. The resulting reduction in dose to these organs can be as much as a hundred-fold. A variety of devices is available for this purpose.

COLLIMATION DEVICES

Devices commonly used to limit beam size include manual collimators and positive beam limitation (automatic) collimators installed on all modern equipment, cones, extension cylinders and aperture diaphragms (Figure 79). The most effective of these devices in providing a sharp border on the x-ray field are those which cause the beam to pass through two apertures rather than one. The collimator and the extension cylinder (commonly misnamed a "cone") provide double apertures (Figure 80). A photograph of a modern collimator attached to a mobile unit is found in the previous Figure 74. The cylinder does so because the radiation must "make it through" both the opening entering into the cylinder and through the opening at the end. Modern collimators utilize a secondary set of shutters for the second "aperture" or opening.

The purpose of a secondary aperture is to absorb *off-focus radiation.* Off-focus radiation is produced in the x-ray tube when a few of the high-speed electrons, as they accelerate toward the anode, veer off-track (usually due to "collisions" with other electrons) and strike the anode somewhere other than at the focal spot. X-rays will be

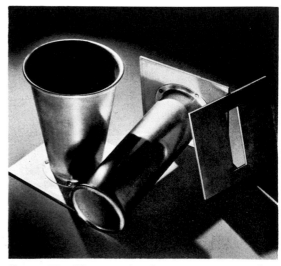

Figure 79. Photograph of cone, extension cylinder and aperture diaphragm, devices used to restrict field size.

Figure 81. Photograph of collimator mechanism, showing upper set of shutters (horizontal white arrow) and lower set of shutters (black arrow). The screw for adjusting the angle of the field light mirror is demarcated by the vertical white arrow.

Figure 80. Diagram showing double-aperture collimation provided by extension cylinders and automatic collimators. The second set of shutters, or the lower aperture, absorbs off-focus radiation (A) and provides a sharper field edge (E).

produced in the anode where these off-focused electrons strike, and a few of these x-rays will be emitted through the window of the x-ray tube along with the primary beam. Off-focus x-rays are *primary* radiation, but they travel in a crooked direction in relation to the rest of the beam, and are thus destructive to the image. Off-focus rays must not be confused with scattered radiation, which originates in the patient rather than in the x-ray tube. Nonetheless, they have similar effects upon the image, reducing contrast. To control this as much as possible, a second set of shutters is employed in collimators (Figure 81).

Since a secondary aperture is closer to the patient it also provides a smaller field with sharper edges (Figure 80). Sharper edges on the x-ray field itself, however,

must not be confused with sharpness of the actual details in the image, which is *not* directly affected by field size limitation.

POSITIVE BEAM LIMITATION

All new x-ray collimators have positive beam limitation or *PBL*, which means that they automatically adjust to the size of the film placed in the Bucky tray. This is both a blessing and a curse. It ensures that the field size will not be larger than the film. But, for those views which should be collimated to a size smaller than the film, it has inadvertently contributed to sloppy practice by radiographers who mistakenly think they no longer need to concern themselves with manual collimation. Every PBL system has an optional *override* which can be set at the collimator. When a "coned-down" view is in order, the radiographer should override the PBL and manually collimate. Failure to do so results in unnecessary exposure to the patient, and defeats the very purpose for which the collimator was built.

OVERCOLLIMATION

The anatomy of interest must always be fully included within the x-ray field. Overzealous collimation can result in "cutting off" essential anatomy from the view and result in a repeated exposure. By so doing, one defeats the most important purpose of collimation—minimizing patient dose.

With experience, the student will come to appreciate that the edges of the actual x-ray beam are not always perfectly aligned with the edges of the projected light field. This is due to the fact that the light field is projected from a light bulb in the side of the collimator and reflected downward from a mirror, while the x-ray beam passes through the mirror from above. The angle of this mirror can be adjusted by a lever inside the collimator, Figure 81, and it is not uncommon for the light field to be projected as much as one-half inch off of the actual x-ray field. In fact, each edge of the light field is only required to be within about one-half inch of the edges of the x-ray field.

With this in mind, a word to the wise would be to *always allow at least one-half inch of light beyond the anatomy of interest,* as long as it does not exceed the film size. For example, when radiographing a hand, allow at least one-half inch of light beyond the fingertips at to each side of the hand shadow. Neglecting this guideline will result in unnecessarily repeated exposures to the patient.

SCATTER RADIATION

Limitation of the size of the x-ray field is extremely important in the control of fog from scattered radiation. When an anatomical area is small, a field should be used that is small enough to include just the area of interest. In limiting the size of the x-ray beam, less tissue is irradiated within the patient, reducing patient dose. Further, the number of different areas within the patient and the table, as well as the number of different angles, from which any given point on the film may receive scattered photons is reduced.

Figure 82 demonstrates this effect. With a wide beam, *A*, scattered radiation may be produced within a large volume of exposed tissue (dashed area). This scattered radiation emanates from various points within the body part, and can reach any point on the film from many different angles. Any one of these scattered rays could strike the

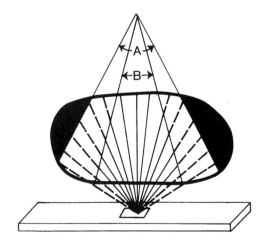

Figure 82. Diagram illustrating how smaller field sizes expose a lesser volume of tissue and a narrower range of angles (solid lines) from which scattered radiation can fog a given area on the film. This reduction in scatter decreases density and increases contrast.

small square area of interest on the film, fogging this area. (Scattered rays are in fact emitted in all directions, and can strike anywhere on the film, but for this demonstration we shall consider a small chosen area.) When the x-ray beam is collimated to a smaller size, *B*, scatter rays can only be produced in the smaller volume of exposed tissue. Also, there are fewer different angles from which this scattered radiation may reach the square on the film. The small square on the film will be more fogged with the wide beam (*A*) than with a narrow beam (*B*).

It is important to remember that *scattered radiation is produced in and from tissue. Literally, the more tissue exposed, the more scatter produced.*

EFFECT ON CONTRAST

In Chapter Four we learned that for image contrast to be changed, the interactions of the x-ray beam must be considered *relative to each other*. We have established that less scatter is produced with narrower x-ray beams, but for this to result in any change in image contrast, we must also show that photoelectric interactions and penetrating x-rays have *not* decreased by the same amount. If this were so, they would cancel out the effect of decreased scatter and overall image contrast would not change.

Figure 83 provides this demonstration, using diagrams of the penetrating and absorbed portions of the primary x-ray beam. Once again, we focus on a small chosen area of the film. Note that the number of penetrating primary beams *striking the small square* is equal regardless of whether the x-ray beam is wide (*A*) or narrow (*B*). In *A*, four x-rays reach the square and one, in the middle, is totally absorbed by photoelectric effect, leaving a small white spot in the middle of the square. In *B*, there are still four x-rays reaching this area. Furthermore, the white spot is unchanged in position and appearance. The *concentration* of penetrating and absorbed rays is not affected by the width of the overall x-ray beam.

The reason that penetrating and absorbed x-rays are *not* affected by beam width is that they are produced in the *x-ray tube*. They follow straight, geometrically predictable paths which do not change, whether in tissue or outside of tissue, just because the location of the edges of the beam is altered (Figure 83).

The reason that the amount of scatter radiation *is* affected by beam width is that scatter is produced in *tissue*, and since it is geometrically unpredictable and random in direction, it can reach the small square on the film from *anywhere* in the exposed tissue (Figure 82).

If scatter radiation, produced by the Compton interaction, decreases, while photoelectric interactions and penetrating rays remain unchanged, then image contrast will change. The Compton/photoelectric ratio has decreased (and so has the "Compton/penetration ratio"), and this means that visible fog in the image will decrease. With this reduction in fog, image contrast will increase.

It is worth noting that the effects of changing field size upon both density and contrast are limited to field sizes less than about 150 square inches, roughly equivalent to an 11 x 14 inch field. With field sizes larger than this, additional scatter radiation is produced at such a distance from our theoretical point of fogging on the film that very few of these additional low-energy scattered rays reach the film and fog it. In other words, changing from an 11 x 14 inch field to a 14 by 17 inch field will not result in a visible change in image density or contrast. *Only when changing to or from field sizes less than 11 x 14 inches are these density and contrast effects noticed.*

Figure 83. Diagram illustrating that field size does not affect the concentration of *primary* radiation nor the occurrence of the photoelectric effect (asterisk). Field size is indicated by bold lines. In (A), four x-rays reach the square area on the film, and one is absorbed by the photoelectric interaction, leaving a white spot on the radiograph. In (B), the edges of the light field are collimated in to obtain a smaller overall field. The square area on the film still receives four x-rays with a white spot in the middle. The effects of field size upon image density and contrast are *entirely* due to changes in the amount of scatter radiation produced within the body, not to any change in the intensity of the primary beam.

EFFECT ON DENSITY

It may be said that the density for any particular area on a radiograph depends on the *concentration* of x-rays striking there. The more concentrated the radiation is, the greater will be the *total* number of x-rays striking within that area. Figures 82 and 83 illustrate the effects of changing field size on the concentration of radiation reaching a small square on the film. In Figure 83, one can see that the same four primary x-rays reach the small square regardless of where the edges of the beam are located. The concentration of *primary* radiation is not affected by the size of the field.

However, as shown in Figure 82, the concentration of *scattered radiation* in this small square area on the film *is changed* by the field size. When the field is collimated to a smaller area, a lesser volume of tissue is exposed and less scatter is produced. There are also fewer angles from which scatter produced in the patient may reach the small square. The amount of scatter rays striking this area is reduced.

In determining the *total* amount of radiation reaching the film, both the primary rays and the scattered rays must be considered. Therefore, even though the concentration of *primary* x-rays is unaffected by field size, the loss of scattered rays results in a reduction in the *total* amount of radiation reaching the small square on the film. There will be less density in the image.

This effect is true for all other small areas on the film, so that the overall density of the radiograph is likewise affected. Smaller field sizes result in lower overall density, because the reduction in scatter radiation leads to a reduction in the total amount of radiation reaching the film. With larger field sizes, overall density is increased, due to additional scatter radiation. These effects are illustrated in Figures 84 and 85.

To maintain image quality, the density effects of field size changes must be compensated for by adjusting technique. It is recommended that such adjustments be made using mAs rather than kVp. Frequently collimation is used for the express purpose of reducing image fog and enhancing contrast. Use of a higher kVp level to compensate would result in more image fog, partially defeating this purpose. Since mAs compensation will not affect contrast, it will not cancel out the desired result, even partially. To maintain a given density, *collimation of the field size to smaller areas requires an increase in mAs from 35 to 50 per cent* (an additional one-third to one-half

the original mAs, depending on how extreme the change in field size is).

Changing from a 10 x 12 inch (24 x 30 cm) field to a typical cylinder or "cone" necessitates a 35 per cent increase. For example, suppose that 30 mAs were used for a good view of the lumbar spine. The radiologist asks for a "coned-down" view of one vertebra. For this exposure, use 40 mAs, an increase of one-third. The most extreme change in field size would be encountered when changing from a 14 x 17 inch (35 x 42 cm) field to a cylinder, such as deriving a technique for a "coned-down" view of the gall bladder from a previous full abdomen exposure. In this case mAs must be increased by 50 per cent or one-half. If the abdomen was exposed at 40 mAs, use 60 mAs for the coned view.

Apparent exceptions to this rule can be attributed to other variables. For example, sinus radiographs are often "coned down" while skull series are not, yet sinus techniques are usually somewhat *less* than skull techniques. In this case, the sinuses are air-filled cavities, very different tissue from the cranium, and much less technique is required. This effect is simply greater than the effect of collimating, so that the net change required is a slight decrease in technique. In the case of the coned-down lateral view of the lumbosacral junction, technique must be increased much more than 50 per cent as compared to the full lateral view, because, in addition to adjusting for coning down, penetration through the iliac bones is required. Radiographers typically increase ten kVp from the full lateral technique for this view, equivalent to almost doubling the mAs. In the absence of other modifying considerations like these, the 35-50 per cent rule of thumb may be applied with confidence to achieve consistent densities. As mentioned in the previous section, changing field size from 11 x 14

Figure 84. Series of radiographs of the hand to demonstrate the influence of the size of cones on the image. Note the enhancement of contrast and the loss of density with smaller cone sizes.

inches to 14 x 17 inches does not require any adjustment, because scatter radiation reaches a "saturation point" at sizes above 11 x 14 inches.

Example: The radiographs in Figures 84 and 85 were produced with the same technique, but progressively smaller field sizes were used. The presence of scatter fogging is apparent in the first of the series, causing an overall grayness and loss of contrast. In Figure 84, the scattered radiation was mostly produced by the tabletop and cassette surrounding the anatomy of interest. As the field size is diminished, it can be clearly seen that the contrast is substantially enhanced. Further, the smaller field sizes demonstrate a significant loss of density. The mAs value should be increased by roughly ¹/₃ of the original to compensate for this density loss, assuming that the original density was desirable.

Ratio of Secondary to Primary Radiation

The ratio of secondary to primary radiation emitted by thin parts, such as the hand, is small, irrespective of the size of the field, because of the small amount of tissue irradiated. This does not hold true for the thicker and more dense structures. This fact is demonstrated in a series of posteroanterior screen radiographs of the frontal sinuses (Figure 85), wherein radiographs A to C were exposed with the same factors.

Figure 85. Series of radiographs of the PA sinuses which were all made using the same technique factors. (A) made without a cone, (B) made with a large cone, (C) and (D) made with progressively smaller cones. Note the dramatic improvement of contrast and lesser density at smaller field sizes.

Radiograph A was made *without* a cone; note the high image density that is largely attributable to fog generated by the neck and shoulder girdle. Radiograph B was made with a large cone and the fog is somewhat reduced because the tissue in the shoulder girdle has not been irradiated.

Radiographs C and D were made with smaller cones and the fog density has been greatly reduced. The visibility of details is greatly improved because the small cone limits the *amount* of tissue irradiated; hence the quantity of secondary radiation is greatly diminished.

EFFECT ON OTHER QUALITIES

While contrast increases and density decreases from smaller x-ray fields, sharpness of recorded detail, magnification and distortion are unaffected. (A common misconception is that scattered radiation affects the sharpness of recorded detail. This is false, and is fully discussed in Chapter

Twelve.) These recognizability functions involve the recording on the film of the edges of the anatomy of interest, all of which lies within the beam, and have nothing to do with the edges of the x-ray beam itself.

CALCULATING FIELD SIZE COVERAGE

The total area of field size coverage is directly proportional to the square of the distance from the x-ray tube target to the film. Any given side of a rectangular field, or the diameter of a circular field, is directly proportional to the SID. This relationship simply follows the laws of similar triangles, where the distances involved represent the height of the triangles and the sides or diameter of the fields represent the bases of the triangles, as illustrated in Figure 86. Where there are two apertures, as in collimators or extension cylinders, it is easiest to always use the diameter of the aperture *farthest away from the tube target* as the base of the smaller triangle. The distance from

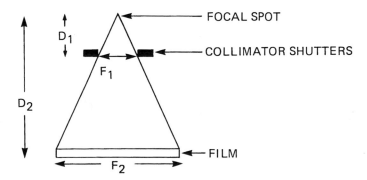

Figure 86. Diagram of similar triangle geometry formed by the x-ray beam. The field size is directly proportional to its distance from the focal spot.

the target to that opening will be the height of the smaller triangle. Either of the two similar triangle formulae below may be used to arrive at a correct answer:

$$(1) \quad \frac{D1}{F1} = \frac{D2}{F2} \quad \text{or} \quad (2) \quad \frac{D1}{D2} = \frac{F1}{F2}$$

Where D is the distance from the tube target, one to the aperture and the second to the film, and F is the side or diameter of the aperture for the first triangle and of the field at the film for the second. In practice, the radiographer should be able to make simple calculations of this type quickly *in his head*, since they are direct proportions. For example, if the distance to the film is twice the distance to the end of a cylinder, the diameter of the round field at the film will be exactly twice the diameter of the end of the cylinder. For a rectangular field, the problem must be worked through two times, once for each dimension of the field—length and width.

Example: Collimator Coverage

A common example of the value of memorizing this relationship is found when the field light in a collimator burns out in surgery. Suppose that the bottom set of collimator shutters are 15 inches from the tube target (which may be estimated at about one inch below the center of the cylindrical tube housing) and the SID being used is about 45 inches. If the two pairs of shutters, which you can see through the window of the collimator, measure three inches apart by four inches apart, the field size at the film will be 9 x 12 inches (15/45 = 3/9 = 4/12). Two other specific variations in applying this principle follow:

Example: Cone Coverage

A new cone has been obtained. The diameter of the cone at its lower rim is 5 inches and the distance from the focal spot to the rim of the cone is 15 inches. What is the diameter of the field coverage at an SID of 36 inches? When the foregoing values are substituted in the formula, the answer may be derived as follows:

Solution: $F2 = \dfrac{36 \times 5}{15}$

$F2 = 12$ inches. Answer.

Example: Diaphragm Size

It is desired to cut an aperture that will limit the x-ray beam to a 10-inch coverage of a 10 x 12- inch film at an SID of 40 inches. The distance from the focal spot to the lead diaphragm is 4 inches. What is the diameter of the aperture to be cut in the lead diaphragm?

Solution: $F1 = \dfrac{10 \times 4}{40}$

$F1 = 1$ inch. Answer.

A little practice will help the student become comfortable with these ratios. Try EXERCISE 15 below, then check your answers from the Appendix.

EXERCISE 15

In the following exercises the "aperture" refers to the diameter or width of the bottom opening of a cone or cylinder, the bottom set of shutters in a collimator, or the device through which the x-ray beam and light field pass before projecting onto the film. Use similar triangle proportions to fill in the missing size or distance:

	Distance from target (focal spot) to Aperture	Source-Image Receptor Distance	Size of Aperture	Field Size at Film
1.	10 inches	40 inches	6 inches	_____
2.	12 inches	36 inches	5 inches	_____
3.	20 inches	50 inches	4 inches	_____
4.	15 inches	60 inches	_____	16 inches
5.	18 inches	36 inches	_____	12 inches
6.	18 inches	45 inches	_____	25 inches
7.	15 inches	_____	5 inches	10 inches
8.	20 inches	_____	4 inches	12 inches
9.	_____	40 inches	6 inches	16 inches
10.	_____	72 inches	3 inches	12 inches

SUMMARY

1. X-ray field size must never be larger than necessary to include the anatomy of interest, or unnecessary patient *dose* will occur in addition to the destruction of image quality.
2. Restriction of field size enhances image *contrast*, by reducing the volume of tissue available to produce scatter fogging.
3. Field size restriction also reduces image *density*, which may need to be compensated for by increasing mAs up to 50 per cent.
4. Field size has no relation to the geometrical *recognizability* functions in the image—sharpness of recorded detail, magnification, or distortion—because the penumbral geometry at the anatomy of interest is not changed.
5. Changes in field size are directly proportional to changes in the SID/SOD ratio when the "object" is considered to be the final aperture through which the x-ray beam passes (the end of the cone, cylinder or collimator).
6. Double-aperture collimators reduce *off-focus radiation.*
7. Positive beam limiters or *PBL collimators* should be over-ridden whenever a field size smaller than the film is appropriate.
8. Always allow $1/2$-inch of field light beyond the anatomy of interest, unless it exceeds the film size.

REVIEW QUESTIONS

1. Which image quality is increased by reducing field size?
2. Explain why reducing field size reduces image density:
3. The lower shutters in a collimator are 12 inches from the focal spot. If these shutters are opened to a 4 inch square, how big will the x-ray beam be at 42 inches from the focal spot?
4. The end of a 6-inch diameter extension cylinder is 15 inches from the focal spot. At what distance from the focal spot will you get a circular field with an 18-inch diameter?
5. To compensate image density for converting from a 14 x 17 film to a 5-inch square, by what percentage must you increase mAs?
6. Why do collimators have two sets of shutters?
7. Even though collimation improves image quality, what is the *most* important reason to use it?
8. When should a PBL collimator be over-ridden?
9. Always allow _____-inch of field light beyond the anatomy of interest, unless it exceeds the film size.
10. Scatter radiation reaches a saturation level at field sizes above:

Chapter 10

PATIENT STATUS AND CONTRAST AGENTS

The relative differences in the composition and thickness of tissue components of a body part exert great influence on the radiation traversing it. This applies not alone to different parts of the same body, but also the same parts of different bodies.

Absorption is intimately associated with the atomic number of the tissue elements being irradiated. Bone is less penetrable than the surrounding soft tissue. Body fluids possess about the same absorption characteristics as soft tissue. The pathologic and physiologic states of the tissues are also important when considering absorption differences. Selection and alteration of exposure factors must be made with these facts in mind.

PHYSIQUE

No two human physiques are identical. Not only do they differ in their general family and racial physical characteristics but individual parts vary widely in size, shape, and tissue density. Naturally, gradations between types of physiques do occur.

In radiography, therefore, any x-ray exposure system should encompass all of the body deviations with sufficient latitude so that radiographs of diagnostic utility can be produced with some measure of standardization.

BODY HABITUS

The analysis of a living body for radiographic purposes requires its classification into one of four types, or more pertinently, somatotypes. Also, some discernment as to the physiology of the body should be made as well as an estimate as to the influence of disease or trauma on the tissues. There are four general types of physique classified under the term habitus–hypersthenic,

sthenic, hyposthenic, and asthenic.

The characteristics of each type resolve into states wherein they can be generally separated almost as an entity from each other. It is not possible to strike much of an average in classification because the features of all body types are extensively interrelated. By study of the extremes of each type, however, a definite understanding of the variables in physique that must be met in radiography can be achieved and exposure compromises, usually of a low order, can be effected.

Hypersthenic

The hypersthenic type is characterized by softness and roundness throughout the various bodily regions. The tissues tend to be flabby with an excess of subcutaneous fat. The torso is barrel-like. The anteroposterior and lateral thicknesses are quite comparable in the head, neck, trunk, and limbs. Abdominal and thoracic volume is predominant as compared to the head and extremities. The well developed chest is relatively short and wide at the base. The neck is short and thick and the waistline is high. The vertebral column is relatively straight when viewed laterally and the back is usually well padded with fat.

This type tends to become obese and is often a victim of hypertension. Degenerative diseases of the heart, arteries and kidneys are common to the type.

Sthenic

The sthenic type is strong and active. The joints and bones are large. The physique is heavy in muscle and bone and relatively rectangular in shape. The skin is thick with an abundance of underlying connective tissue. These persons are physically well balanced.

The anteroposterior trunk thicknesses are less than those in the hypersthenic type. The well-developed chest is larger than the abdomen. The trunk is long and the pectoral area is wide; the waist is slender and low. The neck is long. The clavicles are heavy and prominent.

Asthenic

The asthenic type exhibits a sense of linearity and delicacy of body. The neck is long and slender and projects forward. Small bones and stringy muscles prevail. The thorax is long, flat and narrow. The ribs are thin and prominent and the shoulders are narrow without muscle relief. The shoulder girdle lacks muscular support and the scapulae tend to protrude posteriorly. The trunk is short and the limbs long. The abdomen is flat and shallow in depth. The, abdominal viscera tend to be ptosed. The lumbar curve is flat and the thoracic curve is often prominent.

Hyposthenic

The hyposthenic body habitus is not as extreme a variation as the hypersthenic or asthenic. In body size, it lies somewhere between the sthenic and the asthenic types, but may be described as very thin. The primary distinction between the asthenic habitus and the hyposthenic habitus is not in size but in condition: While the asthenic patient is physically weak and emaciated from pathological conditions, appears sickly, and is often advanced in age, the hyposthenic patient is young, active, and relatively strong but is definitely underweight for his height and extremely thin compared to the average.

In spite of their small size, hyposthenic patients have a body composition with muscle/fat tissue ratios similar to sthenic patients, and, therefore, technique may be adjusted entirely in accordance with their size without further consideration as to condition. A technique chart with small enough part measurements may be followed.

The foregoing physical characteristics are of course the extreme variants of the four somatotypes. The body being an intermixture of all types may exhibit in a more or less dominant manner special characteristics of one or the other type. Knowing the general characteristics of the extremes makes the analysis of the patient a little easier for radiographic purposes.

BODY TISSUES

For radiographic purposes, body tissues may be divided roughly into two groups: those consisting largely of *organic* materials (soft tissue) and those containing organic materials impregnated with *inorganic* substances (bone).

Organic Tissue

Organic tissue generally constitutes the soft tissues or flesh and comprises skin, fat, muscle, cartilage, tendon, nerve trunks, brain, blood vessels, viscera, etc., which all contain a large amount of fluid when compared to inorganic tissues. Organic tissues are composed of carbon, hydrogen, nitrogen, and oxygen, and possess low x-ray absorption properties. Muscle tissue contains approximately 75 to 80 per cent fluid; fat stores little fluid–about 20 per cent. Pulmonary tissue contains a large quantity of moisture-laden air in the living state.

Soft Tissues

Radiographically, soft tissues may be generally grouped as follows: solid and hollow viscera; viscera surrounded by fat; intramuscular inclusions such as fat, air, or mineral salts; pools or body fluids, such as blood; musculature; and, fat. Soft tissues that are not demarcated by fat (or air), such as the stomach, cannot always be delineated, and it is then necessary to introduce a suitable contrast medium. The x-ray absorption properties of individual soft tissues vary; muscles, body fluids, connective tissue, and solid viscera have about the same degree of absorption as water whereas fat and air-laden pulmonary tissue offer considerably less absorption.

Fat

Females and young children have more body fat than males. Alteration in the fat content is probably the most important single variable, other than disease, that determines the water content of the body at any specific period in its life. For example, a malignancy may cause a patient to lose weight. If the weight loss is principally fat, the water content remains unchanged. However, the body water may be expected to increase upon disappearance of the fat. Endocrine disturbances are often evidenced by fat accumulation. Aged obese persons exhibit a wide disproportion between muscle and fat, the latter predominating.

Living Bone

The normal adult bony and cartilaginous skeleton comprises approximately 20 per cent of the total body weight.

Living bone is a versatile tissue possessing an organic matrix (collagen) upon which mineral salts have been deposited. It furnishes the supporting framework of the body. It is soft in young persons and hard in the older. It bears most of the blood cells; it stores minerals and releases them to various parts of the body as they are needed. It is capable of repairing itself after injury and of growing like other tissues until the body reaches adulthood: The minerals in bone are calcium phosphate and calcium carbonate in a ratio of 2:1.

Infants' bones are seldom as well delineated radiographically as those of an adult because their mineral content is less than that in the normal adult bone. The radiographic appearance of bone is directly related to its mineral content. Normal adult bone possesses high x-ray absorption characteristics.

Bone marrow is widely dispersed in the human body; its function is to form blood. The space within the bone is filled with blood-forming tissues. The total marrow space is greater in the adult male than the female and its average volume is about 168 cubic inches. The volume increases in elderly persons because of the aging process perhaps at the expense of cortical bone.

Bone is in a constant state of building up and tearing down a little at a time. In growth, bone is built by erosion (by osteoclasts) of the inside of the bone (medulla) thereby enlarging the medullary cavity while bone forming cells (osteoblasts) build up the bone externally. Bone fractures are repaired by the laying down of a soft fibrous tissue called callus that largely originates in the periosteum and joins the ends of the fractured segments. The callus is replaced gradually with hard, new bone due to the action of the osteoblasts. The jagged edges that might interfere with function and also any excess bone produced during the repair process are smoothed away by the osteoclasts.

Growth in length of the bone is a bit different. In childhood each bone contains a disk of cartilage (epiphysis) at its ends. As growth takes place, the cartilage disk extends itself and the part nearest the bone absorbs calcium to make bone. When the bone reaches its normal length the cartilage is entirely replaced by bone.

Body Fluids

Human body fluids comprise approximately 62 per cent of body weight distributed throughout all of the tissues. The range in males may be 55 to 70 per cent; in females, 46 to 60 per cent. Bodies of the lean muscular type may contain approximately 70 per cent fluids; whereas obese bodies may contain as little as 42 per cent fluid. Fluid content is a major factor in the generation of secondary radiation by the body tissues.

Fluids exist in localized quantities in the urinary, gastrointestinal, and biliary tracts, the circulatory vessels, joint spaces, glands, spinal cord, and intraventricular spaces of the brain. If body fluids are to be differentiated from the body structures, they must be surrounded by, or infused with, some medium that will provide the necessary differential contrast.

EVALUATION OF PATIENT

The radiographer must continually train his eyes and mind in evaluating the patient for radiographic purposes. He should try to view the body as a physiologic or pathologic entity; each part is pulsating with blood or other fluids; it is composed of muscle, fat, bone, etc., which may be normal or affected by various degrees of nutrition, trauma, disease, or hydration.

Evaluation should be based upon the patient's physique and upon the clinical situation. In general, it is the objective in examining new patients to make, initially, survey radiographs that will record all details of the anatomical area in question. The radiographer should be able after some clinical experience to recognize deviations from the normal, since these changes intimately affect the choice of exposure factors. The influence of disease, trauma, age, and nourishment, should be recognized early. For example, the short obese person might possess 35 per cent or more of body fat; 65 per cent of the body weight may consist of skeleton and lean body tissues containing about 73 per cent water.

These tissues in a lean, well-trained athlete might contain approximately 20 per cent more water. Hence more radiation would be absorbed by the tissues and more secondary radiation produced. Obviously, the obese person would not absorb as much x-radiation as the muscular type.

INFLUENCE OF AGE

During the early months of a child's life, the gain in weight is rapid. Usually the child's weight doubles in the first six months and triples at the end of a year. Thence the gain in weight is slow but steady until the eighteenth year. Throughout life there is a constant flux in the mineral content of bone. During the growth period, bone formation occurs at a greater rate than bone resorption. In middle life, bone formation and resorption is in balance. The rate of bone resorption exceeds bone growth in old age. Mineralization of average living bone decreases with age. Dehydration of tissues assumes major radiographic importance in the aged since chemical as well as structural osseous changes take place. Such changes may be generally described by the term *atrophy* and are manifested by a reduction in body water and a mineral loss. The soft tissues of infants contain a greater quantity of body fluid than the adult and the aged less than the younger adult.

Pediatric techniques are often derived by modifying adult techniques according to the proportions of the anatomy. It is well to note the proportionate differences in the growth of various body parts throughout our physical development. The femur (thigh) represents the extreme in growth—It is over five times longer and thicker in an adult than in an infant. On the other hand, the human skull expands less than three times its original diameter from infancy. This means that the pediatric technique for a skull will be roughly one-third to one-half that of an adult skull technique, while the pediatric technique for a femur will likely be as little as one-fifth that of an adult.

ANTHROPOLOGICAL FACTORS

There are physical differences in the mass, density, and shape of various bones for different human races, which are often substantial enough to require adjustments in radiographic technique. This is particularly true for skull radiography. A workable rule of thumb cannot be stated for any particular anthropological group, for at-least two reasons: First, there is too much variation within a racial group, and second, racial groups have become widely intermixed. However, an observant radiographer will recognize those patients whose skull appears to have greater bony mass than average, and *increase techniques by approximately one-third of the average mAs.*

There are three anthropological categories for skull shapes: *Mesocephalic* skulls are roundly oval in cross-section, with an angle of approximately 47 degrees between the mid-sagittal plane and the petrous ridges. These represent an average insofar as radiographic techniques are concerned. *Dolichocephalic* skulls are extremely oval, narrow side-to-side, and long front-to-back, with a petrous angle of roughly 40 degrees. There will be a greater difference in technique when changing from the AP projection to the lateral projection, and the lateral may require a slight decrease in technique as compared to the average skull. *Brachiocephalic* skulls are very round and broad, with a typical petrous angle of 54 degrees. These types of skulls frequently present a thicker bony mass as well as a broader shape, and may require up to one-third more mAs for all views.

SOFT TISSUE–BONE RELATION

The proportion of bone to soft tissue is fairly static for a given anatomic part. If the part is naturally large, the probabilities are that the bone is large and has a proportionate amount of soft tissue covering it. The radiographer must judge whether the part is *naturally* small, average, or large. The aggregate of the tissues possesses a certain thickness-density ratio that influences the degree of x-ray absorption that will take place. This fact must be considered when determining the amount of penetration that is necessary to overcome within a reasonably short exposure time, the absorbing power of the part. This penetration level dictates a minimum kVp requirement for each body part, regardless of variable thicknesses between patients. Table IV in Chapter Six lists the optimum kVp levels for each body part.

BODY THICKNESS

Human beings are dissimilar in their thickness characteristics. These tend to change in varying degrees during life and in health and disease. Despite these human differences, it is possible to establish certain pattern measurements for radiographic purposes that conform to what may be termed *average* thickness ranges. Such measurements can be standardized just as anthropologists have standardized indices of human measurement. They are an important means toward standardization of exposure factors.

METHOD FOR MEASURING THICKNESS OF PART

The type of calipers to be used for mensuration is illustrated in Figure 87. Be sure the calipers are always in good repair. All measurements should be made along the course of the projected central ray. In general the nonmovable leg of the calipers is placed opposite the body entrance or exit of the central ray and the movable leg closed so that it just makes contact with the skin. The calipers should not be squeezed for tissue will be displaced and a true dimension will not be obtained. This method should be employed in measuring

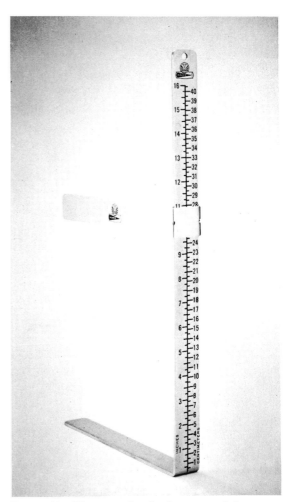

Figure 87. Photograph of calipers used for measurement of body parts.

the head and the upper and lower extremities.

Chest measurements should normally be made with the patient standing or sitting erect in a neutral or resting state. Respiration should be normal. When the central ray enters or leaves the body in the median plane, it is most important that the thickness of the tissue in the pectoral area be included. Therefore, the measurements should be made with the calipers horizontal and at the level of the seventh thoracic vertebra.

For anteroposterior projections of the abdominal structures, measurements are normally made with the patient supine and at rest. The nonmovable leg of the calipers is placed in a horizontal plane next to the skin posteriorly; the movable arm is then closed so that it just touches the anterior wall of the abdomen. With this measurement gentle palpation of the abdomen should be made to determine the presence of an unusual amount of gas or fluid. When present the radiographer should make allowances in the use of the mAs factor.

When making abdominal measurements with the patient erect or semierect, it should be recognized that the abdominal viscera gravitate to the pelvis thereby increasing the density of the tissues accumulated in the pelvic region.

THICKNESS RANGES

The young adult conforms to a definite physical standard and may be considered as basic for establishing average thickness ranges. For that reason, a series of average-thickness ranges has been established.

Determination of Average Thickness Ranges

Statistically, the frequency with which adult patients conform to a fairly average-thickness range for a given projection is relatively high. Since the x-ray absorption properties of human tissues are *unpredictable*, some latitude in compensating for this fact can be made. Thousands of accurate measurements of tissue thickness were made for various projections.[*] The thickness of the tissue to be traversed by the x-ray beam was always determined in the same manner and it was measured along the course of the central ray. The tissues were never compressed by the measuring calipers. In each case, the thickness of tissue was tabulated. The frequency with which various thicknesses appeared for a given projection was then statistically determined, Table VII. The higher thickness frequencies for a given projection were then grouped into an *average-thickness range*, to which could be applied a common group of exposure factors with the assurance that satisfactory radiographic quality would be rendered in more than 85 per cent of cases. It should be stated at this point that patient weight and patient height are not reliable indices of x-ray absorption and cannot be used as guides in formulating or standardizing an exposure for a given projection.

The implications of Table VII for radiographic technique are very significant indeed. First, these statistics show that techniques can be usefully standardized, because relatively high percentages of patients fall within an "average range" of thickness. Note that for most distal extremities and skulls, more than 90 per cent of all adult patients will conform to a single "average" technique. The lowest percentage in Table VII is for the AP projection of the lumbar spine at 69 per cent. This fig-

---

[*]Fuchs, A. W.: The Optimum Kilovoltage Technique in Military Roentgenography. *Am. J. Roentgenol., 50: 358-365, 1943.*

TABLE VII

Table Listing Average Thickness Ranges for Various Projections and the Frequency with Which the Adult Patient Dimensions Fall into Each Average Range

Region		Average Thickness Adult—Cms.			Per Cent Frequency
		AP	PA	LAT	
Thumb, fingers, toes		1.5-4			99
Hand		3-5			99
				7-10	93
Wrist		3-6			99
				5-8	98
Forearm		6-8			94
				7-9	92
Elbow		6-8			96
				7-9	87
Arm		7-10			95
				7-10	94
Shoulder		12-16			79
Clavicle			13-17		82
Foot		6-8			92
				7-9	91
Ankle		8-10			86
				6-9	96
Leg		10-12			85
				9-11	89
Knee		10-13			92
				9-12	92
Thigh		14-17			77
				13-16	76
Hip		17-21			76
Cervical	C1-3	12-14			77
Vertebrae	C4-7	11-14			98
	C1-7			10-13	90
Thoracic		20-24			76
Vertebrae				28-32	81
Lumbar		18-22			69
Vertebrae				27-32	77
Pelvis		19-23			78
Skull			18-21		96
				14-17	88
Sinuses Frontal			18-21		97
Maxillary			18-22		88
				13-17	96
Mandible				10-12	82
			20-25		82
Chest		OBL		27-32	84
		24-30			83

ure can be deduced for abdominal procedures in general, including studies of the urinary system and gastrointestinal tract. Even for abdominal procedures, it can be said that two out of three patients will conform to a single "average" technique. Therefore, radiographic technique can be confidently approached in a systematic way.

Second, the radiography student can extrapolate average thicknesses to memorize from Table VII. These provide an essential starting point from which to derive techniques for various thicknesses of body parts. Note that, combining the figures for the chest, thoracic spine, lumbar spine, and pelvis, *average thicknesses for the adult torso in general may be stated as 22 centimeters (about 8 and 1/2 inches) in AP projection, and 30 centimeters (about 12 inches) in lateral projection.* You should memorize these two measurements so that technique adjustments can be made for various torso thicknesses.

Part thickness affects the absorption of x-ray photons in an exponential fashion, that is, small changes in thickness cause great changes in the absorption of photons. Radiographers must become adept at adjusting the mAs in exponential proportion to body thickness variations between patients. A very workable rule of thumb for this relationship is: *Every four centimeters of thickness affects density by a factor of two.* A patient measuring 26 cm, then, through the torso would absorb twice as much radiation, and result in half as dark a radiographic density (when not compensated for), than the average 22-cm patient.

A corollary to this rule of thumb would be that *every four centimeters of thickness requires a change in mAs by a factor of two.* Thus, an 18-cm patient would require one-half the mAs of the average 22-cm patient, and a 26-cm patient would require twice the mAs. This rule is not only useful on a daily basis but can also be applied effectively in developing technique charts to standardize and control exposure to patients (Chapter 27).

Try the following brief exercise to practice the four-centimeter rule, and check your answers from the Appendix.

EXERCISE 16

For each of the following problems, list the actual mAs you would use based on the part thickness rule:

Part	Technique Chart mAs	Technique Chart Thickness	Actual Part Thickness	mAs Used
1. Elbow	5	6 cm	10 cm	_____
2. Femur	10	17 cm	13 cm	_____
3. UGI AP	7.5	20 cm	25 cm	_____
4. L-Spine AP	30	24 cm	16 cm	_____
5. Chest	10	22 cm	24 cm	_____

Scatter Radiation

The problem of scatter radiation fog increases in proportion to the thickness of the part. It has been found that the radiation emerging from a tissue thickness of 6 inches may assume a ratio of scatter radiation to primary radiation of 5 to 1, and with greater thicknesses it may rise to 10 to 1.

Also, larger patients attenuate more of the primary x-ran photons and there is less useful exposure to the film. Radiographic density decreases, and, at the same time, since the ratio of scattered radiation to primary radiation has increased, radiographic contrast is reduced.

MOLECULAR COMPOSITION

Apart from the thickness of a part, the degree of absorption of x-rays in the patient is primarily determined by two molecular factors: (1) the average atomic number of the tissue and (2) the average physical density of the tissue. Attenuation (absorption) of x-ray photons is affected by the atomic number of atoms through which they pass in an exponential way. Relatively small differences in atomic number between tissues will result in large differences in the penetration of the x-ray beam. Specifically, photon attenuation is roughly proportional to the cube of the atomic number. For example, the average atomic number of bone is around 20 and that of soft tissue, which is mostly water, is about 7.4. Cubing each number yields 8000 and roughly 405,

respectively. By dividing 400 into 8000, it can be found that bone is approximately 20 times more effective in attenuating x-ray photons than is soft tissue by virtue of its larger atomic nuclei (calcium, phosphorus, etc.).

The physical density of the molecules in a particular tissue (how *tightly packed* they are) is directly proportional to x-ray absorption. Bone tissue is about twice as dense as soft tissue and will therefore absorb roughly twice as many x-ray photons by virtue of its density.

Comparing the exponential effect of atomic number with the proportional effect of physical tissue density, it can be clearly seen that the major molecular factor bearing on the penetration of the x-ray beam is atomic number. This is further supported by the fact that atomic numbers in the human body vary much more than most tissue densities. Most tissues are close to water density. This is why the stomach is not normally contrasty against the surrounding muscle.

There are, however, two exceptions: lung tissue and fat tissue. In the exceptional case of the lungs, the density of the air with which they are insufflated is about 0.001, while the physical density of the surrounding soft tissues is about 1.0. This is such a dramatic ratio of difference, 1000 to 1, that the contrast of the air in the lungs against the surrounding soft tissue is attributed to the density difference, rather than the atomic number difference which is very slight: Air has an average atomic number of about 7.6, while soft tissue is about 7.4. Fat is also substantially less dense than other soft tissues. (Fat is only 20% fluid, while other soft tissues are about 80% fluid). This is enough of a difference fat to show up slightly darker than muscles and organs on a radiograph. Careful scrutiny of an abdomen radiograph (Figure 90) demonstrates that the kidneys would not be distinctly visible against the background densities of muscles and other organs, if it were not for the fact that the kidneys are encapsulated in thick layers of fat which create a darker density outlining each kidney on the radiograph. For differences in the physical density of tissues to produce subject contrast, they must be very great differences.

There are basically only five types of materials visible on standard radiographs: Gas, fat, fluid, bone and metal. All soft tissues are of fluid density, equal to water radiographically. Barium and iodine compounds are, chemically, metals. Using soft tissue or fluid as a background, gas (air) and fat are demonstrated against it because of extreme differences in their physical density. On the other hand, bone and metals including contrast agents are demonstrated because of their atomic numbers (large atoms).

MAGNITUDE OF ABSORPTION VARIABLES

In radiography there are a number of unpredictable absorption variables in body tissues that are influenced by physiologic or pathologic changes and they may be disregarded in some measure if the exposure system provides enough latitude. Generally, small deviations from the normal in tissue density or thickness can be ignored. Recognizable abnormal conditions, of course, may be easily compensated by adjustment of the variable exposure factor selected, usually the mAs.

Large Absorption Differences

When structural tissue details are widely different, each presents wide differences in absorbing power and wide differences in tone value will exist in the radiograph. Where a body part contains thick heavy bone surrounded by a large quantity of muscle and fat, as in the lumbar vertebral region, x-ray absorption differences become relatively wide (Figure 88). The image of a calcified body (Figure 89), outlined by the darker adjacent densities of its containing tissues also exhibits great tonal differences and provides easy visibility. As a rule, such parts provide little difficulty in recording even though large errors in exposure may be made.

Small Absorption Differences

At times, absorption differences between some tissues may be very small and differentiation becomes difficult. The kidney, gallbladder and liver areas are typical

Figure 88. (Above-*Left*) Screen-grid radiograph of AP abdomen, showing wide absorption differences between tissues and contrast agent.

Figure 89. (*Above*) Portion of PA chest radiograph showing a calcification of medium contrast against a background of pulmonary tissues.

Figure 90. (*Left*) Screen-grid AP radiograph of kidney region that exhibits small differences in density between tissues of comparable physical density and atomic number.

examples in which the x-ray absorbing power of the tissues is almost the same (Figure 90). The tonal differentiation of a small portion of lymphatic tissue within its surrounding tissues, also, cannot be as distinctive against its background density as could a calculus because of the small tissue absorption differences. A shorter gray scale in the image would therefore be helpful and perhaps necessary.

USE OF CONTRAST AGENTS

Contrast agents are employed to render high subject contrast in a viscus that normally has very low subject contrast. These agents comprise various nontoxic chemical preparations that have high x-ray absorption properties. They are either injected or ingested into the viscus before radiography is performed. air is also very useful on occasions because of its very low x-ray absorption properties. The alimentary

Figure 91. Radiographs in which contrast agents have been employed to delineate anatomic structures: (A) stomach and small intestine, (C) kidneys and ureters, (D) colon, and (F) gall bladder.

tract normally cannot be differentiated from surrounding tissues and it must be filled with a "test meal" containing barium sulfate of high purity (A), Figure 91. Study of the urinary tract function requires the absorption of a contrast medium by the body and upon excretion by the kidneys, details of the urinary tract can be radiographically delineated. This type of radi-

ograph is called an intravenous pyelogram. Study of the urinary tract can also be accomplished by inserting radiopaque catheters into the ureters and injecting a contrast agent into the pelvis of the kidney (C). This type of radiograph is known as a retrograde pyelogram. Air is often injected into the large intestine to augment the contrast properties of the barium sulfate meal or enema (B). To study the function of the gallbladder, a harmless dye is injected into a vein. This substance is carried to the liver by the blood stream and is secreted with the bile into the gallbladder. Since the dye in the bile is opaque to x-rays, an image of the gallbladder and its contents can be visualized (D).

Contrast agents may be categorized in several ways. The broadest division is that between those agents which attenuate x-rays much more than soft tissue does and those agents which allow many more x-rays to penetrate through to the film than soft tissue does. Contrast agents which attenuate x-rays, resulting in a low density or clear area on the radiograph, are called *positive* contrast agents. Positive contrast agents are normally fluids, and these may be further subdivided into injectables, ingestibles and oily-viscous media. Contrast agents which allow x-rays to penetrate through, resulting in a darker density on the radiograph, are referred to as *negative* contrast agents. Negative contrast agents are gaseous. Common examples include normal room air, carbon dioxide and nitrous oxide.

Although there are many types and brand names of positive contrast agents, each having different specific chemical formulae, they are all based on either the element *iodine* or the element *barium* bound into molecules with organic salts to make them non-toxic. These two elements are used on account of their very high atomic numbers. The viscosity, density or weight of these fluids has virtually nothing to do with their ability to attenuate x-rays. As discussed in the section on molecular composition of tissues within the patient, atomic number (the *size* of the atoms used) is the single most significant control of x-ray absorption. The atomic number of iodine is 53 and that of barium is 56. Since the

absorption of x-rays is proportional to the cube of the atomic number, these elements in their pure form are hundreds of times more absorbing than soft tissue with its atomic number of 7.4. Their content in a contrast agent is diluted somewhat by the other organic salts and water that make up the agent.

For maximum radiographic information, it is essential to be able to see *through* the bolus of a positive contrast agent. This means that x-rays in the beam must be of sufficient energy to penetrate through the agent and record information on the film. Otherwise, the radiologist will only be able to observe the tangential edges of the bolus, that is, only a small portion of the outermost lining of the organ of interest (Figure 62). The middle portions of the organ, filled with contrast agent, will appear as a blank white density on the radiograph with no information. In order for the beam to penetrate through the agent and record information on the film, a certain minimum kVp level is required. The *optimum* kVp's recommended for penetration of iodine and barium procedures are:

Iodine: At least 80 kVp
Barium: At least 110 kVp (except for esophagrams and air-contrast studies at 90 kVp)

If these kVp levels are used, the typical thickness of the bolus of contrast agent for barium and iodine procedures will be penetrated and the procedure will be of diagnostic value.

Negative contrast agents, which are always gasses, do not have a significantly different average atomic number than soft tissue or water (air Z# = 7.6, soft tissue Z# = 7.4). Therefore, their ability to produce contrast is not related to the ratio of photoelectric interactions to Compton interactions. Rather, because they have such an extremely different physical density (1/1000

Figure 92. Screen radiographs of PA chest, (A) made upon inspiration, (B and C) upon expiration. All were taken at 80 kVp and the same distance; A and B: 2.5 mAs, C: 3.3 mAs.

that of soft tissue), all interactions, photo-electric and Compton, are so reduced that the majority of the beam penetrates through and substantially darkens the film, in comparison with the soft-tissue areas.

INFLUENCE OF RESPIRATION

In radiography of the thorax, the influence of the phase of respiration on the overall image density should be recognized. The great permeability of air-containing tissues to x-rays is well known and generally offers no great exposure problem. However, when the patient is not correctly instructed as to the phase of respiration in which the radiograph is to be made, confusing results are often obtained.

Effect on Density

For an initial posteroanterior radiograph of the lungs, the exposure should be made when the patient suspends respiration upon full inspiration. If the same exposure is made at expiration or partial expiration, the resulting consolidation of pulmonary tissue will cause underexposure and a loss in radiographic density. Hence, when an exposure of the lungs is to be made at the expiratory phase, an approximate mAs increase of one-third is necessary to approximate the original density.

Example 1. These conditions may be illustrated by three posteroanterior radiographs of the chest, Figure 92. Radiograph A was exposed at the inspiratory phase and radiograph B, at the expiratory phase; the exposure factors being identical. Note that a definite loss of over-all image density occurred in radiograph B. Radiograph C was then made using an approximate increase of one-third in mAs to equal the density shown in radiograph A. Note the change in position of the heart silhouette between radiographs A and C.

Example 2. To demonstrate the appearance of the image obtained in both respiratory phases in lateral radiography of the chest, two radiographs were made, Figure 93. Radiograph A was made at inspiration; radiograph B, made on expiration, was exposed with approximately a one-third increase in the mAs so as to compensate for the increase in density of the consolidated pulmonary tissues.

RULE. In radiography of the chest, the mAs value always should be adjusted to the

Figure 93. Screen radiographs of lateral chest demonstrating influence of respiration on density: (A) made at inspiration, (B) at expiration. Both were taken at 85 kVp and the same distance, A: l0 mAs, B: 13.3 mAs.

respiratory phase in which the exposure is to be made. The mAs should be increased approximately one-third when exposure occurs at the expiratory phase if pulmonary densities are to be equalized.

EFFECTS ON OTHER QUALITIES

The condition of the patient and the use of contrast media affect density and contrast, the visibility functions in the image. They do not, however, make details which are already visible any sharper, less magnified nor distorted. These geometrical functions are not directly affected by patient status. Nonetheless, there can be *indirect* relationships between patient status and the geometrical image qualities: First, large patient thicknesses may result in increased object-to-film distance for a particular part of interest. By changing the patient position from PA to AP or vice versa, this problem can be partially alleviated. But, remember that it is the OID rather than the patient condition which is directly responsible for these effects. Secondly, patient motion can destroy sharpness of detail. The effects of motion are discussed in Chapter 23.

SUMMARY

1. Average thickness ranges have been established which apply to more than 85 per cent of all patients for all body parts. Standardized *technique charts* are therefore applicable to a high percentage of patients and should be used by radiographers.

2. Although average techniques are facilitated by the use of standardized technique charts, each patient must be individually evaluated by the radiographer for fine *technique adjustments* based upon body habitus, condition including disease, sex and race characteristics, age, etc.

3. Hypersthenic and very large, muscular patients present a special problem with reduced image *contrast* due to scatter, and density loss, so that other technique factors must be manipulated to compensate and restore these qualities to some degree.

4. Technique should be adjusted by a factor of two for every four centimeters change in body *thickness.*

5. *Subject contrast* between body tissues is primarily a function of average atomic number, because it has an exponential effect on the occurrence of photoelectric interactions. One exception to this rule is in the lungs, where tissue density becomes the controlling factor.

6. *Positive contrast* agents work to produce high subject contrast because their high atomic numbers (large atomic nuclei) multiply the occurrence of photoelectric interactions, not because of viscosity, weight or density.

7. *Negative contrast* agents are always gasses and produce subject contrast because of their extremely low density.

8. The penetration necessary for a body part depends upon the ratio of one tissue type, or different average atomic number, to another. Therefore, *optimum kVp* levels have been established for each body part and for contrast media procedures.

9. *Expiration* chests require at least a one-third increase in technique from the inspiration technique.

10. Patient status and contrast media have no direct relation to the geometrical functions—sharpness of detail, magnification and distortion. They may, however, indirectly affect these qualities if they result in geometrical changes, such as uncorrectable distance increases from the film.

11. The average torso thicknesses are 22 cm in AP or PA projection, and 30 cm in lateral projection.

12. Greater increases in technique are required for large muscular or fluid-distended patients than for fatty, obese patients.

REVIEW QUESTIONS

1. Define Hypersthenic:
2. Define Asthenic:
3. On which two types of body habitue can a regular technique chart be followed without adjusting technique for anything but body part thickness:
4. Define atrophy:

5. What technique adjustment is required for a chest radiograph in *expiration*?

What percentage or proportion of adult patients fall within the "average" thickness category for technique purposes, for the following procedures:

6. Lumbar Spine AP:

7. Sinuses PA:
8. Foot AP:
9. Barium Enema AP:
10. Why do positive contrast media work?
11. Your technique chart lists 200 mA at $1/4$ second for a 24-cm L-spine. You are doing an L-spine on a very thin 16-cm patient. What *total mAs* should you use:
12. On the above patient, what new mAs would you use for a *lateral* view, assuming that the above mAs was correct for the AP view:
13. What is the optimum kVp for penetrating Iodine:
14. What is the optimum kVp for penetrating barium?
15. Why do large patients reduce contrast?
16. What are the average measurements in cm for the torso in AP and lateral projections?
17. List the five general types of materials that are demonstrated on radiographs. Muscular patients require (more, less or equal) technique when compared to fatty patients of the same size.
18. Muscular patients require _____ (more, less or equal) technique when compared to fatty patients of the same size.

Chapter 11

PATHOLOGY AND CASTS

The condition of the patient is the greatest variable the radiographer faces in producing quality radiographs. In addition to being aware of the normal variations in body habitus, tissue composition, age, bony structure, stage of respiration, presence of contrast agents and thickness of body parts discussed in the last chapter, one must also be conscious of abnormal changes due to pathology or medical intervention.

The radiographer must determine the image details that are to be accentuated and, if necessary, make suitable adjustment in the exposure factors. No matter what departures from the normal there may be in the radiographic density of these details, they must be clearly demonstrated if a correct radiologic identification is to be made of existing disease or trauma. When an abnormal *increase* in tissue absorption takes place, the radiographic density *decreases* from the normal value. When a *decrease* in tissue absorption occurs, a corresponding *increase* over the normal in radiographic density takes place.

The radiographer should ascertain the reason that each procedure was ordered, because this knowledge often includes information that bears upon technique selection and can thus prevent repeated exposures. To obtain this information, the radiographer should review the x-ray requisition prior to every procedure, and also obtain a brief verbal history from the patient, if possible. In situations that are unclear, additional information may be obtained from the patient's chart. Radiographers should have at least a rudimentary ability to interpret patient charts. Careful observation of patients frequently provides readily apparent signs of conditions that bear on technique selection. It should be emphasized that obtaining pertinent patient history and assessing conditions that affect radiographic technique are the responsibility of the *radiographer*, not the referring physician or radiologist.

Not all diseases are radiographically visible. Many do not appreciably affect the densities present in the image, and are therefore of no concern in determining techniques. For a pathological condition to require a technique adjustment, it must substantially alter the presence and amount of one of the five radiographically demonstrable materials: Air, fat, fluid, bone, or metals.

ADDITIVE DISEASES

Abnormal conditions which lead to an increase in *fluid, bone,* or *metal* are, for radiographic purposes, generally considered as *additive conditions.* They require added exposure, or increased technique factors, in order to be properly demonstrated. In the case of excessive bone tissue or metals, the increase in technique is necessitated mostly

164

because of their high average atomic "numbers (large atoms). For fluid accumulation in the lungs (Figure 94), an increase in factors is required because the fluid is nearly a thousand times more dense than the air which is normally present (there are one-thousand molecules of fluid for every molecule of air). Fluid distention of the abdomen, on the other hand, does not substantially change atomic numbers nor tissue density, but results in an increase in part thickness, and requires strict adherence to the *four-centimeter rule*, doubling the technique for every four centimeters of added thickness. In each of these cases, more x-ray photons are absorbed by the body tissues, and if an increase in technical factors is not effected, an underexposed, light radiograph will result.

For additive diseases, technique may need to be increased from 35 per cent (1/3) to over 100 per cent (doubling) if the disease is in an advanced stage. *As a rule of thumb, additive diseases require a 50 per cent increase in overall technique.* Since many of these diseases change the content of minerals in the tissue, a change in penetration is indicated. In such cases, the kVp should be altered using the 15 per cent rule, rather than increasing mAs. An 8 per cent increase in kVp will be equivalent to a 50 per cent increase in mAs.

Table VIII lists those diseases which are commonly encountered in radiography and which may require substantial increases in technique. The recommended adjustment is given for each, *assuming that the disease is well advanced.* Naturally, the radiog-

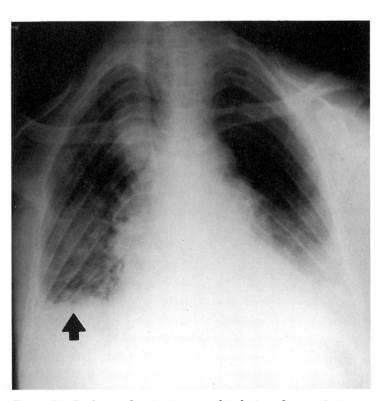

Figure 94. Radiograph using increased technique for a patient presenting with cardiomegaly (enlarged heart) as well as pulmonary edema, (note fluid level at base of right lung).

TABLE VIII
Additive Diseases Requiring Increased Technique

Acromegaly: 8-10% kVp	Osteochondroma: 8% kVp
Actinomycosis: 50% mAs	Osteopetrosis: 8-12% kVp
Ascites: 50-75% mAs	Paget's Disease: 8% kVp
Carcinomas, fibrous: 50% mAs	Pleural Effusion: 35% mAs
Cardiomegaly: 50% mAs	Pneumoconiosis: 50% mAs
Cirrhosis: 50% mAs	Pneumonia: 50% mAs
Edema, pulmonary: 50% mAs	Syphilis: 50% mAs
Hydrocephalus: 50-75% mAs	Tuberculosis, pulmonary: 50% mAs
Hydropneumothorax: 50% mAs	
Osteoarthritis (Degenerative Joint Disease): 8% kVp	

rapher must modify this recommended change upward or downward upon assessing each individual patient.

Acromegaly, osteoarthritis, osteochondroma, osteopetrosis, osteomyelitis, Paget's disease, and advanced syphilis involve either excessive bone growth or the replacement of cartilaginous tissues with bone. In the case of osteoarthritis, even though there is degeneration within the bones themselves, bony spurs grow into the joints and bone tissue replaces normal cartilage and fluid in the joints, necessitating a net increase in technique. In the case of actinomycosis, fibrous carcinomas, cardiomegaly (Figure 94), cirrhosis, pneumoconiosis and pulmonary tuberculosis, the growth or overexpansion of dense fibrous tissues replaces normal tissue. For ascites, pulmonary edema, hydrocephalus, hydropneumothorax, pleural effusion and pneumonia, the accumulation of abnormal amounts of body fluids or the displacement of aerated tissues in the lungs with fluid

requires greater radiographic exposure.

It is well to reiterate the difference between fluid distention of the abdomen and obesity. When the abdomen is truly distended due to ascites or severe infection, the skin is tight and rather hard to the touch. The technique required may be slightly more than the *four centimeter rule* dictates. The radiographer should begin by measuring the abdomen and increasing technique from average according to the rule. If the distention is pronounced, an additional 25 per cent increase in the resulting mAs is called for. For hypersthenic patients with very loose, flaccid skin that is soft to the touch, technique increases due to measured thickness will be somewhat less than the *four centimeter rule* dictates. This rule is an average and applies to variations in thickness which are attributable to mixtures of additional musculature, fluid and fat. The skin of these patients may be somewhat loose, but will not feel overly soft on palpation.

DESTRUCTIVE DISEASES

Abnormal conditions which lead to an increase in *air* or *fat,* or to a *decrease* in normal body fluid or bone, are radiographically considered as *destructive conditions.* These

require a reduction from typical exposure techniques in order to be properly demonstrated. Both air and fat are significantly less dense than fluid, and absorb fewer

TABLE IX

Destructive Diseases Requiring Decreased Technique

Aseptic Necrosis: 8% kVp	Hyperparathyroidism: 8% kVp
Blastomycosis: 8% kVp	
Bowel Obstruction: 8% kVp	Osteitis Fibrosa Cystica: 8% kVp
Cancers, osteolytic: 8% kVp	Osteomalacia: 8% kVp
	Osteomyelitis: 8% kVp
Emphysema: 8% kVp	Osteoporosis: 8% kVp
Ewing's Tumor: 8% kVp	Pneumothorax: 8% kVp
Exostosis: 8% kVp	Rheumatoid Arthritis: 8% kVp
Gout: 8% kVp	
Hodgkin's Disease: 8% kVp	

x-ray photons.

For destructive diseases, overall technique may need to be reduced by 30 to 50 per cent. *As a rule of thumb, destructive diseases require a 30 per cent decrease in mAs, or a 5 per cent reduction in kVp.* Table IX lists destructive diseases commonly found in radiography, and the recommended technique reduction for each.

Aseptic necrosis, various bone carcinomas, Ewing's tumor, exostosis, gout, Hodgkin's disease, hyperparathyroidism, osteitis fibrosa cystica, osteoporosis, osteomalacia, osteomyelitis and rheumatoid arthritis result in either a demineralization of bone or an invasive destruction of the bone tissue. Less penetration is required to

Figure 95. Radiograph using decreased technique for a patient with emphysema, (note overdistention of lungs with air).

secure optimum image contrast, so generally the kVp should be reduced for these diseases. In blastomycosis, yeast-like fungi produce gas pockets within tissues, while bowel obstructions, emphysema (Figure 95) and pneumothorax are processes which essentially "trap" air or gas within body cavities. Due to their extremely low physical densities, gasses are radiolucent and allow radiation to pass through to the film. Dark radiographs result unless technique is reduced.

TRAUMA

The challenges in determining optimum radiographic techniques for most trauma patients relate to the above discussion of disease conditions, particularly as regards the presence of excess fluids or gasses within the tissues. For example, pneumothoraces are common to trauma patients and, due to excessive aeration, require a reduced technique. Internal bleeding in the abdomen or hematomas in the brain may require a 30 per cent increase in mAs, while blood pooling in the lungs can necessitate increases from 30 to 100 per cent more than normal.

POSTMORTEM RADIOGRAPHY

Experienced radiographers learn to expect considerable pooling of blood and fluids in dead bodies, particularly in the head, thorax and abdomen. An increase in technique, typically about 35 per cent increase in mAs, may be anticipated. Even shortly after death, blood and fluids will begin to pool in the lungs, and since postmortem radiographs are taken with the body recumbent, the fluids will pool across the entire lung field. In addition, bear in mind that postmortem radiography is by definition an *expiration* chest technique. Without the normal air insufflation of the lungs, an increase in technique is indicated. *Postmortem chest techniques must be increased by at least 35 per cent (one-third)*, and may require a 50 per cent increase, depending on the amount of time since death. This, 35 per cent rule should be applied on the first exposure attempted, or a repeated exposure will very likely be needed.

SOFT-TISSUE TECHNIQUE

Normally, bullets and metallic foreign bodies do not need to be penetrated by the x-ray beam for radiographic localization. Any increase in technique would merely reduce the radiographic visualization of tissues around the foreign object. However, many small foreign bodies such as slivers of wood, glass or metal, or swallowed bones are better visualized by using a reduced *soft tissue technique*.

Metal and most types of glass are actually highly radiopaque, but very small slivers of the same can be difficult to detect. Chicken bones or similar objects which may become lodged in the laryngopharynx are often not very dense in cortical bone and have only slight radiographic contrast. Wood splinters are especially troublesome: Because of the air pockets they contain, they may show up early on as a slightly *darker* density, radiolucent against a soft tissue background. But in a brief period of time wood splinters will absorb fluid from the surrounding tissues and become very difficult indeed to distinguish from tissue. The technique employed must be tailored to demonstrate soft tissue, rather than the usual bone tissue.

Figure 96. Soft tissue technique used to demonstrate a sliver of glass (arrow) in the neck. From a cervical spine technique, the kVP was decreased from the usual 76 kVp to 64 kVp, all other factors unchanged (15 mAs, 3-phase machine, 200-speed screens).

To maximize the visualization of these small foreign objects, image contrast must be enhanced and overall density must be lightened up. A reduction in kVp will accomplish both of these objectives (Figure 96). There should be no attempt to "compensate" for the drop in kVp by adjusting mAs. As a rule of thumb, *for soft tissue techniques, subtract 15 per cent of the kVp from the average technique without changing mAs.* In addition to demonstrating small foreign bodies, such techniques show any damage to soft tissues. Soft tissue visualization is most frequently called for in radiography of the hands and of the neck.

CASTS AND SPLINTS

Radiographic techniques must certainly be adjusted upward for most casts and splints. But to determine the extent of this increase, one must take into consideration the composition of the materials used, their thickness and configuration, and whether they are wet or dry. Radiographs taken after a limb of the body has been set and casted are called *postreduction radiographs.*

Full plaster casts require a minimum doubling of overall exposure factors from the usual technique for that body part. This can be accomplished either by doubling the mAs or by increasing kVp by 15 per cent. For example, suppose that 5 mAs at 60 kVp secured a proper exposure for the AP view of a normal foot. The same foot in a dry plaster cast would require 10 mAs at 60 kVp, or, alternatively, 5 mAs at 69 kVp (using the 15 per cent rule).

Full plaster casts which are still wet, having just been applied, require *three* times the overall technique (Figure 97). To achieve this, the mAs may be tripled, the kVp may be increased by about 22 per cent, or a combination of the two may be employed such as doubling the mAs with an additional 8 per cent increase in kVp.

Unusually thick plaster may be applied around the femur or the torso. A full cast of this type which is dry will require a *tripling* of the usual technique. A plaster cast of this thickness which is still wet can require as much as *four times* the original technique.

Often, "half-casts" are secured to a limb by wrapping a partial cast with an Ace™ bandage. For this situation, use a *50 per cent* increase in technique. That is, half again as much mAs, or approximately 8 per cent

Figure 97. Bilateral radiographs of the feet taken during surgery on the same patient, demonstrating wet plaster cast technique adjustment. (A) was taken of the uncasted left foot using 10 mAs at 62 kVp. The right foot (B) had just been casted in thick, wet plaster. Technique used for (B) was 16 mAs at 70 kVp, an overall increase in *total technique* of approximately three times that of the uncasted foot. (The nearly 15% increase in kVp equivalent to a doubling, plus a mAs increase about half-way to another doubling.)

more kVp. Remember to employ the increase only when the projection of the part of interest passes through the cast material. For example, on a lateral view of a forearm in a half-cast, the bones may not be covered by the cast, and a normal technique may be used.

Fiberglass mesh has become popular as a casting medium. Fiberglass is very radiolucent, allowing the x-ray beam to pass through it virtually unaffected. Normal techniques may be used in most cases. If the fiberglass is thick, a slight increase, not to exceed 30 per cent in mAs or 5 per cent in kVp, may be in order.

Fiberglass may be mixed in roughly equal proportions with plaster. For casts of this type, a general rule of thumb is to increase mAs by *50 per cent* or kVp by 8 per cent (Figure 98). Plastic materials may require increases from 30 to 50 per cent.

Projections must sometimes be made through splints of wood or aluminum. Such splints may require from 35 to 65 per cent increases in overall technique. Whether the splint is applied to one side or to both sides of the limb, the radiographer must assess the *total thickness* of material to be traversed by the x-ray beam. For example, the mAs should be increased by 35 per cent (1/3) for one- half inch of wood, or by 50 per cent (1/2) for one inch. As a rule of thumb, *increase mAs by 50 per cent for wood or aluminum splints.* Solid plastics are similar to wood. Air splints, however, require no adjustment in technique.

The radiographer should be thoroughly familiar with these technique rules for splints and casts, and commit them to memory. For assistance, they are summarized in Table X.

Figure 98. Radiograph of distal leg in a mixed fiberglass/plaster cast, using 50% more mAs than usual for an uncasted leg. Factors: 66 kVp, chart technique (uncasted): 6.8 mAs, actual mAs used: 10 mAs.

TABLE X
Technique Increases for Casts and Splints

Material	Technique Increase
Dry Plaster: medium:	2 x mAs OR add 15% kVp
large:	3 x mAs OR add 22% kVp
Wet Plaster: medium:	3 x mAs OR add 22% kVp
large:	4 x mAs OR add 30% kVp
Half-Cast, Plaster:	Add 50% mAs OR 8% kVp
Fiberglass/Plaster:	Add 50% mAs OR 8% kVp
Plastic Cast:	Add 50% mAs OR 8% kVp
Wood, 3/4-1 Inch:	Add 50% mAs OR 8% kVp
Fiberglass, pure:	No change

SUMMARY

1. Radiographers are responsible for using x-ray requisitions, patient charts, verbal histories and careful observation to acquire *preliminary information* which may bear upon technique selection.
2. *Additive diseases* require an increase in technique, typically 50 per cent, while destructive diseases require a decrease, usually 30 per cent.
3. *Fluid* distention or pooling of fluids, such as in post-mortem cases, require increased techniques, usually from 30 to 50 per cent greater than usual.
4. For *soft tissue techniques*, decrease kVp 15 per cent from the normal, without any other compensation.
5. Plaster *casts* require at least double the usual technique, but can require much more. Half-casts, fiberglass-plaster combinations, and wood splints usually require a 50 per cent increase in technique. See Table X.

REVIEW QUESTIONS

1. How much would you increase your total technique from the chart technique for a humerus in a dry plaster cast:
2. What technique change would be required for a lateral projection of a femur splinted with two $1/2$-inch thick pieces of wood?
3. What technique change is required for an extremity in a fiberglass cast:

For each of the following pathologies, state whether the kVp should be increased for more penetration, or decreased for less penetration:

4. Osteoarthritis (degenerative joint disease):
5. Hyperparathyroidism:
6. Osteochondroma:
7. Hydrocephalus:
8. Emphysema:
9. Hydropneumothorax:
10. Pneumoconiosis:
11. Ascites:
12. A fluid-distended abdomen requires _____ (more, less or equal) technique than a fatty abdomen of the same thickness.
13. Postmortem chest radiographs require _____ (more, less or equal) technique than normal.
14. If the usual technique for a lateral cervical spine is 15 mAs at 76 kVp, what mAs and kVp would be used for a *soft tissue* lateral neck?

Chapter 12

SCATTERED RADIATION AND IMAGE FOG

The effects of scattered radiation are among the most misunderstood concepts in radiography. This chapter will consolidate all of the aspects of this topic covered in other chapters. The relationships of x-ray beam interactions within the patient to the resulting image qualities on the radiograph are rather complicated, and a careful review of Chapters 3 and 4 (Qualities of the Image, and Interactions of X-Rays Within the Patient) may be helpful.

DESIRABLE GRAY SCALE VERSUS FOG

An important concept learned in Chapter 3 is that gray scale is a desirable, *indeed an essential*, component of the radiographic image. Any portion of the image which is blank white presents no information at all (except at its edges), and is diagnostically useless. (Figure 62 in Chapter 6 illustrates such a radiograph, with unpenetrated barium in the stomach.) The same may be said for portions of an image that are pitch black—they are diagnostically useless. The ideal radiograph possesses a range of gray shades from a very dark gray to a very light gray, with no blank areas. This means that every type of tissue depicted must be at least partially penetrated by the x-ray beam.

Optimum kVp results in at least some penetration of the beam through *all* tissues, resulting in a fairly long gray scale. An image with long gray scale has many different shades of gray and depicts many different types of tissue. *Quantitatively, an image with long gray scale has more information in it than a short-scale image.* Of course, gray scale can be *too* long, as described in Chapter 3, but unless all tissues are penetrated to some degree, the gray scale is too short.

Fairly long gray scale is, therefore, desirable. Such images contain much information, but are not immediately appealing to the eye. They have an overall gray appearance. It is important to understand that the apparent "grayness" of such an image is *not due to fog*. Figure 99 compares an unfogged image with long gray scale to a fogged image. Not every "gray" radiograph is a fogged radiograph. Optimally long gray scale is desirable, fog is not.

Gray scale is, by definition, the opposite of contrast. *Image contrast is reduced at a higher kVp. This would be true whether scattered radiation were present or not.* Fog can, however, *contribute* to lower image contrast in a very destructive way. There are several ways in which an image can be fogged, but the most important one to the radiographer is scatter radiation.

Figure 99. Radiographs demonstrating gray scale versus fog. From (A) to (B), increased "grayness" is due to a desirable increase in penetration and gray scale, with no fog present. From (C) to (D), increased "grayness" is due to fog.

SECONDARY VERSUS SCATTER RADIATION

Secondary radiation is radiation produced when the primary x-ray beam interacts with atoms in the body, tabletop or other objects, and emitted *by the object*, not by the x-ray tube. In physics, *secondary* radiation and *scattered* radiation are often synonymous. But, for medical imaging, a distinction must be made.

Even when grids are used, much of the radiation reaching the film is *secondary* radiation, which is emitted from within the body. Grids only eliminate that secondary radiation which has been *scattered* significantly, which has *changed direction* enough to be visibly destructive to the image.

Not all secondary radiation is significantly scattered. Some is emitted in a forward direction, close enough to the original direction of the primary beam that it does not *visibly* change the image. Such radiation will pass through a grid, and may be considered as constructive to the visible image. For imaging purposes, *scatter* radiation should be considered as only those rays which have *significantly changed direction* from the primary beam and are visibly destructive to the image.

CAUSES OF SCATTER FOG

Almost all scatter radiation is caused by the Compton interaction described in Chapter 4. Let us briefly consider each of the three factors that increase the amount of scatter radiation reaching the film. They are:

1. High kVp levels (Chapter 6)
2. Large field sizes (Chapter 9)
3. Large tissue thicknesses (Chapters 10 and 11)

1. HIGH KVP LEVELS: At high kilovoltages, slightly *less* scattering interactions occur in the patient (Chapter 4, Figure 43). However, that scattered radiation which is produced has higher energy, and it is emitted in a more forward direction. With an increased proportion of the scattered rays penetrating through to the film, and with an increased proportion of them directed toward the film, *the net result is an increase in scatter radiation reaching the film, increasing image fog*, (Chapter 6).

But, high kVp settings are required to obtain adequate *penetration* for the radi-ographic studies using contrast agents and for those body parts with high proportions of bone tissue. Furthermore, high kVp is frequently desirable in order to produce longer *gray scale* in the image. In most cases, these two benefits outweigh the gradual increase in fog at higher kilovoltages. Therefore, the selection of kVp should be based primarily upon the penetration and gray scale desired, with scatter radiation only as a secondary consideration.

2. LARGE FIELD SIZES: Chapter 9 describes how larger field sizes allow greater amounts of exposed tissue to generate more scatter radiation (Figure 82), while the concentration of the primary radiation is unaffected (Figure 83). Excessive proportions of scatter radiation are also produced in the x-ray table any time the light field is allowed to extend well beyond the anatomy. As long as the field size is adequate to include all anatomy of interest, there is *no benefit* to further increasing the field size, and no reason for accepting an image fogged in this manner.

3. LARGE TISSUE THICKNESSES: Larger patients or larger body parts present more exposed tissue to generate scatter radiation, even while the primary beam is further attenuated (Chapter 10). The loss of useful rays combined with the increased scatter results in a dramatic increase in visible image fog.

For some procedures, (particularly fluoroscopic procedures), the radiographer or radiologist may be able to reduce tissue thickness by using a *compression paddle* or similar compression device. But for the most part, tissue thickness is outside the control of the radiographer.

Of these three causes of scatter radiation then, high kVp levels have advantages which outweigh the fog produced, and tissue thicknesses are not usually under the radiographer's control, leaving *field size limitation (collimation) as the primary method of preventing scatter radiation.*

Two methods are available to help eliminate scatter radiation *after it has been produced,* but before it reaches the film and fogs it. These are the use of grids, discussed in the next chapter, and the use of the "air gap technique," discussed in Chapter 19.

EFFECTS ON DENSITY AND CONTRAST

Scattering is a *random* event, and therefore, when it occurs in sufficient quantity, it results in a relatively *even density deposit* across an area of the film, if not across the entire film. (Of course, by inverse square law, this deposit will gradually decrease at greater distances from the scattering source; nonetheless, a silver deposit will result both directly under the scattering object and under adjacent structures.)

Figure 100 is a density trace diagram (see Chapter 24) showing the "blanket" effect of scatter fogging. The diagram is a cross-section of the thickness of the silver deposit on the x-ray film. A thicker silver deposit

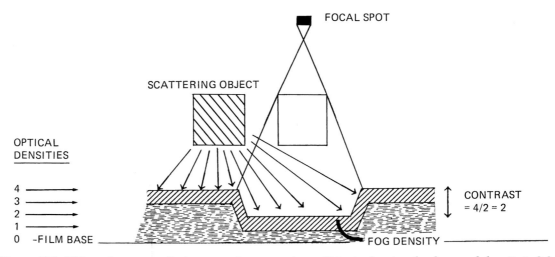

Figure 100. Effect of scatter radiation upon image contrast. Prior to fogging, background density is 3.0, density under object of interest is 1.0, and contrast is 3/1 = 3. After scatter radiation lays down additional "blanket" density of 1.0, background density is now 4.0 and image density is 2.0. Contrast for this fogged image is 4/2 = 2, reduced from the original contrast of 3.

would be seen as a darker density. The white box represents a high-contrast object, such as a bone, being projected onto the film and showing a lighter density. Contrast is measured as the *ratio* of the background density to the density under the object of interest. In this diagram, the background density would normally be 3, and the image density 1. The normal contrast would be $3/1 = 3$.

However, if a scattering object is placed within the x-ray beam near to the object of interest, the scatter radiation produced lays down a blanket of density across the film, covering *both* the area directly under itself and adjacent areas under other structures. In the diagram this added density has a value of 1. The background density is increased to 4, and the image density is increased to 2. The image contrast after fogging is $4/2 = 2$. Contrast has been reduced by scatter fog.

Fog increases density anywhere it occurs on the film. The addition of fog density to those areas depicted as dark grays may be sufficient to turn them pitch black, resulting in a loss of radiographic information. Fog increases density, but in a destructive way, reducing image quality.

It is possible for a radiograph to be both *light* and *fogged* (Figure 101). This frequently occurs with very large patients. The large volume of tissue results in excessive scattered radiation, which would normally

Figure 101. Radiograph of a large patient demonstrating both fog and underexposure. An image can be light and yet fogged.

fog and darken the film, but, at the same time, such thicknesses of tissue reduce the amount of primary radiation reaching the film. The total exposure to the film is reduced, yet a greater *proportion* of that exposure is attributable to fog densities. The result is a "washed out" appearance, underexposed and gray at the same time. Such radiographs are of little diagnostic value.

FOG VERSUS BLUR

There is also a common misconception that scattered radiation "undercuts the edge" of an image, causing it to become "blurred." It has even been asserted that grids reduce blur by eliminating scatter. These are false and misleading statements. As described in Chapters 3 and 24, the *resolution* of details (the ability to distinguish them as separate from each other) is reduced by a loss of contrast, but this is due to less *visibility*, not to a lack of geometrical integrity. The sharpness of the edges of an image depends on the width of the *penumbra*. Anything which does not change the spread of the penumbra cannot be said to affect sharpness.

Scatter is a completely random phenom-enon. It does not "select" the edges of an image to affect, but lays down a blanket of density over the *entire* image. Blurring, on the other hand, is geometrically predictable through penumbra and absorption dia-grams and relates specifically to the edges of the image. Scatter, emanating from the patient, cannot and does not affect the alignment of the primary rays projected from the x-ray tube.

To develop this concept, let us separate a fogging event and the projection of the original image in time. A film may certain-ly be fogged before or after it is used for an exposure. For example, it may be fogged in the dark room during storage. Would such a fogging affect the way that image

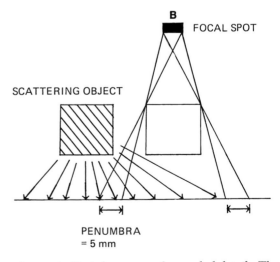

Figure 102. Diagram illustrating that scatter radiation does not affect sharpness of recorded detail. The spread of the penumbral shadow is 5 mm prior to fogging (A), and is still 5 mm after fogging (B). Although *visibility* is reduced by the scatter, blur is unchanged and sharpness is equal.

edges are projected onto the film during an exposure taken at a later time? Clearly the answer is no. The visibility of the image would be compromised because of the fogging, but the projection of the penumbra and umbra of the image during regular exposure is affected only by primary beam geometry.

Figure 102 illustrates that scatter radiation is a phenomenon separate from the geometry of penumbra formation, and does not change image sharpness or blur. Figure 34 in Chapter 3 demonstrates that images can be fogged without blur, or blurred without fog. Because scatter is random in nature, it cannot affect *any* of the geometrical factors in the image—sharpness, magnification or distortion.

Scatter does affect *all three* of the *visibility* functions in the image: It increases density, increases image noise and reduces image contrast. Thus, the overall resolution of the image is destroyed.

Image fog is properly classified as a form of noise, because it is an extraneous density that impedes the visibility of the desired image, just as any artifact would "get in the way." In the hierarchy of image qualities (Figure 37), fog should be listed as a visibility factor under "noise."

SCATTER AND RADIATION EXPOSURE

While it is not within the scope of this text to fully discuss all of the implications of scatter radiation exposure and protection methods, it is important to point out that scattered radiation is the main source of occupational exposure to the radiographer, as well as a substantial portion of the dose received by the patient. Therefore, the reduction and control of scatter production is essential not only for image quality, but also for protection purposes.

Equipment operators must use the three cardinal principles of protection from scatter radiation: minimize exposure time, maximize distance, and use appropriate shielding. Also, remember that the least amount of scatter radiation produced is emitted at right angles to the central ray. *The safest location to stand in an exposed area is to the side of the x-ray beam*, not behind it.

SUMMARY

1. Optimally long *gray scale* is desirable in an image and should not be confused with fogging.
2. Not all *secondary radiation* should be considered as "scatter," only that which has substantially changed direction.
3. The three *causes of scatter radiation* are high kVp levels, large field sizes and large tissue thicknesses. Of these, only *field size* should be considered as a controlling factor.
4. Scatter radiation creates a relatively even density deposit across the entire film area called *fog*. This fog density reduces image *contrast*.
5. *Fog* generally increases the overall *density* of an image. Nonetheless, by gross underexposure it is possible for an image to be both light and fogged.
6. Fog has no relationship to blur or *sharpness*. However, it does reduce the *visibility* of image edges because of the destruction of contrast, and the overall *resolution* of the image is degraded.

7. Scatter fog is a form of image *noise,* impeding image visibility.
8. Scatter radiation is the main source of occupational exposure to the radiographer, and an important part of patient dose.

REVIEW QUESTIONS

1. An image can appear gray overall and still be of high quality if the grayness is due to _____.
2. List the three causes of scatter radiation:
3. Which of these is the most important way for the radiographer to prevent excessive scatter production?
4. List the two methods by which scatter radiation can be reduced or eliminated *after* it has been produced.
5. High kVp levels actually result in *less* scattering interactions in the patient. Give *two* reasons why image fog increases anyway with high kVp:

6. What method can sometimes be used to reduce scatter production due to tissue thickness:
7. Fog always has what effect upon image contrast:
8. What is the relationship between scatter fog and image sharpness?
9. Fog _____ (increases, decreases, or has no effect on) image resolution.
10. In the hierarchy of image qualities, fog is classified as a type of _____.
11. Where is the safest location to stand in relation to the x-ray beam during a mobile procedure?

Chapter 13

GRIDS

UNTIL GUSTAV BUCKY invented the grid diaphragm in 1913, the only control for scatter radiation was by means of various shaped single- and double-aperture diaphragms and cones inserted at the portal of the x-ray tube. Although these devices proved of value, large amounts of scatter radiation could not adequately be controlled in radiography of thick body tissues.

The grid as Dr. Bucky invented it was not too practical at first because it was used in a stationary position and the grid pattern on the radiograph was quite coarse. However, it was for Dr. Hollis Potter of Chicago to solve the problem and place the Bucky grid on a practical basis. This was accomplished by *moving* the grid during the exposure and making the grid strips thinner. By moving the grid during the exposure, all grid lines were blurred out of the image. The first commercial moving grid was announced in 1920 and became known as the Potter-Bucky diaphragm. The necessity for elimination of scatter radiation fog from the radiograph with its resultant improvement in contrast and enhancement in diagnostic quality was ably presented by R. B. Wilsey of the Kodak Research Laboratories. His data presented in 1920 provided the scientific basis for the application of the Potter-Bucky diaphragm to practical radiography. Wilsey's data and Potter's diaphragm marked one of the few milestones in the search for better radiographic results.

The function of the Bucky grid is to absorb scatter radiation emitted by body tissues before it reaches the film. This required that the grid be placed *between* the patient and the film. The grid is composed of alternate strips of lead separated by a radiotransparent substance; the strips are approximately 0.005 inch thick. In use, the focused remnant radiation passes *between* the strips to reach the film (Figure 103). Since scattered radiation is unfocused and is emitted in all directions, it is largely absorbed when it strikes the lead strips.

Types of Grids

There are two types of grids: stationary and moving. The latter is known as a Potter-Bucky diaphragm. When a modern stationary grid is used, an image of the grid strips appears on the radiograph as a number of evenly spaced fine lines. In grids containing 60-80 lines to the inch, the grid lines are barely perceptible at normal viewing distances. However, recent improvements in design have made possible grids containing 110 lines to the inch which are virtually invisible at similar viewing distances. They offer little or no problem from a diagnostic standpoint. The moving grid is used extensively for routine radiography. The stationary grid is more frequently employed in those situations where it is difficult or impossible to use the moving grid.

Among modern moving grids in the Potter-Bucky mechanism, there are two

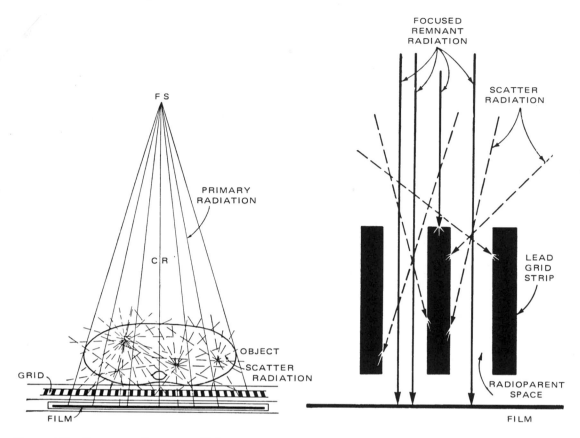

Figure 103. Diagrams illustrating (*left*) function of Potter-Bucky diaphragm in absorbing scatter radiation before it reaches the film; (*right*) details of grid construction.

types of movements used. The *reciprocating* grid uses a motor which drives the grid back and forth during exposure, and the *oscillating* grid mechanism moves it in a circular motion. Either way, the grid lines are effectively blurred out, reducing noise and increasing the amount of visible information in the image.

GRID RATIO

The efficiency of the grid in absorbing scatter radiation is determined by the *grid ratio* which is the relation of the depth of the radiotransparent space between the lead strips, to its width. For example, an 8:1 grid ratio means that the spaces are tall and narrow and that the depth is 8 times the width. The 8:1 ratio grid has great efficiency because only secondary radiation that is traveling approximately parallel to the primary radiation can reach the film; in most instances, this amount is relatively small. In general, a grid ratio of 16:1 is still more efficient, but it requires great accuracy in positioning the patient and x-ray tube to the grid and care in selecting the correct source-image distance. With lower grid ratios, less fog is eliminated but greater latitude in positioning and SID is permissible.

Effect on Image Density

When the grid is employed, it is necessary to increase the mAs over that employed when a grid is *not* used, because the density effect of the secondary radiation is lost and some absorption by the grid of the primary radiation takes place. The amount of increase in mAs is dependent upon the grid ratio, and the approximate increase required ranges from 2 to 5 times the initial mAs value.

EFFECT ON CONTRAST

Image contrast is reduced by scatter radiation fog and is increased in proportion to the amount of scatter radiation eliminated. Employment of a grid normally shortens the gray scale so that images are produced exhibiting higher contrast; the greater the grid ratio, the higher is the contrast obtained. For example, a radiograph made with a 4:1 grid ratio has lower contrast than one made with an 8:1 ratio because of the lower efficiency of the 4:1 grid in fog cleanup.

EXAMPLES OF FOG CONTROL EMPLOYING GRIDS

Demonstration No. 1.

The manner in which contrast is affected when using a stationary grid is illustrated (Figure 104). Radiograph A exhibits some evidence of fog even though a field of correct size and 80 kVp were employed with 5 mAs. Effective reduction of the fog, radiograph B, was obtained by using a stationary-type grid, 100 kVp and 5 mAs for this radiograph.

Figure 104. Two screen radiographs of a 22-cm PA chest demonstrating the elimination of fog and contrast improvement attained with a stationary grid (B).

Demonstration No. 2.

Posteroanterior screen radiographs of the frontal sinuses (Figure 105), were made. Radiograph A was made with a large cone—the high density is due to excessive scatter radiation fog. Radiograph B was made with a small cone of correct size—definite improvement in image quality is apparent. For radiograph C, a cone of correct size and a stationary grid was employed—the cone reduced the amount of tissue irradiated, thereby reducing the scatter radiation produced and the grid absorbed most of the scatter radiation that might have reached the film. This teamwork resulted in good radiographic quality.

INDICATIONS FOR GRID USE

Since scattered radiation is generated both by high kVp's and by large thicknesses of tissue, both of these considerations determine when a grid should be used. Body parts of thicknesses greater than about 12 cm typically produce enough scattered photons to visibly fog the film. This is the size of a large knee, and although some radiologists prefer tabletop non-grid techniques for knees and others prefer grid techniques, all femurs should be done with grids. The shoulder is slightly larger than the knee and is usually done with a grid. Only extremities smaller than the shoulder or the knee produce a small enough level of scatter that the use of grids is never a consideration. Further, consulting Table IV in Chapter 6, it is found that kVp levels in the 70 to 80 range are needed to adequately penetrate the largest extremities such as the femur and shoulder. A related rule of thumb for grid use is that grids should generally be used on any procedure utilizing 70 kVp or more.

The particular grid ratio selected depends primarily upon the typical kVp levels used on a radiographic unit, or in other words, upon the types of procedures most commonly done with a radiographic unit. For procedures typically done in the range 70-80 kVp, a 5:1 or 6:1 grid is recommended. At the other extreme, 15:1 or 16:1 ratios should be used on dedicated chest units using 110-120 kVp. For most general procedures done with the cassette in the Bucky tray of a standard radiograph-

Figure 105. Screen radiographs of the frontal sinuses demonstrating contrast enhancement. Factors: 70 kVp; Radiographs A and B: 15 mAs; radiograph C: 62.5 mAs, stationary grid.

ic table, typical kVp levels range from about 76 kVp to 90 kVp. Therefore, most radiology departments install grids with an 8:1 or 10:1 ratio in the Potter-Bucky mechanisms of each standard radiographic room. The detailed recommendations for grid ratios according to kVp are listed in Table XI.

Grid Efficiency

There are several related factors and measurements for grid efficiency. Some, such as the "Bucky factor," are obsolete and will not be discussed here. The most important factor is the grid ratio just described. Closely related to this is *grid frequency*. Grid frequency is the number of lead strips counted per inch when scanning transversely across the grid. Generally, the more lead strips there are, the more efficient the grid.

However, this is true primarily because the increase in frequency normally results in an increased ratio: To fit more lead strips per inch, the spaces inbetween the strips must be narrower. Making these interspaces narrower will increase the grid ratio, unless the height of the lead strips is also reduced. If the height of the strips is reduced proportionately, no difference in efficiency will occur. Lead content is also frequently cited in terms of efficiency, but the total amount of lead in the grid is partially dependent upon the grid frequency.

If the frequency of a grid can be increased by making the *lead strips themselves* thinner, then efficiency is enhanced while grid lines are reduced. In this case, the grid ratio may be maintained and yet the higher frequency grid would be more effective. But most changes in lead content or frequency affect the clean-up only because they result in changes in grid ratio.

A general statement can be made that increased lead content, increased grid frequency, or increased grid ratio will enhance the efficiency of the grid.

GRID RATIOS AND DENSITY COMPENSATION

As discussed earlier, grids with smaller spacing between the lead strips, in relation to the height of the strips, are more *selective*, that is, the slits through which the radiation must pass are narrower, and, therefore, only those secondary photons which are emitted from the patient in a direction very close to the original direction of the primary beam will be able to pass through the spaces without striking a lead strip. To minimize the number of primary photons being attenuated, the high-ratio grid must be more perfectly centered and aligned with the central ray. Even when this is done, the high-ratio grid will absorb so much more radiation that technique increases are necessitated to maintain image density. The radiographer must

know what magnitude of adjustments are required for each ratio.

This can be a controversial subject, and there seem to be as many formulae for grid conversion techniques as there are authors. One item that must be considered is that grids have evolved somewhat over the years, primarily in regard to the materials used for the interspaces between the lead strips. Progress has been made in reducing the absorption of the x-ray beam by these interspace materials, so that workable technique conversions for modern grids are of less magnitude than many older publications suggest. Experiments have demonstrated that even though interspace material may vary between brand names on occasion, the density change factors and tech-

Figure 106. Radiographs of a PA skull demonstrating the accuracy of the "grid conversion factors" in Table XI in maintaining image density at various grid ratios. The increasing contrast at higher grid ratios must not be confused with average density: To properly evaluate these images, compare a medium density area such as the intra-orbital density marked by the black arrow. (A) was exposed nongrid with 4 mAs at 76 kVp. Correct factors used include: (B) 6:1 grid: *Double* to 8 mAs, 76 kVp, (C) 8:1 grid: *Triple* to 12 mAs, 76 kVp, (E) 12:1 grid: *Four times* original technique: 14 mAs, 80 kVp, and (F) 15:1 grid: *Five times* original technique: 20 mAs, 76 kVp. *Note*: Older textbooks recommend 4X technique for a 10:1 grid, 5X for a 12:1, and 6X for a 15:1. These factors are too high for modern grids–Note that in (D) the technique was increased by 4 times for a 10:1 grid, showing excessive density within the orbit (arrow), as compared to the other five exposures.

nique conversion factors presented in Table XI are accurate for the vast majority of modern grids, which use aluminum interspacing and frequencies of 80-110 lines (lead strips) per inch.

Most authors agree on the technique conversion factors for the lower 6:1 and 8:1 grid ratios. Older texts recommend a 4-fold increase for the 10:1 grid, a 5-fold increase for the 12:1 grid, and a 6-fold increase for the 15:1 or 16:1 grid. Repeated experiments have demonstrated that these figures are *too high* for modern grids with aluminum or plastic interspacers, and result in dark radiographs, as shown in (D) in

Figure 106. The figures listed in Table XI should be committed to memory for use in daily clinical practice. Note that moving grids, such as the Bucky mechanism grid, absorb slightly more radiation than stationary grids of the same ratio. This difference is too slight, however, to warrant a separate list of conversion factors.

The most commonly used grid ratios for Potter-Bucky mechanisms are 8:1 and 10:1. Hence, *as a rule, changing from the tabletop non-grid technique to the Bucky tray will normally require an increase in mAs of about 3 times.* Conversely, changing from the Bucky tray to the tabletop will require a

TABLE XI
Technique Conversion and
Density Factors by Grid Ratio

Grid Ratio	mAs Conversion Factor	Density Factor	Recommended kVp Range
Non-Grid	1	1	Less than 70
5:1 or 6:1	2	$1/2$	70-80
8:1	3	$1/3$	80-90
10:1	3.5	$1/3$	80-100
12:1	4	$1/4$	90-110
15:1 or 16:1	5	$1/5$	110-120

reduction in mAs to about $1/3$ the original.

A more complicated problem is presented when changing from one grid ratio to another. Once the conversion factors are memorized, all that is needed is to make a fraction or ratio out of the two factors involved, always keeping the grid you are changing *to* as the numerator and the grid you are changing *from* as the denominator. For example, when changing from a 6:1 grid to a 12:1 grid, you would need:

$$\frac{TO}{FROM} = \frac{12:1 \text{ Factor}}{6:1 \text{ Factor}} = \frac{4}{2} = 2$$

(2 times the original mAs is needed)

Another example, reducing the ratio this time, would be changing from a 16:1 grid to an 8:1 grid, resolved as follows:

$$\frac{TO}{FROM} = \frac{8:1 \text{ Factor}}{16:1 \text{ Factor}} = \frac{3}{5}$$

($3/5$ the original mAs is needed)

Milliampere-seconds should generally be used to compensate for density loss during the application of grids. Changes in kilovoltage will slightly alter the contrast of the radiograph, which is precisely what you are trying to control in using the grid.

Figure 106 demonstrates the effect of employing the above technique conversion factors to compensate for various grid ratios in maintaining image density.

Be careful not to confuse technique con-

version factors with density change factors. For any density problem, you simply invert the result of the technique factor formula (placing the grid you are changing *from* on top as the numerator and the grid you are changing *to* as the denominator). The following examples demonstrate this concept:

Example 1: Change from tabletop non-grid to Bucky grid without compensation:

Solution: $\dfrac{FROM}{TO} = \dfrac{NG}{12:1} = \dfrac{1}{4}$

New density will be $1/4$ of the original density.

Example 2: Change from 6:1 grid to 12:1 grid without compensating:

Solution: $\dfrac{FROM}{TO} = \dfrac{6:1}{12:1} = \dfrac{2}{4} = \dfrac{1}{2}$

New density will be $1/2$ of the original density.

Example 3: Change from 16:1 grid to 8:1 grid without compensating:

Solution: $\dfrac{FROM}{TO} = \dfrac{16:1}{8:1} = \dfrac{5}{3} = 1\,2/3$

New density will be $2/3$ more, or about 67 per cent more, than original density.

Try the following exercise for practice, and check your answers from the Appendix.

EXERCISE 17

What would your new *density* be if technique is unchanged and the grid ratio is changed from:

1. Non-grid to 6:1 =
2. Non-grid to 16:1 =
3. 8:1 to 15:1 =
4. 10:1 to 6:1 =
5. Bucky to Tabletop =

What would be your new *technique* factor compared to the original in order to maintain image density when changing the grid ratio from:

6. Non-grid to 5:1 =
7. 10:1 to Non-grid =
8. 15:1 to 5:1 =
9. 15:1 to 12:1 =
10. 12:1 to 8:1 =

EFFECTS ON OTHER QUALITIES

Sharpness of detail and the other recognizability functions are based upon geometry—distances, areas, directions, etc. But, as discussed in the previous chapter, scattered radiation is generated at random distances from the film and in random directions and, therefore, can have no predictable geometrical effect upon the image. Scatter reduces the *visibility* of edges of details in the image by destroying contrast but does not affect the *sharpness* of those edges. (A perfectly sharp image does not have to be a visible image. For example, a sharply defined picture may be posted on a billboard, but without any light you could not see it.)

Because scattered radiation can play no geometrical role in image formation, the use of grids, designed only to absorb scatter, cannot have a geometrical effect on the image. The direction of the *primary* radiation is not altered as it passes through a grid.

Neither are magnification nor distortion of shape affected directly by the use of a grid. Grids should be considered to affect only the visibility functions of the image. However, an indirect problem arises when Potter-Bucky diaphragms are used: Since the Bucky tray holds the film normally 2 inches below the tabletop and the patient (and as much as 4 to 5 inches on some tomography units), an increased object-image receptor distance is created which then reduces sharpness and increases magnification as described in Chapter Seventeen. These geometric effects are due to the OID, not to the use of the grid.

GRID CUTOFF

As previously mentioned, the lead strips in a grid absorb some of the primary x-rays as well as many of the scattered rays. With a stationary grid, this absorption will leave white lines of no density on the film, called *grid lines*, where a loss of information occurs. Although these grid lines can be minimized by the use of proper alignment and distance, they can never be completely eliminated when stationary grids are used. The employment of a Potter-Bucky diaphragm blurs out the grid lines, but there is still a loss of density called *grid cutoff*, caused by their absorption of the remnant radiation. Special care must be taken when using stationary *wafer* grids and *grid cassettes* to keep the interference of grid lines to a minimum. When improper distances are used or when the beam is not properly aligned to stationary grids, the

Figure 107. Radiograph of a knee with the central ray off-centered laterally 2 inches using a 12:1 stationary grid. Thin, vertical white lines are grid lines, most visible in the middle of the film.

grid lines recorded become much wider than necessary, obscuring larger amounts of information in the image (Figure 107).

GRID RADIUS

Due to the fact that x-ray beams diverge or spread out as they approach the film, most grids in modern use are *focused* (that is, the lead strips are tilted more as they move away from the center of the grid) so that they are always pointing toward the source of the x-rays—the x-ray tube target (Figure 103, left). This tilt of the lead strips is called *canting.*

With a focused grid, the *grid radius* is that distance from the grid at which lines drawn from the lead strips, with their various degrees of tilt, would converge to a focal point or *convergent point.* Since there is some margin for error, actual grid radii are given as ranges rather than as one specific number. The two most common such ranges are 36-42 inches and 66-74 inches, obviously designed for the two commonly used source-image receptor distances of 40 inches and 72 inches. The target of the x-ray tube must be placed at a distance from the grid within the radius designated. If it is not, excessive grid cutoff will occur, with the lead strips absorbing much more *primary* radiation than desired and creating grid cutoff on the radiograph. This occurs because peripheral x-rays strike the grid strips broadside. Placing the x-ray tube either too close to the grid or too far away

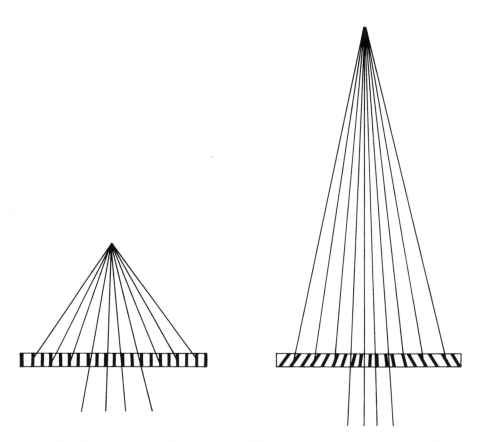

Figure 108. Diagram illustrating grid cut-off from placing the x-ray tube too close to a parallel grid (*left*), or outside the grid radius on a focused grid (*right*).

from the grid will result in the same grid lines and loss of information (Figure 108).

Parallel grids have no canting of the lead strips. Each strip points straight up. Therefore, parallel grids have a radius of infinity—the further the x-ray tube is away from the grid, the more parallel the primary rays will be to the lead strips. For this reason, grid cutoff problems never occur by having the tube too far away from a parallel grid. Placing the x-ray tube too close to a parallel grid, however, causes the beam divergence to be great, an inordinate amount of primary radiation is absorbed toward the periphery, and severe grid lines with a loss of information occurs (Figure 108).

Any time the SID used is not within the grid radius, the density pattern resulting on the radiograph will be a darker strip of density down the middle of the lengthwise axis of the film, with a loss of density toward both lateral sides equally, as long as other factors and centering were correct (Figure 109).

Demonstration No. 1

The radiograph in Figure 109 was produced without using a phantom or patient in the beam, and with a somewhat exaggerated distance change, in order to demonstrate better the effects of using improper source-image receptor distances that are not within the grid radius. The ratio of the grid used was 15:1, focused grid, 85 lines per inch, with a radius of 36-42 inches. The SID used was 20 inches (too close to the grid). Note that density is lost equally toward both lateral sides of the film. Upon close examination, it is seen that the density loss is due entirely to severe grid lines where no information is recorded under the lead strips. It can also be surmised that the grid cutoff created is

Figure 109. Radiograph demonstrating grid cut-off from placing the x-ray tube at 20 inches SID with a 12:1 40-inch radius focused grid.

more severe for the higher-ratio grid than for the lower-ratio grid even though the distances used were the same. This describes the factor of *selectivity* in grids. Grids with high ratios have shorter ranges for their grid radii, within which the SID used must fall, so that the distance used must be more exact. The same types of mistakes will cause more severe grid cutoff and information losses with higher-ratio grids.

The proper placement of the stationary grid is also critical in minimizing grid cut off and information loss. With wafer grids, a common error is to place the grid upside down over the film cassette. With a focused grid, the effect is to obliterate the densities toward both lateral sides of the film equally. This effect is similar to placing the x-ray tube outside of the grid radius, but much more severe (Figure 110).

Figure 110. Diagram and radiograph showing the grid cut-off caused by placing a focused stationary grid upside down.

ALIGNMENT OF THE
BEAM AND GRID

When performing portable radiographs with stationary grids, two other common problems are placing the grid and film tilted so that they are not perpendicular to the central ray (equivalent to angling the central ray across the lead strips) and off-centering the central ray or grid in relation to each other. Off-centering or angling across the lead strips have the same effect. While there may be some loss of density toward both lateral sides of the film, the loss will be much greater toward one side than the other, as illustrated in Figure 111 and demonstrated in Figure 112. Again, these problems become more severe when working with selective, higher grid ratios than with lower grid ratios.

Only when off-centering or angling the central ray *across* the lead strips (in a direction perpendicular to the strips) do visible grid cutoff problems occur. Tube angles and off-centering can be used when done

along the long axis of the strips. It is for this reason that the x-ray tube may be angled lengthwise along the table when using the Potter-Bucky diaphragm but must not be angled across the table. A typical application of this concept occurs in mobile radiography of skull injuries, as shown in Figure 113. Often, the patient is on their back and a lateral radiograph of the skull must be taken *cross-table* with a horizontal beam. If a 10-x-12-inch stationary grid or grid cassette is placed in the normal fashion relative to the skull, the lead strips will be running vertically. With the grid in this position, note that the central ray must be perfectly centered superiorly-to-inferiorly on the patient, otherwise it will be off-centered across the strips and cause grid lines. But, in building the head up on a sponge to ensure that the occipital bone is included on the radiograph, the central ray may be purposely off-centered along the strips, vertically, in order to center properly to the anatomy.

Figure 112. Radiograph demonstrating the grid cut-off caused by off-centering the central ray by two inches across the strips of a 15:1 stationary grid. The effect of angling the beam or tilting the grid would be similar.

Figure 111. Diagram illustrating grid cut-off from angling or off-centering the x-ray beam across the grid strips, or by tilting the grid crosswise.

SPECIAL GRIDS

In mobile radiography, a device of considerable help is the grid cassette, a cassette with a grid built in. These cassettes are very expensive and care must be taken not to drop them, which can easily damage the grid or the screens inside. When using grid cassettes, the centering and angling considerations just discussed must be carefully followed.

The crosshatch grid and the closely related rhombic grid (Figure 114) are occasion-ally used during biplane angiography or similar procedures, where there is a high level of cross-scattering radiation from film changers and the table. If such a grid is constructed with all lead strips in the same plane, the *moiré grid artifact* occurs, where there is a loss of density under each intersection of the strips. To avoid this artifact, these grids are constructed as two linear grids, one placed above the other.

Figure 114. Diagram of crosshatch and rhombic grid patterns.

Figure 113. Diagram of centering problems encountered in portable cross-table grid-cassette radiography of the skull. The CR must be centered to the grid crosswise even thought this may place it off-centered to the skull in a superoinferior direction. The CR may be centered to the anatomy, however, in a posteroanterior direction even though doing so places it off-centered to the grid lengthwise.

SUMMARY

1. Grids should be used on anatomy thicker than 12 cm or when 70 kVp or more is employed in order to remove severely *scattered x-rays* from the remnant beam, reducing image *noise.*

2. Since scatter radiation fogs the film, its removal by grids contributes to increased image *contrast.* The higher the grid ratio, the greater the contrast increase.

3. Grids also cause a loss in *density* which must be compensated for by increasing mAs from 2 to 5 times. The higher the grid ratio, the greater the loss of density and the more technique adjustment is needed.

4. *Technique* adjustments for changing grid ratios, nongrid to grid, or grid to nongrid, may be calculated by making a ratio out of the two corresponding conversion factors—from 1 for nongrid and up to 5 for a 16:1 grid (see Table XI).

5. Grids have no effect upon the *recognizability* functions in the image—sharpness of detail, magnification or distortion. Scatter radiation reduces image visibility, but it is random and therefore its removal by grids cannot have any effect upon the sharpness of the image carried by the focused remnant beam.

6. Grids must be placed facing up, perfectly centered to the beam crosswise across the strips, kept perpendicular to the beam, and the x-ray tube must be placed at a distance within the grid radius. Failure to do any of these four things results in severe grid cutoff and loss of density. The higher the grid ratio, the more *selective* it is and the more critical these four alignment factors become.

REVIEW QUESTIONS

1. What is the purpose of a grid, in regard to image quality:

2. A grid has a frequency of 40 lines per cm. It is 1 mm ($^1/10$ cm) thick. What is the grid ratio?

3. What is the purpose of the Potter-Bucky Diaphragm?

4. Your original mAs was 60. Changing from 12:1 grid to a 6:1 grid, what should your new technique be to maintain density?

5. Explain the difference between grid ratio and grid radius:

6. Using a stationary grid, your radiograph shows grid cut-off (decreased density) and thicker grid lines toward one side of the film. Name *two* possible causes:

7. When changing from the tabletop to the Bucky tray, assuming a Bucky grid ratio of 12:1, what would your new density be compared to the original density if you did not adjust technique:

8. If you performed a portable cross-table lateral skull on a grid cassette with a focused grid in it, you placed the grid with lines running vertically, you were centered to the grid horizontally but not vertically since you raised the patient's head considerably on a sponge to avoid cutting off the back and then centered properly to the head, the grid had a radius of 40 inches and a ratio of 8:1, and you used approximately 55 inches distance in the emergency room to get around equipment; describe what problem would appear in your finished radiograph:

9. What material is most commonly used for grid interspacers?

10. At what kVp level should you generally begin using grids?

11. Explain Grid "selectivity":

12. What is a "linear" grid:

13. What factor is used to measure the efficiency of a grid?

14. When changing from a 10:1 grid to a 15:1 grid, and adjusting your mAs to maintain the original density, exactly what will happen, and by how much to *patient skin dose*?

15. If grids remove poorly-directed scattered x-rays, why don't they improve the sharpness of the image?

16. Grid efficiency can be enhanced by increasing what three factors?

17. Define "convergent point":

Chapter 14

INTENSIFYING SCREENS

X–RAY INTENSIFYING screens are radiographically indispensable. Although they introduce some measure of detail unsharpness in the image, their value in radically reducing patient exposure and reducing motion unsharpness is of prime importance. Less than 1 per cent of the x-rays striking an x-ray film is absorbed by the emulsion to expose it; the balance fails to perform any useful radiographic work. The absorption of the x-rays by the emulsion primarily governs the formation of the latent image. It is obvious, therefore, that a means for fully utilizing this small percentage of energy is desirable. This may be accomplished by the use of x-ray intensifying screens that serve to increase the effect of the x-radiation on the sensitized emulsion by means of fluorescence, thereby reducing the exposure. Certain chemicals have the ability to absorb x-rays and instantaneously emit light. This property is called *fluorescence*.

HISTORICAL

Fluorescence was first systematically studied by Sir George Gabriel Stokes of Cambridge, England, in 1852. He showed that a large number of solid bodies and solutions possess the power of absorbing radiation of various wave lengths and then transforming and emitting it in such a manner that an increase in the wave length occurs. (Remember that an increase in wave length indicates a lower energy. Therefore, these materials simply "break" the absorbed radiation into "pieces" of lower energy and then emit these low energy waves.) For example, a solution of quinine sulfate was found to absorb ultraviolet rays and then emit them as visible blue rays. As might naturally be expected–and which later proved to be true in Röntgen's discovery–the extremely short wave length of the rays above the visible violet of the spectrum caused them to be absorbed by most fluorescent bodies and to be emitted as visible light rays of longer wave length. Stokes applied this principle in other experiments by employing a sheet of paper coated with a paint made from pulverized crystals of barium platinocyanide–another fluorescent chemical. There were a number of other investigations conducted with fluorescent materials from this time up to discovery of the x-rays, but little knowledge was added to the discoveries made by Stokes.

At the time of his discovery, Röntgen was searching for light rays beyond the visible spectrum, and the nature of the experiment which he was making at the time with low-pressure discharge tubes in a darkened room led him to cover the tube completely with black paper. When the tube was excited, he noticed that a barium platinocyanide fluorescent screen lying on a table a few feet away glowed brightly.

The covered discharge tube precluded any possibility of the effect being due to ordinary or ultraviolet light, and he reasoned that there must be some strange radiation emanating from the tube. Objects that were interposed between the energized tube and the screen caused images to appear. Since this strange light caused the screen to fluoresce, it became possible to photograph and record the images. Röntgen then made those first radiographs, which have become very familiar to us.

Development of Fluorescent Chemicals

Röntgen's discovery of x-rays by means of the fluorescent screen served as a new means to further intensive research in the study of fluorescent compounds. In fact, subsequent experimental work with x-rays and various fluorescent crystals finally led Becquerel to the discovery that uranium or its compounds constantly emitted radiations which were very similar to x-rays in that they penetrated opaque objects, ionized gases, and also caused fluorescence.

To understand more fully the development of the fluoroscopic and intensifying screen, some knowledge relative to the modern conception of fluorescent compounds is necessary.

Edison's Work

In the period, January to March, 1896, Thomas Alva Edison ambitiously tested some 8,500 different materials in his efforts to build a new incandescent lamp. Finally, from among 1,800 which fluoresced, he discovered that the fluorescence of calcium tungstate crystals has approximately six times more intensity than barium platinocyanide. He then recommended the use of this salt for x-ray fluoroscopic screens in March of 1896. Edison prepared

Figure 115. First radiograph of the hand using a fluorescent screen to enhance the x-ray exposure, made in 1896 by Professor Michael Pupin.

his calcium tungstate screens by mixing the crystals with collodion and spreading a thick layer upon paper; later, cardboard was employed, and on occasion, thin sheets of aluminum.

FIRST USE OF INTENSIFYING SCREENS

At the time of the discovery of x-rays, Professor Michael Pupin of Columbia University had been keenly interested in the work conducted in Germany on discharge-tube phenomena; consequently he was one of the few persons in 1896 who had any equipment adequate to produce x-rays. Pupin immediately began to study these rays and accomplished a tremendous amount of experimental work. In addition, a large number of patients were sent to him for examination by the local physicians.

The exposures necessary for him to employ were very long and he made every effort to increase the efficiency of his apparatus so that he could shorten the exposure. This he accomplished in February of 1896 by sandwiching together a photographic plate and a fluorescent screen that Thomas Edison had sent to him. He then made an exposure of a hand in a few seconds that formerly had required an hour's exposure.

A large number of buckshot were revealed in the image (Figure 115). Subsequent improvement in fluorescing power of the fluoroscopic screen by Edison, and its application to radiography by Pupin, meant much to radiology, for it made possible shorter exposures and consequently increased the life of those fragile, unstable x-ray tubes then in use.

SCREEN AND CASSETTE CONSTRUCTION

THE INTENSIFYING SCREEN

In modern intensifying screens, the fluorescent crystals used are suspended throughout a layer of plastic similar to the way that film emulsion suspends crystals of silver bromide. This "emulsion" of phosphor crystals is finely coated onto sheets of flexible polyester. The screens may be mounted in pairs in the top and bottom of light-proof cassettes, so that radiographic film can be sandwiched between them. Each screen consists of the plastic *base*, a *reflective layer*, the *phosphor layer*, and a *protective coat* of thin, clear plastic to prevent scratches, Figure 116. The total thickness of modern intensifying screens is about 0.4 mm.

Base

The polyester plastic base of the intensifying screen ranges in thickness, depending on the brand, from 180 to 250 micrometers, roughly one-quarter of a millimeter. The base must be durable, yet flexible enough to allow good contact across the entire surface of the film. It must be homogeneously radiolucent to the x-ray beam so that no artifacts are created in the image. It must also be chemically inert so that there

is no chance of it discoloring the emulsion in contact with it. Such discoloration of the emulsion would interfere with the light emission of the screen.

Reflective Layer

Light produced by the phosphor crystals in the emulsion is emitted isotropically, in all directions. Although much of the light is emitted toward the film, light emitted "sideways" and "backwards" away from the film is lost and lowers efficiency. For general-use screens, a very thin layer of titanium dioxide or a similar white, reflective substance is spread over the screen base. This layer acts as a mirror, reflecting the light that is emitted in a direction away from the film back toward the film, maximizing the benefit of fluorescence.

Unfortunately, light reflected from this layer has a longer distance to travel before reaching the film, so it spreads out slightly more than the light emitted directly toward the film and contributes to penumbra or *blur*. (See Figure 125 demonstrating variations of the crossover effect.) For this reason, some brands of "fine" screens or "extremity cassettes" designed for high resolution of detail do not employ the reflective layer.

Figure 116. Diagram of the components of an intensifying screen and cassette.

Phosphor Layer

The *phosphor layer* consists of fluorescent crystals suspended uniformly within a plastic *binder* solution which is coated onto the base and allowed to dry. This is the "active layer," the primary functional part, of the intensifying screen. The phosphor crystals used must be efficient at absorbing x-rays and re-emitting that energy as visible light. Several specific phosphors are used, and these will be discussed in detail later. The phosphor layer must be durable and flexible. Its thickness varies considerably with the "speed" or intended used of the screen, and may range from 80 to as much as 250 micrometers.

Protective Coat

A thin protective super-coating of tough plastic, sometimes called the *T-coat* or *tough-coat*, about 20 to 25 micrometers thick, serves two functions: It gives some protection to the delicate phosphor layer from damage during the loading of films, handling and cleaning, and it helps to prevent artifacts caused by static electricity discharges from friction during film loading. The T-coat must be clear and transparent to the light emitted by the phosphor crystals, and must be very thin. Therefore, great care must be taken in handling screens, since abrasive cleaners, fingernails, and film edges can all still easily penetrate this layer and damage the phosphor layer.

THE CASSETTE

The *Cassette* is designed to be a light-proof case for the radiographic film and to hold the film and intensifying screens in proper placement to each other. It must be thin and light-weight for easy handling, yet it must have a sturdy, durable frame and rigid, inflexible covers so that the contact of the flat surfaces of film and screens inside it is protected. Care must be taken not to drop cassettes, as the resulting damage can lead to warped backing and consequent poor film/screen contact, which destroys the sharpness of the image and can render the cassette useless.

The front of the cassette must made of material that is as uniformly radiolucent as possible, yet sturdy. New graphite carbon-fiber and plastic materials have proven ideal for these needs, especially in low-kilovoltage mammography. Older cassettes may have bakelite or aluminum fronts. The back of the cassette is the "lid" one opens to load and unload film, and includes latches for secure closure of the cassette. The cassette back is frequently made of a stronger material than the cassette front, since radiolucency is not essential "behind" the film. In most cassettes, the back cover includes a thin sheet of lead or copper foil (Figure 116). The purpose of this foil is to absorb *backscatter* radiation which is produced in the bucky tray, film holder, table or wall immediately behind the cassette. Backscatter radiation from these sources behind the cassette can fog the radiograph, especially during exposures of large body parts.

Many modern cassettes are made with a slight curvature to the lid which can be seen when it is opened, a concave bending away from the open cassette. As the cassette is closed on a film, the effect of the curve is to squeegee out any air pockets to better ensure uniform film/screen contact. Intensifying screens may be mounted inside the front and the back of the cassette. Fine-detail or slow-speed cassettes may have a screen mounted on only one side, usually the back or lid. For regular dual-screen cassettes, some manufacturers designate which screen is to be mounted in front and which in back by labeling them along the edge. This indicates that the back screen is thicker than the front. Since some of the radiation is absorbed by the front screen, the actual exposure to the back screen is always less. To compensate for this and ensure identical radiographic den-sities on both sides of the film, the back screen is slightly faster than the front one by making it thicker. Some manufacturers make the two screens in the pair identical. But, for those who make them different thicknesses, it is essential to mount them correctly as labelled.

Pressure Pad

Wherever an intensifying screen is mounted, there will be a felt or foam rub-ber pressure pad between the screen and the cover. The *pressure pad* or *supportive backing* is of critical importance: Its func-tion is to guarantee sufficient, uniform pres-sure when the cassette is closed to assure complete contact of the screens with the film across their entire surfaces. Figure 116 shows a cross-sectional diagram of the var-ious layers within a typical screen cassette, including both the screen and the cassette itself.

EFFICIENCY OF THE PHOSPHOR LAYER

To produce density on the radiographic film, an intensifying screen must perform the following three operations in order: (1) absorb x-rays; (2) convert the energy from these x-rays into visible light rays that will expose the film, rather than dispersing it as some other form of energy; and (3) suc-cessfully emit the produced light out of the phosphor layer and to the film. In measur-ing the efficiency of intensifying screens, radiographic physics textbooks categorize these processes using various terms: For example, "Intrinsic efficiency" has been used to describe the ability to both absorb and convert the x-ray energy, while "screen efficiency" has been used to describe the ratio of light produced which escapes the screen (emission). "Quantum detection efficiency" and "attenuation coefficient" are both terms used to describe absorption. To simplify the following discussion for the student, we shall use only three terms, strictly defined by each of the three essen-tial processes:

Absorption Efficiency: The ability of the phosphor layer to absorb x-rays

Conversion Efficiency: The inherent ability of the phosphor chemical to convert x-ray energy into visible light rays, rather than dispersing it as some other form of energy that does not significantly affect the film

Emission Efficiency: The ability of the produced light to escape the phosphor layer and reach the film to expose it

Let us now examine the various characteristics of the intensifying screen phosphor layer, how they affect each of these three processes, and the results in overall screen efficiency:

THICKNESS OF THE PHOSPHOR LAYER

A common method used by manufacturers to produce screens of different *speeds* (efficiencies) is to make the phosphor layer thicker or thinner. For a particular phosphor type or screen brand, thicker phosphor layers are the main method for achieving higher speeds. Which of the three processes defined in the previous section are affected by phosphor layer thickness? Just as thicker patients absorb more radiation, so thicker phosphor layers will absorb more x-rays, and more light will then be produced by the screen. This is simply due to the fact that more atoms have been placed "in the way" of the x-ray beam, and so the likelihood that a particular x-ray will be absorbed increases. Absorption efficiency increases.

Note that with a thicker phosphor layer, some of the produced light will have to travel farther to escape the screen itself - this light may "run into" other phosphor crystals on its way out. Since it is more difficult for produced light to penetrate out of the phosphor layer and reach the film, the *emission efficiency* is slightly lowered. This effect is very minor, however, when compared with the great increase in *absorption efficiency*. The net result is that thicker phosphor layers emit much more light, because of increased x-ray absorption.

PHOSPHOR DENSITY

The configuration (shape) of some types of phosphor molecules allows them to be packed more tightly together within a crystal. Thus, there will be a higher *concentration* of molecules in each crystal. This is described as a higher molecular density or physical density (mass per volume of space). There are simply more atoms *per cubic millimeter* for the x-rays to "run into," and absorption goes up proportionately. The physical density of the phosphor molecules is an important reason why "rare earth" screens were such an improvement over the old technology.

Interestingly, manufacturers have recently developed new gross shapes of the entire *crystals themselves*, such as *flat-shaped* crystals. In this way, it is sometimes possible to pack the crystals closer together within the binder substance, and still maintain a good uniform distribution. This may be thought of as the "crystal density" of the phosphor layer, and it has the effect of proportionately increasing the absorption of x-rays. Whether packing the crystals closer together, or packing the molecules within each crystal closer together, an increase in phosphor density enhances the *absorption efficiency* of the screen.

ATOMIC NUMBER OF PHOSPHOR ELEMENTS

"Large" atoms, those with a high atomic number (Z#), have many more electrons in their "shells." However, their actual *diameter* as measured across the outermost shell only increases very slightly when compared to atoms of low atomic number. This is because, as protons are added to the

TABLE XII
Highest Atomic Number Elements Used in Screen Phosphors

Phosphor Molecule	Highest Z# Element:	Atomic Number
Barium Fluorochloride	Barium	56
Lanthanum Oxybromide	Lanthanum	57
Gadolinium Oxysulfide	Gadolinium	64
Calcium Tungstate	Tungsten	74
(Various Activators:	Niobium- Terbium	41-65)

nucleus and electrons added to shells, the shells collapse in closer and closer to the nucleus. In other words, atoms with a high atomic number are not so much "larger" as they are more "concentrated." This increased concentration of electrons within the space around the nucleus is referred to as the atom's *electron density*. Atoms of high atomic number have a more *dense cloud of electrons* around them. This means that an x-ray passing through the space of such an atom will be much more likely to strike an electron and be absorbed by it. Thus, high atomic number elements absorb x-rays much more efficiently than low atomic number elements. It is for this reason that high atomic number elements are sought after as phosphors for intensifying screens.

Table XII lists the highest atomic number element used in each of the most common types of intensifying screens for comparison–note that these are all elements "high up" on the periodic chart, with 56 or more electrons. The use of high atomic number elements increases the *absorption efficiency* of the screen.

K-EDGE EFFECT: Directly related to the atomic number is the binding energy of the K-shell in these atoms. The K-edge effect may be thought of as an *exception* to rule that higher atomic numbers increase absorption. Ironically, if the atomic number is *too high*, as is the case with calcium tungstate, so that the K-edge binding ener-

gy is well above the average x-ray beam energies, then absorption due to the photoelectric effect may be *lost*. This is fully explained in a following section, but is mentioned here because it is directly related to the atomic number of the elements used in the phosphor layer.

CRYSTAL SIZE

Historically, larger crystals were sometimes used to increase the *absorption* efficiency of a screen. However, this method increased mottle effects and caused a loss of resolution of fine details, and it is no longer employed because of these limitations.

CHEMICAL COMPOUND USED FOR PHOSPHOR MOLECULE

Thomas Edison tested hundreds of chemical compounds to determine which was most efficient at *converting* x-ray energy into visible light. He concluded that calcium tungstate, with its intense emission of blue light, was best suited for use in radiographic intensifying screens to expose film. This compound was the standard for many decades, well into the 1970s. With enhanced chemical technology and knowledge, it was found that several "rare earth" elements when treated with trace amounts of terbium, thulium, europium or niobium as chemical activators (catalysts), were *2 to*

Figure 117. Diagram of the effect of adding dye to the binder of high-detail intensifying screens. On average, light only penetrates through the dye a limited distance, indicated by the length of the arrows. Only the light traveling most directly downward toward the film escapes, thus reducing penumbra and increasing sharpness of detail. Since overall light output is reduced, screen speed is lowered, and increased techniques are required.

4 times more efficient than calcium tungstate in converting x-ray energy into fluorescent light. Thus, if two phosphor layers of equal thickness are compared, the activated rare earth chemical will produce more light than the calcium tungstate. This is a higher *conversion efficiency,* and is due entirely to the chemical properties of the molecules. Several types of phosphor compounds are now used in different brands of intensifying screens, each having a different intrinsic conversion efficiency.

ADDITION OF DYES TO PHOSPHOR LAYER

A color dye may be added to the phosphor binder in order to reduce the amount of light reaching the film from distant points within the phosphor layer and improve sharpness of detail. The diffuse light which produces penumbra (blur) around a detail is emitted at a greater angle and must travel a greater distance to reach the film than light which is emitted directly toward the film. When just the right amount of dye is added, direct light will just escape the screen while much of the diffuse light will be absorbed by the dye before escaping and reaching the film

(Figure 117). Thus, penumbra is reduced and sharpness enhanced.

However, a price is paid for the improved resolution: The speed of the intensifying screen is substantially reduced, since less total light is reaching the film. In turn, this necessitates increased techniques which result in higher exposures to the patient. This increased exposure is acceptable when used on distal extremities. Cassettes with these types of screens used to be called "detail" cassettes because of the enhanced sharpness of details they produced. They are now generally referred to as "extremity cassettes."

Under normal room lighting, one can open a detail or extremity cassette and easily recognize the yellow or gray appearance of a screen with such a dye added. Which of the three types of efficiency do added dyes affect? The answer is the *emission efficiency* of the screen, since they reduce the amount of produced light that escapes from the screen.

THE REFLECTIVE LAYER

When a reflective layer is added behind the phosphor layer in an intensifying screen, or when the reflectivity of this layer is somehow improved, more of the produced light will reach the film. Improved reflectivity, then, also increases the *emission efficiency* of a screen.

KVP DEPENDENCE AND K-EDGE EFFECT

At some time in your life you have likely seen how some types of rocks glow in the dark or *phosphoresce.* Each different phosphorescent mineral emits its own characteristic color of light - one emits green light, another yellow, and so on. A particular mineral always emits the same color of light. The same holds true for the *fluorescence* of the phosphor crystals used in intensifying screens - each chemical emits a characteristic *color* or *wave length of light.* The nature of these phosphor chemicals is to always emit the *same wave length* of light. The wave length of a ray of light (its color) is a direct manifestation of its energy, so we might re-phrase this to say that a particular phosphor always emits light photons of the same *energy.*

This is the very key to how intensifying screens work: The energy of a single incoming x-ray photon will be *split* by the phosphor into hundreds of light photons, each one having exactly the same energy. For example, a calcium tungstate screen always emits blue-violet light rays having about 3 volts of energy each. How much light will be produced from a single x-ray photon of 30 kilovolts? The 30 kilovolts of energy, or 30,000 volts, will be *split* into units of 3 volts each. The law of conservation of energy requires that the *total* amount of energy after this event be equal to the original amount (10,000 photons at 3 volts each equals 30,000 volts total). Theoretically, then, some 10,000 blue light rays will be emitted from this single x-ray!

In reality, the above calculation is over-simplified, because it assumes a 100 per cent conversion efficiency for the phosphor chemical. The real conversion efficiency for various phosphors is much less, from 5 per cent to 20 per cent. The remaining energy is dispersed as heat. Assuming a 5 per cent conversion efficiency for calcium tungstate, the actual amount of light emitted would be 10,000 X 5 per cent = 500 light rays. Further, remember that this light is emitted isotropically in all directions from the phosphor crystal, and only a portion of it is directed toward the film, even with the use of a reflective backing in the screen. Also, some of the light is absorbed

before it escapes the screen, and some penetrates through the film without being absorbed. Perhaps 100 light photons will ultimately expose the film due to each single x-ray photon striking the intensifying screen. Still, this is a very impressive increase in overall efficiency. The invention of intensifying screens in 1896 reduced patient exposures a *hundred-fold,* and was truly an historic event in medical imaging.

This same phenomenon, that a screen always emits the same energy of light regardless of the energy of the incoming x-ray photon, causes the output of the screen to be *kVp-dependent.* Figure 118 illustrates this effect. When a higher keV x-ray photon strikes a phosphor crystal, the crystal will split that energy into *more* light photons, all with the same energy, rather than emitting higher-energy light rays, which would change their color. Whereas a 30-keV x-ray would be split into 10,000 light rays of 3 volts each, a *60-keV* x-ray would be split into *20,000* light rays, still at 3 volts each. Therefore, as kVp rises, the intensifying screen increases its actual output of light and glows brighter. This can be demonstrated easily by opening any screen cassette in the laboratory, exposing it to various kVp levels at equal mAs, and observing the brightness and color of the light emitted. The color of the light does not change, but the higher the kVp, the brighter the screen glows. While converting x-rays into light, the screen has converted *energy differences* into *intensity differences* (as if the mAs had been increased rather than the kVp). The film is exposed to more light photons, rather than higher energy photons. The kVp-dependence effect is classified as a change in the *conversion efficiency* of the screen.

The kVp-dependence effect is *slightly* offset by the fact that at higher kVp levels, the x-ray beam is more penetrating and less

Figure 118. Diagram of the kVp-dependence effect of intensifying screens. The energy of a single x-ray is "split" by the phosphor crystal into tens of thousands of light photons, always of the same color and same energy. Note that if the keV of the single incoming x-ray is doubled, the *amount* of light photons emitted will double, resulting in a greater exposure to the film.

x-rays are absorbed by the screen. There is a drop in *absorption efficiency* at higher kilovoltages, but the increase in conversion efficiency due to kVp-dependence is much greater. Because the increased *conversion efficiency* at higher kVp levels is so much greater than the loss of absorption and K-edge effects, the *net change in screen speed is a dramatic increase at higher kilovoltages, resulting in darker radiographic densities.*

Radiologic physics textbooks use absorption graphs to depict an irregularity in the absorption of x- rays by intensifying screens known as the *K-edge* effect. As kVp is increased, there can be-a sudden surge in the screen's absorption of x-rays just when the kVp surpasses the binding energy of the K-shell electrons in the screen. (Binding energy is how "tightly" the electrons are held in orbit.) Intensifying screens absorb x-rays primarily by the photoelectric effect (Chapter 4). This surge in absorption is due to the fact that the photoelectric effect is prevalent when the x-ray beam energy is just slightly above the K-shell binding energy. Generally, as kVp is increased, there is more penetration and

Figure 119. Graph of the K-edge effect for tungsten in calcium tungstate screens (solid curve) with the, x-ray spectrum for a 100 kVp beam added (dashed curve.) Note that at this kVp, most x- rays are produced in a range of 20 to 50 keV, where the absorption of the screen is quite poor (and less than the K-edge absorption.) At the K-edge of tungsten, where absorption suddenly spikes to a high level, there are only a few x-rays being produced. Thus, the absorption of the screen is poorly matched to the actually energies of the x-rays.

less absorption. The K-edge effect is an *exception* to this rule. Figure 119 graphs this relationship: Note that the absorption curve steadily drops as keV increases, *except when the keV crosses the K-edge for tungsten.*

In the older calcium tungstate screens, this "surge" of increased absorption occurred at about 69 keV, the K-shell binding energy for the element tungsten. This might have caused havoc with technique selection, except for the fact that the *average* energies within the x-ray beam are well below this K-edge energy. Recall from Chapter 1 that the *average* energy of the Bremsstrahlung x-rays in the beam is about one-third of the set kVp. The Bremsstrahlung spectrum is added (dotted line) in Figure 119 to show that *most* of the x-rays even in a 100-kVp beam have energies averaging around 35 keV and ranging from 20 to 50 keV, well below the K-edge. Only a small portion of the beam, those few x-rays above 69 keV, are subjected to this "sudden surge of absorption." Thus, the K-edge effect for calcium tungstate screens was only noticeable at very high kVp's and generally of little consequence in setting techniques. It did, however, mean that the overall absorption of radiation by calcium tungstate screens was not very efficient.

SUMMARY

Besides all of the factors just discussed, *anything* which increases the *exposure rate* to the intensifying screen will, of course, result in more light output from that screen. The key word here is the *rate* of exposure, since the apparent brightness of a glowing screen is in reality the *rate* of light emission from it.

The milliampere station selected by the radiographer controls the rate of exposure, and higher mA values will cause the screens to glow brighter. Increased exposure time has no effect on the output rate of the screen—it glows with the same steady brightness. But, naturally, since the screen would glow for a longer period of time, the exposure time must be factored into the end *total* of light exposure to the film. The effects of kVp-dependence have just been discussed; in addition to these effects, recall that within the x-ray tube itself, higher kVp's result in the production of greater amounts of Bremsstrahlung radiation. This means that at higher kVp's, the rate of x-ray exposure to the screens has also increased and this results in even more light output from those screens.

Having covered the variables that bear upon the actual light *output* of a screen, we should observe that only those characteristics which are inherent to the screen structure itself ought to be considered as affecting the *screen speed*. The speed of a screen is published by the manufacturer as a numerical value, 100, 200, and so on. If screen B has twice the speed of screen A, then screen B will be expected to emit twice as much light *under identical exposure conditions.* When factors that alter the exposure *to* the screen are considered, such as increased mA, bear in mind that even though the light *output* of the screen may increase or decrease accordingly, this does not constitute a change in the inherent *speed* of the screen. Table XIII summarizes all of the variables affecting the output of intensifying screens, and is helpful in clarifying these relationships.

TABLE XIII
Variables Affecting Intensifying Screen Output

I. Inherent Screen Speed
    A. Absorption Efficiency
        1. Thickness of Phosphor Layer
        2. Physical Density of Phosphor Layer
        3. Average Atomic Number (Z) of Phosphor
        4. K-Edge of Phosphor
    B. Conversion Efficiency
        1. Chemical Compound Used as Phosphor
    C. Emission Efficiency
        1. Reflective Backing (use of, effectiveness of)
        2. Added Dye (use of, effectiveness of)
        3. Thickness of Phosphor Layer (binder material)
II. Exposure Factors (affecting remnant beam)
    A. kVp
    B. mA
    C. All Beam Attenuators (filters, patient, grid)

EFFICIENCY OF RARE EARTH SCREENS

The *rare earth screen* made its debut in the 1970s and has since become the standard of practice, much more commonly used now than calcium tungstate screens. Rare earth screens are so named because in most cases the phosphors utilized are based upon elements with atomic numbers between 57 and 71 on the periodic chart of the elements, known as the *rare earth elements*. Various compounds of yttrium, lanthanum, gadolinium, and barium have been used. When special "activators" such as the elements niobium, thulium, or terbium are added to these compounds, a maximum fluorescent response is achieved upon exposure to x-rays. The two most widely used compounds in screens are thulium-activated lanthanum oxybromide and terbium-activated gadolinium oxysulfide.

Table XII lists the highest atomic numbers of the elements in several of these compounds. Note that the first three of these compounds, marketed as rare earth screens, all have atomic numbers *lower* than that of the old calcium tungstate screens. If screen speed were solely dependent upon the atomic number of the material, we would expect the rare earth screens to be *less* efficient than the older calcium tungstate screens. Clearly, in rare earth screens, there must be other factors which compensate for these lower atomic numbers, and then beyond compensating, go on to result in a faster overall speed. Indeed, there are at least *three* such factors. They are the K-edge effect, phosphor density, and inherent conversion efficiency.

K-Edge Effect

Ironically, the lower atomic number of the rare earth elements places their K-edge at a lower energy as well. As shown in Figure 120, this actually *improves* overall absorption: To demonstrate, consider the fate of those photons having 40 kV of energy. The beam spectrum curve in both Figures 119 and 120 shows that there are

Figure 120. Graph of the K-edge effect for lanthanum in a rare earth screen (solid curve) with the x-ray spectrum for a 100 kVp beam added (dashed curve.) Note that the K-edge for lanthanum is much more closely matched to the peak of the x-ray beam than the K-edge of tungsten shown in Figure 119. Those x-rays produced between 39 and 69 keV (shaded area representing the two different K-edges) are much better absorbed than they were in tungsten. Gadolinium, yttrium and terbium also have lower K-edges similar to this one.

many more photons at this energy than, say, at 80 kV. (Remember that *most* x-rays in the beam average only about one-third the energy of the kVp.) If more of these 40-kV photons can be captured by the screen, efficiency will improve dramatically. Compare the position of the K-edge for calcium tungstate in Figure 119 to that for Lanthanum Oxybromide in Figure 120. In the calcium tungstate, there is *no* photoelectric absorption of 40-kV x-rays by the *K-shell*. In Figure 119, the absorption curve at 40 kV represents photoelectric interactions occurring primarily in the *L-Shell.* (The K-shell is absorbing x-rays above 69 keV, but there are only a few x-rays at

these energies.)

For lanthanum oxybromide, Figure 120 shows that 40-kV x-rays are slightly above the K-edge. This is the ideal situation for photoelectric interactions to occur in the K-shell. These x-rays have just enough energy to knock K-shell electrons out of their shell without any left-over scatter radiation, and so they will be completely absorbed by the K-shell electrons. With the addition of K-shell absorption, the overall absorption curve spikes sharply upward. At *40 kV,* more photons are absorbed by lanthanum than by tungsten, even though lanthanum has a lower atomic number. The same is generally true for all photon energies in the shaded area of the beam spectrum in Figure 120. Compared to calcium tungstate, there will be increased absorption of those x-rays ranging in energy from 39 kV to 69 kV.

Phosphor Density

The configuration (or "shape") of rare earth molecules allows for the phosphor molecules to be more "tightly packed" together. They are more concentrated within a volume of space than the calcium tungstate molecules can be. Clearly, this will result in additional absorption of x-rays, as there are simply more molecules per cubic millimeter for the x-rays to "run into."

Conversion Efficiency

Calcium tungstate has an inherent conversion efficiency of only 5 per cent. Only 5 per cent of x-ray energy is converted into emitted visible light, the rest is dispersed as heat. Gadolinium and lanthanum compounds have a conversion efficiency of almost 20 per cent, nearly four times that of calcium tungstate. This improvement is

TABLE XIV
Why Rare Earth Screens Are Faster

Screen Type	Absorption Efficiency	Conversion Efficiency
CaWO$_4$ Par	20%	5%
CaWO$_4$ High	40%	5%
Rare Earth Phosphors	60%	20%

simply characteristic of the chemical molecules used.

Table XIV compares the absorption efficiency and conversion efficiency of two different thicknesses of calcium tungstate screens and a typical rare earth screen. In comparing the two calcium tungstate screens, note that the *absorption efficiency* is doubled for the "high-speed" screen; the only difference between these two screens is that the high-speed screen is *thicker*, which affects its absorption. Since the same chemical is used, conversion efficiency is equal. The rare earth screen, however, shows a dramatic increase in *both* absorption efficiency (60%) and conversion efficiency (20%). The improved absorption is due to both the K-edge effect and increased phosphor density. These two improvements are so effective that they compensate for the lower atomic number of the rare earth elements, and go well beyond that to bring about a net increase in absorption. The very high conversion efficiency multiplies these factors still further,

resulting in a family of intensifying screens that are *two* to *eight* times faster than calcium tungstate. This improvement has dramatically reduced patient exposures in modern radiography.

SPECTRAL MATCHING

Radiographic films are designed to be most sensitive to specific colors of light. The old calcium tungstate screens emitted blue-violet light, and film was designed to be most sensitive to this color. Most rare earth screens emit light wave lengths that are centered in the *green* portion of the spectrum. Special film was designed for use with these screens, which is most sensitive to green light. Any mis-matching of screen emission with film sensitivity, placing blue-sensitive film in a green-emitting screen, or green-sensitive film in a blue-emitting screen, will result in some loss of efficiency and the resulting radiograph will turn out *underexposed.*

Some barium and lanthanum compounds emit blue light rather than green. Barium is not a true rare earth element, but barium compounds are frequently marketed as "rare earth" screens. Therefore, one must be careful to determine the color of light emission and film requirements when considering the purchase of any "rare earth" imaging system.

SCREEN SPEEDS AND DENSITY

The function of the intensifying screen is to intensify the effect of x-ray exposure upon image density. *Speed* refers to a screen's ability to produce density with a given exposure to x-rays. The higher the speed of the screen, the more density will be produced at a given exposure. Higher

speeds reduce the patient dose, since lower exposure settings will produce adequate radiographic density.

The speed of an intensifying screen is derived from the *intensification factor*, the factor by which exposure can be reduced to obtain a similar density when using the screen. The intensification factor is mathematically expressed as:

$$IF = \frac{\text{Exposure required without screen}}{\text{Exposure required with screen}}$$

For example, if a direct, non-screen exposure required 300 mAs to produce a density of 2.0, and an exposure with *Screen A* required 10 mAs to produce the same density, the intensification factor for *Screen A* would be 300/10 = 30. The *speed* of *Screen A*, then, is 30 times faster than direct exposure.

TABLE XV
Traditional Image Receptors
(Calcium Tungstate & Direct Exposure)
Technique Conversion Factors and
Density Factors by Screen Speed

Screen Speed	Descriptive Names	mAs Conversion Factor	Density Factor
3.3	Direct Exposure Holder (No Screen)	30 x	1/30
30-50	Slow or Detail Speed	2 x	1/2
100	Par or Medium Speed	1	1
200-250	High Speed	1/2	2
250-300	High-Plus Speed	1/3	3

TABLE XVI
Rare Earth Screens
(Factors Compared to Traditional Par Speed)
Technique Conversion Factors and
Density Factors by Screen Speed

Screen Speed	Descriptive Names	mAs Conversion Factor	Density Factor
50-80	Single Extremity Single Fine	1.5 x	2/3
200-300	Medium Rare Earth	1/2	2
400	Regular Rare Earth	1/4	4
600-800	High Speed or Fast Rare Earth	1/8	8

DENSITY FACTORS

Different brand names of screens are often derived from various descriptive terms to indicate the relative speeds of their screens. A simplified speed factor system can be derived as in Tables XV and XVI. Some of the more common generic variations of speed names are listed below each speed. Although the par-speed calcium tungstate screens are almost out of use in modern radiology departments, defining the par speed as a standard speed factor of 1 allows the other derived factors to be rounded and easily memorized. It must be remembered that these speed factors indicate the relative *density* levels that will be produced when there is no compensation in technique. They are not technique factors as were used in discussing grids. To obtain the necessary technique adjustment factors, simply invert the density factors.

It should be noted that Tables XV and XVI list rounded out conversion factors in order to facilitate memorization. Depending on the brand, rare-earth fine extremity cassettes have speed one-sixth to one-seventh that of the regular rare-earth cassette. The mAs should be increased six to seven times when changing from regular rare-earth to rare-earth fine-extremity cassettes. Fine cassettes are listed in Table XVI as having roughly two-thirds the speed of par.

Depending upon the particular brand name of rare-earth screen used, other speeds will be encountered. The exact speed factors for these screens must be obtained from the individual manufacturers. Although some rare-earth screens boast a speed of 1200 (12 times the par speed), these are rarely used for two important reasons: First, their speed is increased from that of the regular rare-earth screen by using a thicker emulsion, which results in a substantial loss of sharpness in the image. Second, their speed is so excessively high that quantum mottle will become visible on the radiograph from the grossly reduced mAs values used. Because such speeds cannot be recommended for general radiographic use, they are not listed in Tables XV and XVI. Examples of how the density factors in these Tables can be used in solving both density and technique problems follow.

When changing from one screen speed to another, make a ratio out of the two involved factors, placing the screen factor you are changing *to* as the numerator over the screen factor you are changing *from* as the denominator. This formula will indicate the relative change to be expected in density.

Example No. 1: Change from a high-speed calcium tungstate screen to a direct-exposure film holder. What will the density change be?

Solution: $\dfrac{\text{TO} = \text{D.E.} = 1/30}{\text{FROM} = \text{H} = 2} = \dfrac{1}{60}$

The new density will be $1/60$ of the original density.

Example No. 2: Change from a slow screen to a rare earth screen. What will the density change be?

Solution: $\dfrac{\text{TO} = \text{R.E.} = 4}{\text{FROM} = \text{Slow} = 1/2} = 8$

The new density will be 8 times greater than the original density.

To solve the technique problems, simply invert the above formula, placing the screen speed you are changing *from* as the numerator over the screen speed you are changing *to* as the denominator. In example No. 1 above, the technique change required would be to increase the mAs by 60 times. In example No. 2, you would need to reduce the mAs to $1/8$ of the original.

Example No. 3: Change from a rare-earth regular screen to a rare-earth fine-extremity cassette. What change in technique is needed to maintain density?

Solution: $\dfrac{\text{FROM} = \text{R.E. Reg.} = 4}{\text{TO} = \text{R.E. Fine} = 2/3} = 6$

The new technique must be 6 times more than the original.

Example No. 4: Change from a direct-exposure holder to a rare-earth regular screen. What change in technique is required to maintain image density?

Solution: $\dfrac{\text{FROM} = \text{D.E.} = 1/30}{\text{TO} = \text{R.E.} = 4} = 1/120$

Only $1/120$ of the original technique is needed.

The effect of increasing screen speed upon radiographic density and the use of density factors in adjusting technique to maintain density at various screen speeds is demonstrated in Figure 121.

When the actual speeds are known, it is more accurate to simply make ratios out of them in order to derive technique adjustments or predict density results. For example, when changing from a 50-speed screen to a 250-speed screen, the latter is $250/50 = 5$ times faster and will produce 5 times the density at the same technique. To adjust for this change, technique must be cut to $1/5$ $(50/250)$. When changing from an 80-speed screen to a 200-speed screen, in order to maintain density, the technique must be adjusted to $80/200 = 0.4$ times the original, or 40 per cent of the original.

In everyday use, the actual speeds are not often noted on the screen cassettes. Only a descriptive speed name is given, such as "regular" or "high" speed, on the cassette. For this reason, it is worthwhile for the student to study Tables XV and XVI and memorize the rounded out density factors for the various descriptive names.

Figure 121. Radiographs of a knee and step wedge demonstrating the accuracy of the technique factors given in Tables XV and XVI in maintaining overall density with various speeds and types of screens. Note in particular step 5 on the step wedge, a medium density value. All were taken at 70 kVp. Factors: (A) direct exposure using 300 mAs (30 times par), (B) slow screen using 20 mAs (double par), (C) par screen using 10 mAs, (D) high-speed screen using 5 mAs ($^1/_2$ par), (E) high-plus screen using 3.3 mAs ($^1/_3$ par), (F) "regular" rare earth screen using 2.5 mAs ($^1/_4$ par), (G) "medium" rare earth screen using 5 mAs (double "regular"), and (H) rare earth "fine" or "extremity" screen using 18 mAs (6 times "regular").

Try the following exercise for practice, and then check your answers from the Appendix.

EXERCISE 18 :

What would be your new *density* if technique is unchanged and screen speed is changed from:

1. 300-Speed to 75-Speed:
2. Direct Exposure to Slow:
3. High to Rare Earth Regular:
4. Par to Slow:
5. Rare Earth Extremity (fine) to Rare Earth Regular:
6. Regular Rare Earth to Medium Rare Earth:

What would be your new *technique* factor compared to the original in order to maintain image density when changing screen speed from:

7. 50-Speed to 250-Seed:
8. High Plus to Direct Exposure:
9. Rare Earth Regular to Rare Earth Extremity:
10. Slow to Rare Earth Extremity:
11. High to Par:
12. Direct Exposure to Regular Rare Earth:

Influence of Temperature

The fluorescent property of screens excited by x-rays decreases as the temperature increases. At 95° F. screens emit less fluorescent light than at 70° F. One might assume that this fact is important radiographically. Actually, it is not, for the x-ray sensitivity of the x-ray film used with screens increases with the temperature. Since film and screens are used in combination at a given temperature, the screen effect balances the film effect and there is no need to observe the differences from a practical radiographic standpoint.

EFFECT ON CONTRAST

Screen radiography produces higher contrast in the image than can be attained by direct exposure when using the same kilovoltage. The higher contrast is a characteristic response of the emulsion to the fluorescent screen light. Also, the front screen tends to absorb some of the longer wave length secondary radiation emitted by the patient, thereby reducing the level of fog on the image. A comparison between contrasts produced on direct exposure (A) and on screen exposure (B) employing 50 kVp is shown in Figure 122.

The effect of increasing image *contrast* is not very notable from one speed of screen to the next. It is quite visible when comparing screen exposures to direct non-screen exposures. This is due to the fact that x-ray film has a higher inherent contrast when exposed to light rather than when it is exposed to x-rays and also to the

Figure 122. Radiographs of a hand showing the dramatic increase in image contrast when changing from a direct exposure technique (A) to a medium speed intensifying screen with screen-type film (B).

fact that screen output is kVp dependent:

Higher kV x-ray photons result in *more* light being emitted by the screen than low kV photons. Since scatter radiation averages much lower energy than the primary beam, it will not be as effective in producing light when it strikes the intensifying screen. Proportionately less light will be produced by scatter than by primary radiation. Therefore, the effect of scatter radiation on the overall image will be somewhat less notable. With scatter contributing less to the overall image, contrast is increased when screens are used.

EFFECT ON SHARPNESS OF DETAIL

Loss in image sharpness always ensues when screens are employed, because the fluorescent light diffuses across image boundaries within the body of the screen itself. No matter how fine a crystal is used in screens, its fineness does not compare with that of the film emulsion crystals. Any radiograph made with screens cannot compare favorably as to detail sharpness with a radiograph made without screens. However, when screens are not used, patient movement may occur during the longer exposure times required whether the part is immobilized or not. Screens should always be employed whenever there is a possibility of movement, and the exposure time should be as small as possible.

image. For that reason each pair of screens is placed in a rigid holder (cassette) so that they will be in direct contact with the film. Any damage to the cassette from dropping it or otherwise abusing it can bend or dent this structure, causing air-gaps between the screen and film surfaces inside. Any time visible light passes through an *interface* or boundary between two very different media, the light will bend or *refract* (Figure 123). This diffusion of the light is made worse by the increased distance to the film created by the air pocket. The result is a spreading of penumbral edges or blur, and a severe loss of image sharpness.

THICKNESS OF PROTECTIVE COAT

The protective coating of varnish or plastic is necessary to protect the screen emulsion somewhat from scratches. However, the coating adds to the distance through which light from the screen must travel to reach the film, so it must be as thin as practically possible. If the protective coat is thick, the light from the screen will spread out more before it reaches the film, contributing to penumbra and reducing sharpness.

Figure 123. Diagram illustrating the effect of poor film-screen contact from a warped screen. Light refracts as it passes through from the screen into the air bubble, spreading the penumbra. In addition, the increased distance to the film allows further penumbral spread. Sharpness of detail is lost.

SCREEN-FILM CONTACT

Close contact between the active surfaces of the screens and the emulsion surfaces of the film is essential so that sharpness of detail will not be impaired. Poor or uneven contact allows the fluorescent light to spread and produce blurring of the

SCREEN SPEED

Sharpness of detail generally decreases with higher screen speeds. While changing from one screen speed to the next may not cause a notable change, the difference between direct-exposure (non-screen) technique and screen technique, or that

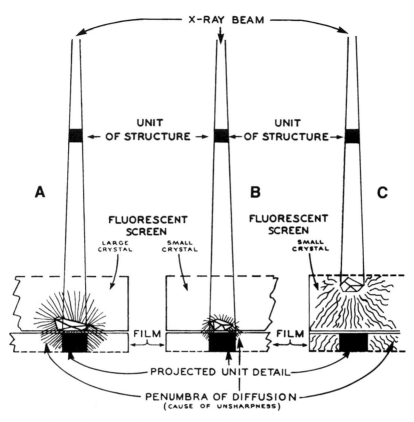

Figure 124. Diagrams illustrating the effects of phosphor crystal size and phosphor layer thickness upon image sharpness: (A) larger phosphor crystals increase penumbra, reducing sharpness, (B) smaller crystals increase sharpness, (C) thicker phosphor layers result in some crystals being located further from the film, allowing more penumbral spread and reducing sharpness.

between a detail or extremity cassette and a high-plus or rare-earth screen, is marked. Most screen speed increases are accomplished by using thicker emulsions. This places some of the crystals farther away from the film (deeper in the emulsion) so that penumbral light from each crystal diverges more before reaching the film. Increasing the size of the phosphor crystals is another method used to increase screen speed. Larger crystals also result in greater penumbral spread of light from the screen to the film. Whether from thicker emulsions or from larger crystals, the result is less distinct edges of the recorded image and sharpness of detail is lost (Figure 124). However, these distances and penumbral changes are microscopic, and in comparison with factors such as OID or focal spot size they are relatively minor. Changing from calcium tungstate to rare-earth screens does not present a problem with detail loss, because the efficiency is achieved by using chemicals such as lanthanum oxybromide, gadolinium oxysulfide or barium fluorochloride, which have higher absorption and conversion efficiency for x-rays, rather than by increasing emulsion thickness.

Binder Dyes

An effective method used to increase the sharpness of intensifying screens (at the expense of speed) is to add a color dye to the binder. Many detail screens have a yellow dye. Just as colored glass stops some light from passing through, this dye prevents those light photons which are diverging more (and thus have a longer distance to travel before escaping the binder) from being emitted. Since the beams escaping are those travelling a straighter course, sharpness is improved (Figure 117).

SCREEN CROSSOVER

When two screens are used, a *crossover* effect occurs whereby light from one screen may pass through the film base to the opposite emulsion, or even on through to the other screen's reflective backing and then reflect back to the film emulsion. This increases penumbral divergence of the light and thus reduces detail. For this reason, some extremity cassettes or other high resolution cassettes have only one screen so as to improve sharpness of recorded detail by eliminating crossover (Figure 125).

Some manufacturers have recently added a layer of color dye just under the protective coating of the newer screens, which aids in reducing some of the crossover effect.

Figure 125. Diagram of geometry of screen light emission and crossover effects: (A) direct emission of light from phosphor crystal to nearest film emulsion minimizes penumbral spread, (B) light reflected off reflective layer in screen spreads more before reaching film, reducing sharpness, (C) cross-over effect with light passing through film base to opposite emulsion increases penumbral spread, (D) cross-over effect with light passing completely through film to opposite screen's reflective backing, then back to film, showing maximum spread and least sharpness.

EFFECTS ON OTHER QUALITIES

Shape distortion and magnification of the *gross* image are not affected by screen speed, because there are no significant distances involved on the microscopic level of individual crystals in the screen and film, which are in direct contact. (It may be said that sharpness of edges is lost because the edges spread out, but this is not the same process as magnifying the gross image, so that you could actually measure a larger image with a ruler.)

Very high screen speeds, particularly the rare-earth speeds, may indirectly lead to quantum mottle in the image by dramatically reducing the mAs needed. As thicknesses and concentrations of crystals are increased in order to produce extremely high speed screens, there is a greater probability that phosphor crystals may clump together, causing an uneven distribution of the crystals throughout the screen. This will also lead to a grainy "mottled" appearance in the final radiographic image, called *material or receptor mottle.* Thus, very high speed screens may lead to two types of image mottle: quantum mottle and material mottle.

SCREEN LAG

As previously mentioned, the property of fluorescence in a substance is its ability to emit radiation of one quality when stimulated by radiation of another quality. A common example is the luminous paint employed on instrument dials to render them visible in darkness. Such paints are excited by tiny quantities of radioactive material included in a paint mixture consisting usually of zinc sulfide or a sulfide of some other metal. *Phosphorescence,* however, is another phenomenon comparable to fluorescence. In a fluorescent material, the glow of light only takes place as long as the substance is excited by radiation. In a phosphorescent chemical, the glow continues for an appreciable period *after* the exciting radiation is cut off. A typical example is the action of x-rays on an intensifying screen showing screen lag or afterglow. In such an example, the glow of light continues after the x- rays are turned off. When screen lag is present, the radiographer cannot reload his cassette immediately for an image made by the previous exposure would be recorded on a fresh unexposed film. The second radiograph might contain two images if the afterglow from the first exposure was sufficiently strong in intensity. It is possible for an afterglow to remain for months after exposure if the screen is of poor quality. Fortunately, the rigid production controls employed in the manufacture of modern screens precludes the use of fluorescent chemicals that exhibit phosphorescence. In good-quality screens, the intensity of fluorescence must rapidly reach its peak as the x-rays strike the crystals and should cease immediately upon termination of the exposure.

A test of persistent screen phosphorescence (test for screen lag) may be made by exposing the lower lumbar vertebral area laterally with 85 kVp and an appropriate mAs value at an SID of 40 inches. The exposed film is removed from the cassette and replaced by another film. The second film is left in the cassette for 10 to 15 minutes, and then processed. If no image is produced, the problem of phosphorescence does not exist with respect to the screens tested.

SPECIAL SCREENS

Special *gradient* screens have been developed which gradually increase speed from one end to the other. This gradation of speed is accomplished by gradually increasing the thickness of the emulsion in most cases. Similar to the use of compensating filtration, such screens are designed for radiography of anatomy which changes in thickness substantially across its length.

The most common application of the gradient screen is in the 36-inch-long cassette for use on thoraco-lumbar spine radiography in evaluation of scoliosis patients. These long cassettes should be marked *high speed* on one end and *par speed* on the other end. They should always be placed in the wall mount, with the par speed or slower-speed end at the top and the high-speed end at the bottom. In this fashion the density at the lumbar spine will be enhanced to an adequate level, while the less sensitive screen emulsion at the upper thoracic spine region will produce less density appropriate to the smaller thoracic vertebrae and thinner shoulder area. Placing this type of cassette upside down will certainly result in a repeated exposure, as the lumbar end of the spine will be grossly underexposed and the thoracic end excessively overexposed. This type of screen is also occasionally used when a single radiograph of the entire leg is needed, placing the high-speed end at the thigh/pelvis region.

CARE OF SCREENS

As screens influence the quality of the radiograph, their proper care is important. The fluorescent light emitted by intensifying screens obeys the laws of light, and any foreign matter on a screen will absorb light during the exposure and cause objectionable marks in the radiograph. Consequently, bits of paper, lint, and dust should be carefully removed and dirt and stains should never be allowed to remain on the surfaces of the screens. To avoid scratches and finger marks, the active surfaces should not be touched or handled except in washing. Cassettes may be stored in the processing room, but they should be kept at a safe distance from chemicals and all other possible sources of contamination or damage. Developer stains cannot be removed from screens. Therefore, as a safeguard, handle cassettes away from chemicals in the processing room. They should be kept closed when not in use.

SUMMARY

1. By converting x-rays into visible light, intensifying screens multiply the exposure effect of the x-ray beam and reduce the required *patient dose* to obtain diagnostic images.
2. As screen speed increases, image *density* is increased for a given exposure. Non-screen direct-exposure techniques require excessive amounts of radiation and, therefore, should only be used on the distal extremities.
3. As screen speed increases, image *contrast* is enhanced. This effect is not very visible from one screen speed to the next, but it is remarkable when changing from direct-exposure film holders to intensifying screens.
4. Increasing screen speed *usually* causes a loss of *sharpness* in image detail, because most speed increases are accomplished with more or thicker emulsion crystals or screens. Changing from calcium tungstate to rare-earth screens is an exception to this rule, because more effective chemicals are used. But changing from one rare-earth speed to a faster rare-earth speed is accomplished by thicker or more emulsion again and, therefore, reduces sharpness.

5. Intensifying screens have no effect upon the *magnification* or *shape distortion* of the gross image, because they are in direct contact with the film.
6. Screen *lag* or phosphorescence occurs in old screens and renders technique uncontrollable.
7. Screen *speed* is measured by the *intensifaction factor*. It increases with *kVp* and decreases with temperature.
8. The light output from a screen is affected by its thickness, phosphor density, the average atomic number of the phosphor, the inherent conversion efficiency of the phosphor chemical used, the addition of dyes, the K-edge of the phosphor, and the kVp used.
9. Rare earth screens are much faster than calcium tungstate screens because (1) they take advantage of the K-edge effect, (2) they have a higher phosphor density, and (3) they have a much higher conversion efficiency.
10. Very high-speed screens can lead to both the appearance of quantum mottle and material mottle in the image.

REVIEW QUESTIONS

1. List the components of an intensifying screen:
2. When an intensifying screen phosphoresces after the x-ray exposure terminates, what is this called?
3. When changing from a cardboard holder direct exposure to a rare earth extremity cassette, to what factor will patient exposure be decreased after the technique has been adjusted?
4. If par speed is assigned a speed number of 100 what is the relative speed for:
   a) "High" speed
   b) "slow" speed
   c) Rare Earth "Regular" speed
5. Why is a high-speed calcium tungstate screen faster than a par-speed calcium tungstate screen?
6. Why is a "extremity" or detail-speed calcium tungstate screen sharper than a par speed calcium tungstate screen if both have the same thickness of emulsion?
7. What is conversion efficiency?
8. Which type of screen efficiency is increased by using a thicker emulsion?
9. What is the cross-over effect?
10. What is the purpose of the pressure pad in a cassette?
11. When changing from a 400 speed rare earth screen to a 1200-speed rare earth screen of the same phosphor, what image quality is *reduced*?
12. Leaving the same technique, how much darker will a high speed screen exposure be than:
    a) a slow-speed screen?
    b) a direct exposure holder?
13. Why must green-sensitive film be used with rare earth screens?
14. How do very high speed screens contribute to image mottle?
15. What is a gradient screen?
16. What is the difference between fluorescence and phosphorescence?
17. What effect does increasing kVp have on screen speed?
18. List the three general types of efficiency for intensifying screens.
19. How can rare earth screens be faster than calcium tungstate screens, when rare earth elements have lower atomic numbers than tungsten?

Chapter 15

IMAGE RECEPTOR SYSTEMS

FILM-SCREEN COMBINATIONS

WHILE AN IMAGE may be formed on film by light, gamma rays, or other forms of radiation including x-rays, the properties of the latter in producing a radiographic image are of a distinct character. For this reason, x-ray film must be distinctly different from that used in photography. It has not been possible to manufacture a film that is solely sensitive to the action of x-rays and not to light. In fact, modern radiography depends greatly upon the use of the visible fluorescent light emitted by x-ray intensifying screens to augment the x-ray action on the film. Two general types of x-ray film are employed in medical radiography, *screen-type* film and *direct-exposure* film.

Screen-Type

Film that is particularly sensitive to the *fluorescent* light of x-ray intensifying screens is known as screen-type x-ray film. The visible fluorescent light from screens amplifies the direct action of the x- rays. When used with intensifying screens, screen-type film is much faster than the direct-exposure type. When screen-type film is used without intensifying screens, however, it is about half as fast as the direct-exposure type. Nonetheless, it is frequently exposed without screens: In radiography of the smaller thicknesses of the body such as the hand, ankle, etc., screen-type film provides a wider range of densities than when it is employed with screens. Because of its lower sensitivity to direct action of the x-rays, the background density of the processed radiograph is usually less than that of the direct-exposure type.

Direct-Exposure Type

Direct-exposure film (no-screen film) is especially sensitive to the *direct* action of the x-rays. It is used only for the thinner body parts. Its silver content is greater and the film has a higher inherent contrast than the screen-type film when directly exposed.

Direct exposure film has such thick emulsion that it cannot be run through the rollers of automatic processors. Since auto-

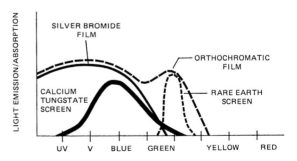

Figure 126. Graph of intensifying screen light emission spectra superimposed upon film sensitivity spectra. Any mismatching results in a loss of density. Note, for example, that rare earth screens are centered over the green portion of the light spectrum, while silver bromide film is centered over the blue-violet portion.

matic processors are nearly universal in medical radiography, direct exposure film has become generally obsolescent, but may still be found for specialized uses.

Orthochromatic Film

The development of intensifying screens utilizing the rare-earth elements as phosphors necessitated the manufacture of a new type of x-ray film. Film emulsion is designed to be chemically sensitive to a specific frequency or wave length of light. Since calcium tungstate screens emit a blue-violet light wave length, regular screen x-ray film emulsion was chemically compounded to be sensitive to this color. True rare-earth elements, however, emit a wave length of light centered mostly in the green portion of the spectrum (Figure 126). *Orthochromatic* x-ray film was developed for use with rare-earth screens in order to efficiently convert this green light into image density.

Since many radiology departments now have both green-sensitive film and blue-sensitive film stored in their darkrooms, it is important for radiographers to take care not to mix screen and film types. If orthochromatic film is used in calcium tungstate screens, or if regular film is used in rare-earth screens, the result will be insufficient density. Uninformed attempts to correct such a situation by increasing techniques will only lead to unnecessary patient exposures until the real error is found.

FILM COMPOSITION

X-ray film consists of an *emulsion* of finely precipitated silver bromide crystals suspended in gelatin that is coated on *both* sides of a transparent blue-tinted polyester support called the *base.*

Film Base

The base furnishes support for the emulsion and provides the correct degree of stiffness for handling.

At various times attempts were made to improve the over-all quality of film by tinting the film. The purpose was to emphasize contrast and thus make it easier to visualize the densities present in the image. The colors used or locally applied were various shades of green, pink, orange, or blue.

The first commercialized (patented) method to be applied to x-ray film in America was described in 1933 by George A. Scanlan and Charles Holzwarth of Parlin, New Jersey who introduced a blue tint in x-ray film. The idea became popular with radiologists because they found that the presence of the blue tint slightly emphasized contrast differences. Modern x-ray film is blue tinted.

SUBCOATING. After the base is made, it is covered on both sides with a thin adhesive-type material so that the sensitive emulsion will adhere to the base. This is called the subcoating and prepares the base for emulsion coating.

Emulsion

The *emulsion* itself starts with gelatin. Next, virgin silver is dissolved in nitric acid to form silver nitrate; then the silver nitrate solution is mixed with potassium bromide and gelatin to produce an emulsion of silver bromide crystals. It is then coated on both sides of the film base. After drying, the surfaces of the emulsion coatings are specifically treated to prevent surface abrasion.

The purpose of the silver emulsion is to *absorb* radiation during an x-ray exposure and produce a latent image. The degree of exposure depends upon the intensity of the radiation *emerging* from the object that is interposed between the focal spot of the x-ray tube and the film, to reach the film.

Since gelatin is a most important constituent of the emulsion, some details regarding its source and characteristics are of interest.

GELATIN. Gelatin is a necessary constituent of the x-ray film emulsion and its properties should be familiar to all radiographers. A most important discovery in the manufacture of photographic sensitive materials occurred many years ago as previously mentioned when gelatin was found to be an ideal medium for suspension of silver salts. Its ability to withstand action of the developer and fixer solutions at the processing temperatures normally employed without affecting the distribution of the silver crystals within it was most important. The fact that it assisted in the sensitization of the emulsion came as an after development.

Gelatin for photographic purposes is extracted from calf or cattle skins. In the early days of photography some gelatin was found to be good and some not. A study of this fact revealed that cattle grazing on pasturage containing mustard plants retained microscopic traces of sulfur in their hides, which in turn was carried in the gelatin obtained from them. Moreover, the silver bromide crystals suspended in this kind of gelatin were much more sensitive to the action of x-rays or light than crystals obtained in gelatin having no trace of sulfur. Film manufacturers obviously cannot depend upon the vagaries of bovine grazing habits when making film, but the problem was solved by adding the proper amount of natural synthetic mustard oil and now, other chemicals, to the emulsion formula.

Chemically, gelatin is a colloid and a very complex substance. Without special treatment, gelatin becomes soft and flexible when soaked in water because it absorbs an amount several times its bulk. An important physical property of gelatin is that in both liquid and solid forms it is clear and transparent so that no optical impairment of the image occurs when it is used in film manufacture. Gelatin immersed in hot water will dissolve to a liquid but it will not dissolve in cold water. This is an advantage for two reasons: (1) the liquid state is necessary for emulsion mixing and coating, and (2) the gelatin should not dissolve at the temperatures employed in processing the x-ray film. In the manufacture of the emulsion the gelatin can be given additional hardness without seriously impairing its porosity or clarity. Another favorable characteristic is the fact that when incorporated in the emulsion, it can swell considerably in a cool solution without dissolving thereby permitting action of the processing chemicals on the silver crystals without altering their places in the emulsion; afterwards the gelatin can be shrunk and hardened in the fixing bath so that the radiograph can be washed and dried. The influence of gelatin on sensitivity varies with different gelatins; therefore the gelatin must be carefully selected. Increased sensitivity can be given to the emulsion by adding certain substances to the gelatin during manufacture.

SILVER SALTS. In the preparation of the emulsion, a solution of potassium bromide is made with water. Pure silver nitrate is made by dissolving virgin silver in nitric acid. The solutions of potassium bromide and silver nitrate are slowly added to the gelatin solution in total darkness. The potassium bromide and silver nitrate solutions combine to form a precipitate of silver bromide in gelatin. This results in a thick, creamy emulsion.

The silver bromide emulsion is now heated to temperatures that vary from 50-80° C. This process is known as digestion and tends to increase the sensitivity of the emulsion. It is next cooled to a thick jelly and cut up into fine shreds which are washed in water for several hours to remove the potassium nitrate and other soluble salts. The washed emulsion is again heated and mixed with additional gelatin. In this state it is ready to be coated on the film base.

Emulsion Coating

In the coating operation, the film base is passed at high speed through a trough containing the sensitive emulsion where it acquires a coating of uniform thickness. The coated film next passes into a chamber of cold air where the emulsion is chilled to a jelly. It then traverses other chambers where it is dried and a nonabrasive coating

is applied. It is then tested and spooled into a huge roll. The finished film is finally cut to the various sizes required by the radiologist. Each emulsion layer is about one-thousandth of an inch in thickness. Since x-rays pass readily through x-ray film—and also through x-ray intensifying screens when used—an emulsion layer is coated on *both* sides of the film base, providing thereby a greater effect upon exposure to x-rays than would be possible with an emulsion coated only on one side.

T–COATING. The emulsion is protected by the very thin, non-abrasive coating of varnish. This "tough-coat" or t-coat guards against emulsion damage from scratches. It must be thin enough, however, to easily wash away upon development. The four main component layers of duplitized x-ray film are illustrated in Figure 16, Chapter 2.

LATENT IMAGE FORMATION

The silver bromide crystals in the emulsion are composed of alternating atoms of silver and bromine with a few "free" silver ions (atoms) mixed in (Figure 127-A.). Exposure to x-rays ionizes the atoms, liberating electrons (negative ions) and breaking the bonds between the atoms (Figure 127-B.).

In manufacture the emulsion is treated with silver sulfide or other chemicals which constitute "impurities" within the silver bromide crystals. These altered molecules reside on the surface of the crystal at sites called *sensitivity specks* (Figure 128-A.). Sensitivity specks have the ability to "trap" electrons, and provide the future sites for the beginning of the development process leading to a visible image. Development only can be continued by the *growth* in size of these specks, and *not* by the formation of new specks. Crystals that do not possess sensitivity specks cannot develop.

The general aspects of latent image formation and visible image development are diagrammatically shown in Figure 128. A complete silver bromide crystal, composed of thousands of atoms, is shown in (A), with sensitivity specks (impurities) on the surface. Exposure to x-rays (B) ionizes atoms, releasing free electrons as also shown in Figure 127-B. Enlarging our view of a sensitivity speck (C), it is seen that it soon traps many of the free electrons (D), acquiring a strong negative charge. Free or "migrant" silver atoms (see Figure 127-A) have a positive charge, and are attracted to the negatively charged sensitivity speck. They move slower than the free electrons, and arrive at the sensitivity speck later, attaching themselves to it, (Figure 128, E), and forming a clump of silver particles (F). The amount of silver deposit depends on the amount of exposure. If sufficient silver accumulates around the speck, it will act as a development center making the entire crystal potentially developable. This constitutes the *latent image (G)*.

Upon chemical development (H), the rest of the crystal is attacked by reducing chemicals that separate the remaining silver and bromine atoms from each other, pulling the bromine out into the developer solution. The remaining silver accumulates around the various sensitivity specks, forming a large clump of black metallic silver (I)

which remains on the film, composing an image. If the quantity of x-rays that strikes the crystal happens to be insufficient, the sensitization speck will not grow to the point where it can break down the entire crystal upon development. The fully exposed crystal will usually develop and be reduced to black metallic silver within the normal time of development at a given temperature.

A.

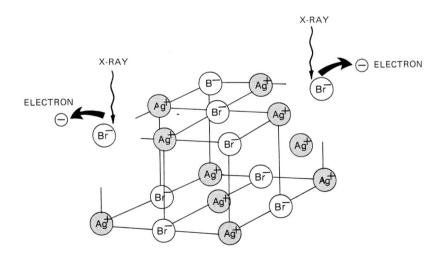

B.

Figure 127. Cubical structure of silver bromide crystal showing (A) alternating atoms of silver and bromine, and a free silver ion. X-rays ionize atoms, breaking the chemical bonds between them and liberating electrons (B). In Figure 128, these liberated electrons are shown as negative charges, and free silver ions as positive charges.

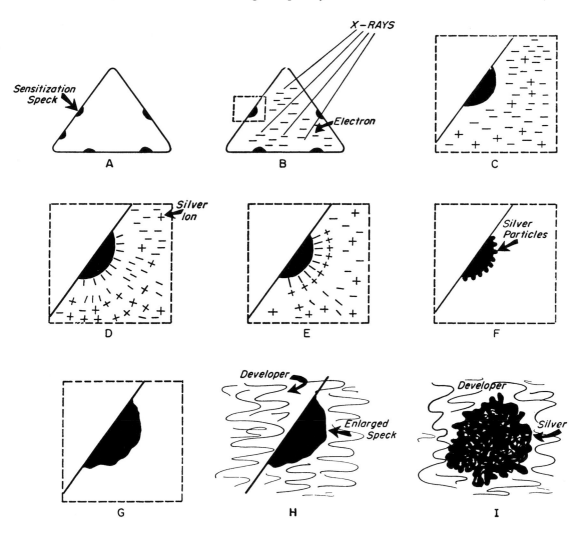

Figure 128. Changes occurring within the silver bromide crystal upon exposure and development. Electrons liberated by exposure (B) accumulate around the positive sensitivity speck (D). Free silver ions then attach to the sensitivity speck (E), forming a clump of silver (F). During processing (H and I), additional silver atoms "broken" from the crystal by developer solution continue to attach to the clump, making it grow in size.

FILM SPEED

The shorter the exposure required in making a high quality radiograph, the faster the film is said to be. As with intensifying screens, films come in various speeds and contrast/gray scale characteristics. Generally, a "high" speed film is about twice as fast as a "medium" speed film. *Relative speeds,* using a value of 100 for "medium," are usually determined using 80 kVp exposures, and accurately compare one film's speed to another. These must be obtained from each film manufacturer.

Since the concentration and size of crystals in the film are optimized for sharpness of detail in most cases, speed differences are usually attained by changing emulsion thickness. Chemical changes may be used to alter speed, contrast and gray scale characteristics. In selecting a film type, its compatibility with the intensifying screens it will be used with must also be taken into account.

Shelf-Life of Film

Faster speed films are more sensitive, not only to regular exposure, but also to scatter radiation, background radiation and other environmental fogging variables such as high temperatures and humidity during storage. Most manufacturers list the expected good *shelf-life* or a recommended expiration date on each box of film. Film stock for a radiology department must be purchased in relatively small quantities over short periods of time for this reason. The longer the film is stored, the greater the background fog present prior to use. High-speed films have a much shorter shelf-life due to their high sensitivity, and must be rotated even more frequently.

IMAGE RECEPTOR SPEED

Films and screens must always be considered together in selecting a receptor system that will produce the desired image characteristics. Some applications are focused on high speed to minimize patient dose, such as in angiography, others emphasize long gray scale such as chest screening radiography, others demand high contrast, and still others focus on maximum sharpness of detail. Each manufacturer provides a selection of different film/screen combinations to fit these various needs.

When considering receptor system speed, especially in view of patient exposure, the *total system speed must be considered by multiplying the film speed by the screen speed and dividing by 100.* For example, if a 100-speed screen were used with a 50 speed film, the overall receptor system speed would be 100 x 50/100 = 50. If a 200-speed screen were used with a 200-speed film, the overall receptor speed would be 200 x 200/100 = 400. What is the overall speed for a 30-speed screen and a 50-speed film? The answer is 15.

Within a particular radiology department, a standardized single speed of film is normally utilized, and only screen speeds are varied. So in making technique adjustments, usually one needs only to consider the screen speed changes. In situations where different speeds of film are used, radiographers should be aware of the technique adjustments required by considering overall receptor speed.

When manufacturers attempt to increase film speeds by using larger crystals or higher concentrations of crystals, the crystals can clump together and cause a *grainy* appearance in the image, called *film mottle*. Such films will always present noise in the image, and should be avoided.

FILM CONTRAST AND LATITUDE

X-ray film is manufactured with inherent contrast characteristics that are most suitable for the type of radiograph it is designed to produce. It is axiomatic that different kinds of x-ray films made by one manufacturer or those made by another manufacturer yield different contrasts even though the same developer and processing procedures are employed. Two general types of medical x-ray film are normally employed that can yield any one of several kinds of radiographic contrast depending upon the manner in which the films are exposed. The use of either type is based primarily on the speed and image defini-

tion requirements for the various projections.

Screen-type film possesses an emulsion that is particularly sensitive to the fluorescent light emitted by x-ray intensifying screens. It is less sensitive to the direct action of x-rays. The characteristics of this film are such that a relatively *higher* contrast is obtained when it is exposed with intensifying screens than when the same film is directly exposed to x-rays at the same kilovoltage.

When two posteroanterior radiographs at 50 kVp and 36" SID are made of a body part such as the hand (Figure 129), one with 1.5 mAs and intensifying screens (*Left*) and the other without them (*Right*) at 40 mAs, the images differ materially in contrast and sharpness of detail. In the case of the screen exposure, bone details exhibit greater contrast, but there is some loss in image sharpness. The soft tissues show higher density and in some areas details cannot be easily visualized because of some opaque densities. The radiograph made *without* screens, however, will show a lower contrast and greater detail sharpness,

Figure 129. Two radiographs of the hand showing increased contrast resulting from use of intensifying screens (*left*), less contrast and higher latitude without screens (*right*).

Figure 130. Radiographs of the foot employing the same kVp, (*left*) with high latitude film, (*right*) with short latitude film. Note the lower contrast with the high latitude film.

while the densities representative of *all* tissues are translucent. However, screens should always be employed in radiography of the heavier body parts and where shortness of exposure is necessary to stop movement.

It should be noted that *high-latitude* films are often recommended to produce long gray scale images, such as in screening chest radiography. These films produce low contrast and long gray scale (Figure 130) to maximize the amount of information recorded. They therefore allow a greater margin for error in setting exposure techniques, that is, they have *high exposure latitude*, which reduces repeat rates.

Solarization

Extreme overexposure of radiographic film can lead to a bizarre *reversal* of the image densities (Figure 131) in which structures such as bone which normally appear "white" will be dark, and the background density lightens. This effect is called *solarization.*

Figure 131. Radiograph exhibiting solarization in the neck area and edges of the shoulders, due to extreme overexposure in a duplicator unit. Note that the bones in these areas are dark.

GEOMETRIC FACTORS

Film with emulsion coated on both sides is called *duplitized* film. When observing the duplitized radiograph, one is actually looking at *two* superimposed images, one in each emulsion, with a microscopic distance between them imposed by the film base. When recorded by an angled beam, one of the two images will be shifted in relation to the other. This shift is known as *parallax.* The double image will result in reduced sharpness of detail.

Thicker film emulsions and larger crystals also result in less sharpness of detail and can contribute to mottling. A thicker film base separates the two emulsions at a greater distance, and thus contributes to *parallax* unsharpness. These effects are *microscopic* in magnitude. They are so minor in comparison with the effects of intensifying screens, focal spot size, distances and motion that the choice of radiographic film is not a serious consideration in controlling sharpness of detail. Film should be selected entirely upon the basis of its speed and contrast characteristics.

The image resides in the film emulsion, and there can be no distances or angles involved therein. Hence, the type of film used has no relation to magnification and shape distortion.

HALATION. Any time light passes from one medium into another, such as from air into water, a certain percentage of the light will be reflected from the surface separating these two media. When exposing an x-ray film in a screen cassette, not all of the light from the screens passes completely through the film. After entering into the film, a small amount is reflected at the back surface rather than passing back into the air. This reflected light comes back to the opposing emulsion, causing a slight "halo" effect around image details. The result is a destructive loss of recorded detail. This slight "halo" effect is termed *Halation.*

Halation is particularly pronounced with single-emulsion film. A special coating is applied to the nonemulsion side of the film to reduce this effect. When using single-screen cassettes with single-emulsion film, the film emulsion must be placed in direct contact with the screen, and the special coating must be placed opposite the screen. The correct sides of the film can be easily identified even in dark room lighting, because the *emulsion side is dull, while the coated side is glossy.* The dull side of the film should always face the intensifying screen.

FILM HOLDERS

All types of film holders serve the primary function of protecting the film from light, and cassettes also provide a support system for intensifying screens that should assure direct film/screen contact across the entire area of the film.

There are many types of special purpose cassettes, including curved cassettes for knee, hip and shoulder radiography, grid cassettes with the grid built into the cassette, and 36-inch cassettes for scoliosis studies or long bone measurement.

The front of the cassette must be rigid and durable, but radiolucent to the x-ray beam. Cassettes with radiolucent (non-metal) backs that include a sheet of lead foil can be placed in reverse position if necessary to reduce scatter radiation much like a grid would. This is actually a *filtration* technique, but since scatter radiation has less energy than the primary beam overall, more scatter than primary radiation will be filtered out by the lead foil and contrast is enhanced. This method is workable for medium-sized anatomy such as skulls, cervical spines and proximal extremities, but should never be used on torso anatomy where only the effectiveness of a high-ratio grid will suffice to clean up the scatter radiation generated.

SUMMARY

1. The use of higher-speed film types results in increased image *density* for a given exposure.
2. Higher film speeds also produce slightly increased *contrast.*
3. Higher film speeds lead to a reduction in *sharpness* of image detail, because more or thicker emulsions or larger crystals are used.
4. Film speed has no effect upon *magnification or distortion* of the gross image, because the image resides within the emulsion.
5. In all of the image qualities, the above effects must never be considered alone but always in connection with the use of intensifying screens. It is the complete screen/film combination, as a *receptor system*, which determines the final image results.
6. Film sensitivity *type* must be properly matched with the screen emission type being used—that is, ortho film with rare-earth screens, regular film with calcium tungstate screens, and direct-exposure film with direct-exposure holders—in order to prevent a loss of density.
7. *Latent image* formation occurs when x-rays ionize silver bromide crystals, releasing free electrons to accumulate at the *sensitivity speck* and attract migrant silver ions.
8. *Halation* is a halo effect caused by reflected light from the back surface of the film, and is most pronounced on single-emulsion films.
9. In loading single emulsion films into cassettes, the *dull* side (the emulsion side) should face the cassette screen.
10. Cassettes must be carefully handled to prevent damage that can lead to poor screen/film contact or light leaks.
11. Placing cassettes backward to reduce scatter should only be done on medium-sized anatomy, not torso anatomy.

REVIEW QUESTIONS

1. Clumping together of large crystals in high-speed films can lead to what type of image noise?
2. What is the total receptor system speed for a 200-speed film in a 300-speed screen?
3. Switching from 50-speed film to 200speed film, how much darker will the image be using the same technique?
4. What effect do faster speed films usually have on image sharpness?
5. How do high-latitude films help reduce repeat rates?
6. What special type of unsharpness is caused by duplitizing film?
7. Define"halation":
8. Why do plastic and fiber cassettes have a sheet of lead foil in the back?
9. Reversing cassettes should never be substituted for a grid when radiographing _____ anatomy.
10. What imperfection must a silver bromide crystal have in it to develop into a silver image?
11. Image density will _____ (increase, decrease, or not be affected) when film is mismatched with screens.
12. What is used as a flexible but firm colloidal suspension for silver bromide crystals in film emulsion?
13. The shelf-life of high speed films is _____ than that of regular speed films.
14. What is solarization, and what causes it.

Part III

GEOMETRICAL FACTORS

Chapter 16

FOCAL SPOT SIZE

THE TERM *focal spot* is normally used to refer to the area on the x-ray tube anode from which x-rays are emitted, as seen from the viewpoint of the film. This area is determined by the width of the beam of electrons striking the anode and by the *bevel* or angle of the surface of the anode where the electrons impact.

The relation of the anode bevel angle to image qualities is discussed in the next chapter. The stream of high-speed electrons from the x-ray tube filament is *focused* onto a small area on the anode surface, hence the name *focal spot*. The focal spot is smaller than a pinhead, and all useful x-rays are emitted from this small area. Because the anode surface is beveled (angled), the apparent size of the focal spot depends upon the direction from which it is observed. For the purposes of this chapter, only the *effective* or *projected* focal spot size will be discussed. This is the size of the focal spot as seen from the viewpoint of the x-ray film or image receptor. Image quality is determined only by the *projected* focal spot size.

EFFECT ON SHARPNESS OF RECORDED DETAIL

The focal spot of the x-ray tube is comparable to the light source employed in shadow formation. The influence of the focal spot on detail is confined to image sharpness. With all other factors constant, *the smaller the focal spot, the sharper the recorded detail. The size of the focal spot is inversely proportional to image sharpness.* A large focal spot, although capable of withstanding high electrical energies, does not produce the sharpness of detail that is characteristic of tubes with a small focal spot. It is advantageous to use, whenever possible, a smaller focal spot with smaller tube capacities or a rotating anode tube.

The effect of focal spot size upon the sharpness of recorded details is illustrated in Figure 132 using a line-pair test pattern.

Note that smaller line pairs can be recognized when using the smaller focal spot. Increasing focal spot size reduces image sharpness because the penumbra at the edges of the details is increased (Figure 133). With more penumbra, a blurry image results. Note in Figure 133 that as penumbra grows from larger focal spots, it spreads *inward* as well as outward, invading the umbral shadow so that the umbra shrinks in size.

When excessively large focal spots are used in conjunction with long object-film distances, it is possible for the umbral shadow to shrink to the point of disappearing entirely, so that a blurry patch of penumbra is the only image left on the film and information is lost.

Figure 132. Radiographs of resolution template exhibiting the.increase in sharpness and greater number of line pairs resolved using a small focal spot (S) as compared to a large focal spot (L).

PENUMBRA

X-rays can be emitted at various angles and from different points within the area of the focal spot, and yet record the same edge of an object on the film. This means that the same edge of the object will actually be recorded several times in various different locations on the film, Figure 134. This "spreading" of the edge constitutes blur or *penumbra*. Figure 134 demonstrates

why penumbra occurs in radiography. Note that all x-rays emitted at the same angle as beam "A" but from other regions of the focal spot (dashed lines) will be absorbed by this object. All x-rays emitted at the same angle as beam "B" but from different regions of the focal spot (dotted lines) will reach the film unattenuated.

Inbetween beams "A" and "B", different amounts of x-rays are absorbed by the object depending on their angle and point

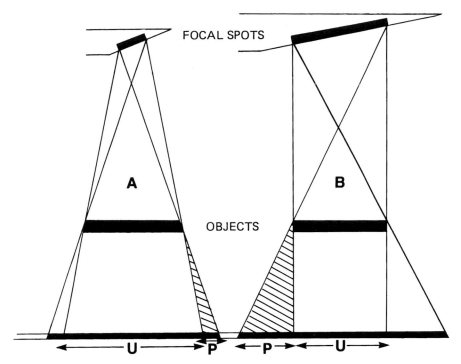

Figure 133. Diagram illustrating that larger focal spot sizes increase penumbral blur (p) but actually shrink the umbra (u). Note that the penumbra is directly proportional to the focal spot size - tripling the focal spot triples the penumbral spread or blur.

Figure 134. Diagram illustrating creation of penumbra. All x-rays parallel to *A* but emitted from the focal spot to the right of it (dashed line) are subject to absorption by the object. None of the beams parallel to *B* but emitted to the left of it (dotted lines) are subject to absorption by the object. Between *A* and *B* some beams are subject to absorption by the object and others are not. This *partial* absorption causes a partial shadow celled *penumbra*.

of origin within the focal spot. In other words, between "A" and "B" absorption of the x-ray beam is *partial,* increasing toward the object. This causes the edge gradient known as geometrical penumbra. Hence, "penumbra" may be thought of as a *partial absorption* process, (bearing in mind that "partial" refers to a portion of the total amount of x-rays which the object in question is capable of absorbing, not to a portion of the total x-ray beam).

Focal spot is directly proportional to penumbra: Doubling the FS doubles the penumbra (Figure 133).

WHEN THE FOCAL SPOT IS GREATER THAN THE OBJECT

Occasionally, an opaque object in the tissues may have a diameter less than that of the tube focal spot. If there is sufficient unsharpness caused by a long OID and a short SID, the object may be visualized as a diffuse grey area. This condition is diagrammatically represented, Figure 135, in which a small object (OB) at an extended object-film distance is shown projected by a larger focal spot (B). If details composed the object, all image details would be blurred and indistinguishable, having only the gross shape of the object. If scatter radiation undercut the object, the blurred details would be superimposed by fog, and any suggestion of image might then be entirely eliminated.

In A, the object is shown projected by a focal spot *smaller* than the diameter of the object. The image would then contain details with small blurred margins.

This effect is of great significance in angiography, because vascular embolisms and other pathology of interest may be smaller than the projected focal spot used and, therefore, would not be visibly recorded on the image, leading to misdiagnosis.

Figure 135. Diagram illustrating disappearance of umbral image when the object of interest is significantly smaller than the focal spot size used.

EFFECT ON MAGNIFICATION

The relationship of focal spot size to magnification of the image is a source of confusion for many radiographers. A review of Figure 133 will illustrate that the penumbral portion of the image spreads outward with larger focal spots, theoretically causing the image to grow in size. This fact has led many to believe that larger focal spots magnify the image. But such a notion ignores the additional fact that the umbra, the clear portion of the image, actually shrinks in size with larger focal spots, also shown in Figure 133.

A quick experiment with changing focal

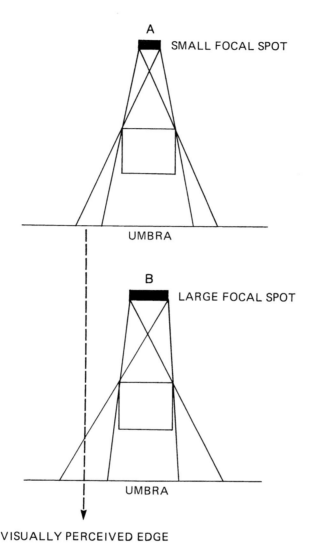

Figure 136. Diagram illustrating how the human eye locates the edge of an image at the mid-point of the penumbra regardless of the amount of penumbral spread. Hence, the apparent *size* of the image does not change with differences in focal spot.

spot sizes will demonstrate that the measured size of the *gross* image of a bone or other anatomical structure does *not* change with focal spots. Magnification of the image should be defined as an expansion of the size of *both* the *umbra* and the *penumbra*. There can be no magnification when the umbra (the most important part of the image) is actually shrinking in size. If both the umbra and the penumbra expand, magnification is present.

A clear understanding of the nature of the penumbra helps explain the apparent contradiction between the diagram in

Figure 133 and the actual results seen on radiographs. Remembering that penumbra is a spreading of the *edge* of an image both outward and inward, it may be surmised that the human eye will tend to locate the edge of the image in the *middle* of the penumbral shadow, Figure 136. Since the penumbra grows inward by an equal amount as it grows outward, its midpoint does not change location. A radiographer measuring the image will line up a ruler at this midpoint in the penumbral edge because the density change in the outer portions of the penumbra is too diffuse to see well. He will thus obtain the same measurement regardless of focal spot size.

To reiterate, focal spot size increases lead to a growth in the blur or penumbra at the edges of an image only. The umbra does not increase in size but actually shrinks. Sharpness of detail is affected, but the magnification of the gross image size is *not*. There is no relation between focal spot size and magnification.

EFFECTS ON OTHER QUALITIES

Focal spot size has no relation to distortion of the shape of the image, because it is not related to alignment or angles.

The focal spot has no controlling effect over the visibility functions of the image—density and contrast. A common misconception is that larger focal spots allow greater tube output, because the larger focal spot sizes are only available with the greater milliamperage settings on the mA knob. Small focal spots may only be used with low milliamperage because the excessive heat created by focusing a large number of electrons into a small area of the anode can damage the anode surface. But at a selected milliamperage, if a larger focal spot were used, *the same number of electrons would still be used to strike the anode.* So the output—the intensity of the x-rays emitted from the tube—remains the same and density is unaffected. Likewise, the focal spot is a geometrical rather than an electrical factor and has no influence on the energy levels in the x-ray beam. Therefore, it can have no effect upon contrast.

Noting that focal spot size affects *only* the sharpness of detail in a radiographic image and does not affect any other image qualities, focal spot size becomes the prime controlling factor over sharpness of detail. While the various distances involved in aligning the x-ray tube, patient and film have an affect upon image sharpness, they also affect other qualities such as magnification, density, contrast and noise. *The focal spot is the only technical factor which exclusively affects sharpness of detail.*

SUMMARY

1. Increasing the focal spot size results in more penumbra at the edges of an image and, therefore, reduces *sharpness* of recorded detail. Focal spot size is a primary control over sharpness, because it affects sharpness exclusively. FS size is directly proportional to blur or penumbra.

2. Focal spot size does *not* affect *magnification* of the gross image. Although penumbra spreads with larger focal spots, the umbra actually shrinks. For magnification to be apparent, the umbra must be enlarged.

3. Focal spot size has no relationship with gross image *distortion*, because it does not relate to alignment nor angles.

4. Focal spot size has no effect upon image *density*, *contrast*, or *noise* because these image qualities are not related to geometry. Focal spot changes are strictly geometrical in nature and cannot bear upon total output or energy of x-rays.

REVIEW QUESTIONS

1. What is the *only* quality that the focal spot size really controls?
2. What is the focal spot?
3. Explain *why* larger focal spots do *not* produce more x-ray intensity in the beam, resulting in a darker film image.
4. *Why* do larger focal spots *not* increase magnification of the gross image size?
5. The smaller the focal spot, the _____ the spread of penumbra.
6. Images of small details can be made to effectively disappear when the focal spot is _____ than the object.
7. Cutting the focal spot size to one-half the original, the amount of image sharpness is exactly _____ .

Chapter 17

THE ANODE BEVEL

THE ANODE *bevel* refers to the angle of the target surface of the anode in relationship to a vertical line drawn perpendicular to the axis of the x-ray tube. The angle of this surface affects both the relative size of the focal spot produced (the *line-focus principle*) and the relative distribution of the intensity of the x-rays within the beam (the *anode heel effect*).

I. LINE-FOCUS PRINCIPLE

The size of the projected effective focal spot is controlled by the width of the beam of electrons striking the anode and the angle of the anode bevel. To control the width of the electron beam, modern x-ray tubes have two different cathodes: large and small. The actual stream of electrons is considerably wider than the resulting projected focal spot.

If the anode bevel angle were exactly 45 degrees, the resulting effective focal spot would be the same width as the beam of electrons impinging on the anode surface. It is desirable, however, to reduce the size of the effective focal spot to achieve finer sharpness of details in the image, as explained in the preceding chapter. This is accomplished by the *line-focus principle*, which states that bevelling the anode at angles steeper, or more nearly vertical,

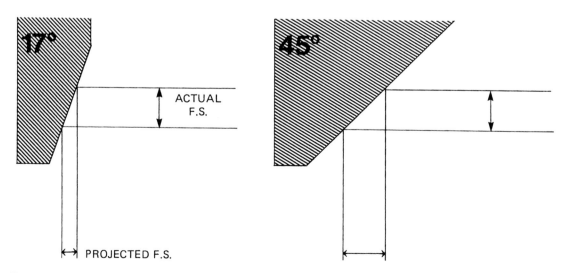

Figure 137. Diagram of the line-focus principle. By using an anode bevel angle much steeper than 45 degrees, projected focal spots much smaller than the actual focal spot can be obtained.

than 45 degrees will cause the effective focal spot to be smaller than the actual focal spot (Figure 137). This procedure allows for greater levels of image sharpness to be achieved, while maintaining adequate dispersal of heat generated over the area of

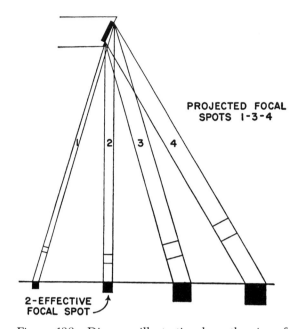

PROJECTED FOCAL SPOTS 1-3-4

2-EFFECTIVE FOCAL SPOT

Figure 138. Diagram illustrating how the size of the focal spot varies with the angle at which it is projected from the target.

the target so that anode damage does not occur. Most target angles are around 15-17 degrees. Angles steeper than this, such as those used in some special procedures tubes, can lead to severe anode heel effect and limitations on film size.

Typical *large* focal spots vary from 1 to 2 millimeters in size, while typical *small* focal spots range from 0.5 to 1 millimeter. *Fractional* focal spots used in special tubes can be as small as 0.3 mm.

From the diagram, Figure 138, it may be seen that the size of the projected focal spot varies with the angle at which it is projected from the target. When the projected focal spot is nearly perpendicular to the face of the target, it is large (4). As the angle decreases toward the central ray, the projected focal spot becomes smaller. The focal spot as projected at the central ray (2) is characteristic of the rated or effective focus of the tube. As the projected focal spot moves anode-wise from the central ray, it becomes smaller (1) until it reaches the limits of the anode side of the beam. Actually, at routine SID's, the differences in sharpness of definition are minimal and are difficult to determine visually.

II. ANODE HEEL EFFECT

Many radiographers have occasionally been puzzled by radiographic density differences which could not always be attributed to the incorrect use of exposure factors. For example, an anteroposterior radiograph of a thoracic spine would show overexposure in the upper thoracic area and underexposure in the lower thoracic area, Figure 142. This regional lack of density balance is often caused by improper alignment of the long axis of the x-ray tube to the body part so that the "heel" effect of the anode was manifested in its worst form. This inherent characteristic of all x-ray

tubes—the "heel" effect—may be employed to advantage in a limited manner to balance radiographic densities in the image.

WHAT "HEEL" EFFECT IS

The "heel" effect is a variation in x-ray intensity output along the longitudinal tube axis (depending upon the angle of x-ray emission from the focal spot). The intensity diminishes fairly rapidly from the central ray toward the *anode* side of the x-ray beam; on the *cathode* side of the beam, the intensity increases over that of the central ray and then slightly diminishes.

X-rays produced at a given point inside the anode have less distance to travel if they exit in a direction perpendicular to the anode bevel surface (toward the cathode) than they do if they exit straight down or toward the anode end of the tube (Figure 139). The anode acts as its own filter. Output is greater towards the cathode end of the tube. Figure 149 in the next chapter demonstrates this actual diminution of intensity toward the anode in the beam of x-rays.

Using average or short SID's (25 to 30 inches) and large film areas, its effect is most advantageous, particularly where decided differences in tissue densities require the balancing of radiographic densities to avoid over- and underexposures within the same image. The "heel" effect is more apparent when using steeper, more acute anode bevel angles than more obtuse

ones. For example, in order to achieve smaller focal spots and greater sharpness in special procedures suites, special x-ray tubes with anode bevel angles of 7-10 degrees from vertical are often employed. Average tube anode angles in the diagnostic department are around 17 degrees from vertical. With the steeper angle used in the special procedures tube, the anode heel effect becomes so severe with large field areas that the maximum film size used must be limited. This is the primary reason that the largest films used in angiography and similar special procedures is the 14-x-14-inch film, rather than the 14-x-17-inch film.

The anode heel effect is also more pronounced with large focal spots than with small ones, because the difference in thickness of anode material through which the x-rays must escape is greater from one end of the focal spot to the other.

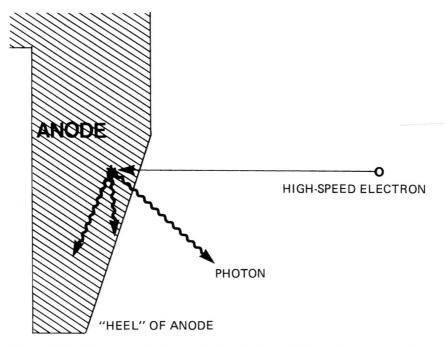

Figure 139. Diagram of the anode heel effect. X-ray photons traveling towards the cathode have less metal to penetrate out of, so beam intensity is greater in this direction.

DISTRIBUTION OF X-RAY INTENSITY OVER FILM AREA

The approximate percentage of x-ray intensity emitted by a tube at various angles of emission may be determined directly from photographic measurements of the radiographic blackening of an x-ray film. For radiographic purposes, this procedure is adequate and gives an indication of the approximate percentage of intensity variation to be expected when the x-ray beam falls on specific areas of different sizes of x-ray films at various SID's.

The mean values of radiographic density measurements obtained from many intensities emitted by various x-ray tubes are graphically shown in Figure 140. This diagram shows radii emanating from the target face, drawn at 4° intervals from 0° to 40° and intercepting horizontal lines representing various SID's. At the termination of the radii at the bottom of the chart, the mean intensity values in percentages are indicated. For convenience, the intensity at the central ray (CR) is assumed to be 100 per cent. To the left, or anode side of the central ray, the intensities diminish in value, while those to the right or cathode side, increase moderately and then decrease slightly.

A radiographic illustration of the differences in intensity is shown in Figure 141. A wire mesh was placed on a 14-x-17-inch film. The long axis of the tube was aligned on the center film axis, and the anode portion of the beam was directed toward the top edge of the film. An exposure at a film distance of 20 inches caused the upper portion of the image of the mesh to have less density than the bottom portion where the cathode portion of the beam exposed the film.

INTENSITY-FILM AREA RELATION

Consulting Figure 140, the vertical dotted lines beginning just below the diagram of the cathode and terminating at the 72-inch SID distance line, indicate various film lengths. Source-image receptor distances are shown as solid horizontal lines. The respective intensity values created by the radiation emitted at various angles of x-ray emission at various SID's is shown at the bottom. For example, on the 48-inch SID line the outermost pair of vertical lines representing the 36-inch length of film passes outside the limits of the x-ray beam. In order to make use of the entire range of intensities on this length of film, it would be necessary to employ a source-image receptor distance of 49 inches. All intensity radii would intercept at this distance; consequently, if an exposure were made, the entire range of intensities would be expected to become evident, let us say, on a radiograph of an entire spine. Since the minimal intensity in the anode portion of the beam, approximately 31 per cent, is emitted in advance to the angle indicated as 0°, it is obvious that the portion of the spine having the least tissue density (the neck) should be exposed by this portion of the beam, and the heavier portion (the lumbar vertebrae) should be exposed by the cathode portion of the beam.

When radiographs on large film are made at relatively short SID's, the percentage distribution of x-ray intensity delivered to a particular size of film at a known source-image receptor distance should be known. This knowledge will aid in correct alignment of the tube and part to the film at the most favorable SID. Radiographic densities cannot be balanced if only the intensity of the central ray is considered.

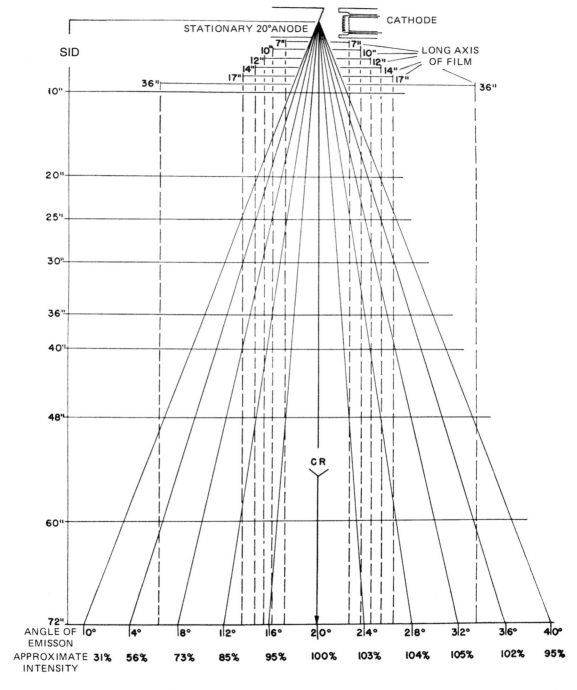

Figure 140. Graphic illustration of the mean values of radiographic density measurements over the x-ray beam at different source-image receptor distances obtained from many intensities emitted by various x-ray tubes.

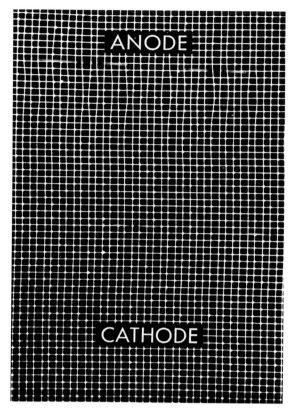

Figure 141. Radiographic illustration of the anode heel effect using a wire mesh image. Note that the cathode end of the film is somewhat darker than the anode end.

Example 1. An example of the "heel" effect is demonstrated by a radiograph, Figure 142, *Left,* of the thoracic vertebrae in which the cathode portion of the beam was directed cephalically. Note the high density in the upper thoracic region and the insufficient density in the lower thoracic vertebrae. By correctly applying the "heel" effect, a radiograph, Figure 142, *Right,* was obtained in which all the densities were properly balanced in the image because the anode portion of the beam was directed cephalically. Note that the densities are less in the upper thoracic region and greater in the lower thoracic area.

Example 2. To demonstrate the influence of the source-image receptor on the "heel" effect, a series of anteroposterior radi-

ographs of the humerus, Figure 143, A-D, were made. Radiograph A was made with a SID of 20 inches and the anode portion of the x-ray beam was directed cephalically. Note the underexposure of the upper portion of the humerus and the overexposure of the distal end. The intensity of the radiation passing to the heavier end of the humerus was insufficient and that portion of the beam passing to the thinner distal end overexposed the area. Radiograph B was made with the same exposure factors after the tube axis was rotated 180°. It may be seen that all densities have been approximately equalized. Radiograph C was made with a 40-inch SID and the anode portion of the beam was directed cephalically.

Note that, because the center portion of the beam only was employed, there was little variation in intensity and all areas have a fairly uniform density. Yet, radiograph D, also made with a 40-inch SID after the tube axis was rotated 180°, shows no improvement over the densities depicted in radiograph C. This example demonstrates that as the SID increases, the "heel" effect diminishes.

RULE. When body parts of unequal thickness or tissue density are to be recorded the following rule should be observed.

Align the long axis of the x-ray tube with the long center axis of the part and film, and direct the cathode portion of the x-ray beam toward the anatomic area of greatest tissue density or thickness.

It should be observed that the "heel" effect diminishes with an increase in the SID and with the use of small size films, since the more uniform intensities of radiation exist in the neighborhood of the central ray. Its greatest effect is observed when the source-image receptor distance is relatively short, when a large film is employed and the body part is unequal in thickness or tissue density.

Figure 142. Screen-grid radiographs of the AP thoracic spine demonstrating the density variation caused by the anode heel effect. (*Left*) cathode portion of beam directed toward the head. (*Right*) cathode portion of beam directed toward the thicker abdomen, resulting in more balanced densities throughout the T-spine.

SUMMARY

1. The line-focus principle demonstrates that the steeper the anode bevel angle, the smaller will be the projected focal spot size, and therefore greater *sharpness* of recorded detail will be obtained and smaller anatomical images may be recorded. A resulting disadvantage is that smaller field sizes may have to be used.

2. The *anode heel effect* demonstrates that the anode acts as its own filter and, due to the anode surface bevel, results in less image density toward the anode end of the radiograph. For this reason, when radiographing anatomy of variable thickness, the thinner end of the anatomy must always be placed toward the anode end of the tube.

3. The anode heel effect is more visible with steeper anode bevel angles, larger focal spots, shorter distances and longer field sizes

Figure 143. Radiographs of humerus illustrating the heel effect at (A and B) 20 inches SID and (C and D) 40 inches SID. Note that the effect is worse at the short 20 inch distance used in (A) and (B). The most balanced view is (D), taken at 40 inches and with the cathode at the thicker end of the humerus.

REVIEW QUESTIONS

1. Using an anode bevel angle of less than 45 degrees causes the projected focal spot to be smaller than the actual focal spot. This relationship is called the _____ .

2. At the "anode-end" of the film the projected focal spot is _____ than the cathode end.

3. In the anode heel effect, explain *why* less x-rays exit the anode toward its own side of the tube than toward the cathode.

4. For an AP thoracic spine radiograph, place the patient with the head toward the _____ end of the x-ray tube.

5. A "fractional" focal spot in a special procedures x-ray tube is usually in what size range?

6. At a shorter SID, the collimator must be opened up to cover the same field size and the anode heel effect is _____ (increased, decreased, or not affected).

Chapter 18

SOURCE-IMAGE RECEPTOR DISTANCE

The distance from the x-ray tube to the film or other image receptor is very important because it has substantial influence upon three image qualities: (1) radiographic image density, (2) magnification of the size of the projected image, and (3) the sharpness of recorded detail. Since this distance is also easily manipulated by the radiographer, it has come to be considered by many as a *fourth* prime factor of radiography, along with mA, exposure time, and kVp.

Source-image receptor distance, abbreviated *SID*, is known by many names. It is sometimes called the *target-film distance* (*TFD*) or the *focus-film distance* (*FFD*). It is measured from the *focal spot* or *target* on the x-ray tube anode to the film holder.

ESTIMATING SID

The source of x-radiation is the surface of the anode within the x-ray tube, located roughly in the middle of the cylindrical tube housing. In mobile radiography or when a measuring tape is not immediately available, the SID may be estimated by extending one arm so that the fingertips are at the middle of the tube housing (not the collimator). *For an average male in the United States, 40 inches will correspond to the distance from the fingertips to the opposite side shoulder of the body.* With the fingertips at the tube, the film or image receptor should be about at the opposite shoulder. *Extending both arms, 72 inches will be slightly more than the distance from fingertip to fingertip.*

For the average U.S. female radiographer, the same guidelines may be used, only measuring to the collimator rather than to the tube. Obviously, one must adjust these rules of thumb if one is much shorter or taller than average, but these guidelines are particularly useful for mobile radiography.

EFFECT ON SHARPNESS OF RECORDED DETAIL

When the x-ray tube is moved farther away from the film and object, the amount of blur or penumbra produced at the edges of the image diminishes. As illustrated in Figure 144, this occurs because those beams recording the edges of the image are more vertical - nearer and more parallel to the central ray. Thus, the SID has a direct effect upon image sharpness: The longer the SID, the sharper the image, and vice versa. As a rule then, the maximum feasible SID should always be used in order to optimize image sharpness.

In practice, several considerations limit the SID we can use: When radiographing patients recumbent on the table with a vertical beam, the technologist cannot reach the tube if it is too high. (When using the upright chest board, in *most* cases one has the option to use 72 inches SID on exposures that would normally be done at 40 inches SID, since the tube can be easily moved horizontally, and the increased sharpness only benefits the image.) The main limitation is that the greater the SID, the more technique is required to maintain image density. For large anatomy, extreme distances would result in high techniques that might damage the x-ray tube. If exposure time is used to increase technique, the probability of unsharpness caused by patient motion increases. Given these constraints, the maximum *feasible* SID should be used.

It is important to understand that, in reality, it is the *source-object distance*, the *SOD*, that is directly responsible for these effects upon image sharpness. Any calculations to predict image sharpness or unsharpness must employ the SOD rather than the SID. The specific geometry controlling image sharpness is discussed in Chapter Twenty. It may be stated that *image sharpness is directly proportional to the SOD.* Any increase in the SID will always result in an increase in the SOD, as long as the distance between an object and the film is maintained. The increased SOD will, in turn, enhance image sharpness as demonstrated in Figure 145.

EFFECT ON MAGNIFICATION

At a set object-image distance, *increasing the SID results in less magnification* of the image size. The diagram in Figure 146 clearly shows that when a longer SID is employed, not only is there less penumbra produced, but the clear umbral portion of the image is reduced in size as well. For all objects which lie at any significant distance from the film, the magnification produced is quite noticeable, Figure 147. For most applications, magnification is undesirable, and generally the maximum practical SID should be used to minimize magnification.

As long as the object is placed directly on the film cassette, as in tabletop radiography, the effects of SID changes become insignificant. But, any anatomy which cannot be placed directly upon the film, such as organs in the middle of the body, will be significantly magnified and blurred by a shorter SID.

The control of magnification by using long source-image distances is of special importance for routine chest radiography. More than one-half of all chest radiographs are ordered primarily to determine heart

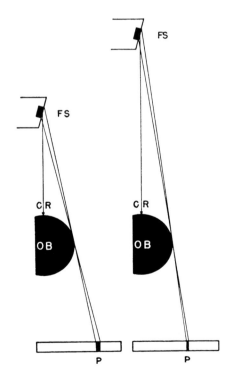

Figure 144. Diagram illustrating that longer source-image distances minimize penumbral shadows and thus improve sharpness of detail.

Figure 145. Radiographs of resolution test template taken with a fixed OID of 8 inches. Arrows demarcate blur points. For Exposure A, 24 inches SID was used to obtain an SOD of 16 inches, resolving 1.23 line pairs per millimeter. For Exposure B, the SID was increased to 40 inches in order to obtain and SOD of 32 inches, resolving 2.46 line pairs per millimeter, and showing a directly proportional relationship between the SOD and image sharpness.

size and condition. Magnification is always present to some degree in radiographic projections. For heart size measurements to be accurate, the magnification of the projected heart "shadow " must be negligible. The heart is relatively anterior in the body, closer to the sternum than to the patient's back. Routine chests are done in posterior-anterior projection in order to place the heart as close as possible to the film, but because a significant distance is still present between the heart and the film, the SID must be increased well beyond the usual 40 inches.

The use of extended distances in order to eliminate visible magnification is referred to as *teleradiography*, meaning "far radiography." Teleradiography should be used for chest series whenever possible–the recommended SID is 96 inches (8 feet), and dedicated chest units are usually installed with the x-ray tube permanently set at 96 inches. When chest series are performed with general radiographic units, 72 inches is con-

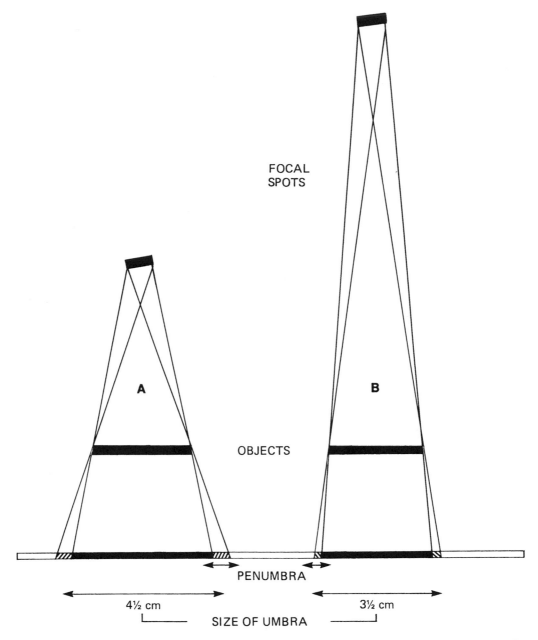

Figure 146. Diagram showing how longer SID's reduce the size of *both* the umbra and the penumbra, reducing magnification of the image. (A) 40 inches SID, (B) 72 inches SID.

ventionally used. Slight visible magnification of the heart is present at 72 inches, but it is at an acceptably low level for most diagnostic purposes.

There are occasions when the magnifica-

tion and blurring effects of a short SID may be used to advantage. A visibility problem is created any time the anatomy of interest is superimposed by contrasty anatomy which is not of interest. This problem can

Figure 147. Radiographs demonstrating magnification of an object from short SID, with a fixed OID of 4 inches. (A) 40 inches SID, (B) 20 inches SID.

often be resolved by using positioning and beam angles to project the image *around* the obstructing anatomy. In the case of the sternoclavicular or temporomandibular joints, the contrasty bones of the upper side of the head present a problem which is not adequately solved by angles. A short SID in the range of 26-30 inches should be used on all such procedures and techniques adjusted appropriately. The short SID will both magnify and blur the upside bones to the extent that the anatomy of interest on the down side, against the film, will be more visible through it. The anatomy of interest which is against the film is affected only in a negligible amount. The combination of positioning, angling the beam and using a short SID will result in the highest-quality radiograph. This technique may also be used in other similar cases such as with the sternoclavicular joints and sternum, which are superimposed by the contrasty spine and ribs.

EFFECT ON SHAPE DISTORTION

Shape distortion is a complex function of the alignment and angling of the x-ray beam and the shape of the object being radiographed. It is thoroughly discussed in Chapter 21. Only effects directly attributable to distance will be discussed at this point.

Figure 147 demonstrates that although

changes in SID will affect the magnification of an image, the shape of the image does *not* change as long as the object is centered in the x-ray beam and the beam is not angled. A circular object will still be circular (not oval) and a square will still be a square (not a rectangle).

Reviewing the definitions of magnification and distortion, it will be recalled that shape distortion only occurs when the measurement of an object in one dimension changes more than that in the opposite dimension—length changes more than width or vice versa. As long as both dimensions, length and width, increase by the same ratio, it may be said that the image is magnified but not distorted. Changes in SID do not distort the shape of an image.

Some confusion has resulted in this area, because an image which is *already* distorted is more obvious when it is also magnified.

Consider a spherical object which is being projected onto the film by an angled beam as an oval-shaped image. Distortion of the shape has already been caused by this tube angle. Reducing the source-image distance will magnify the total image. Both the length and the width of the oval will increase by proportionate amounts. However, the ratio of length/width is still equal, and *shape* has not changed. The distance change is not responsible for any distortion which may be present but only for the magnification of the total image size. Images may be *both* distorted in shape and magnified in size, but each of these problems results from a different cause. Distortion of shape is never *caused* by changes in SID. It may, however, be made more apparent because of the magnification effect of SID changes.

EFFECT ON DENSITY

Intensity directly influences radiographic density; any change in distance will cause a change in density when other factors are constant. *Only a 20 per cent change in distance will cause a visible change in image density and will require an adjustment in technique,* a fact the radiographer must be aware of.

Since x-rays conform to the laws of light, they diverge as they are emitted from the focal spot, and, proceeding in straight paths, cover an increasingly larger area with *lessened* intensity as they travel from their source. This principle is illustrated in the diagram (Figure 148). It is assumed that the intensity of the x-rays emitted at the focal spot (FS) remains the same, and that the x-rays cover an area of 4 square inches on reaching the horizontal plane (C) which is 12 inches from FS. When the source-image distance is increased to 24

inches to plane D or twice the distance between FS and C, the x-rays will cover 16 square inches—an area 4 times as great as that at C. It follows, therefore, that the intensity of the radiation per square inch on the plane at D is only one quarter that at the level C.

The diminution of intensity of the x-ray beam as it travels further and further away from the focal spot in accordance with the inverse square law may be observed in the radiograph (Figure 149). This image was produced by placing one edge of a 14-x -17inch film contained in an exposure holder at the portal of the x-ray tube. An exposure was made and the film processed. The top of the image was at the tube portal. Note the high density in this area. As the radiation coursed downward along the film, the x-ray intensity gradually diminished, hence the loss in radiographic densi-

Figure 149. Flash x-ray exposure with film placed vertically in beam to demonstrate decrease in intensity of radiation as distance increases from the source. The anode heel effect is also noted in this radiograph toward the anode end of the exposure field.

Figure 148. Diagram illustrating the inverse square law. Doubling the distance allows the beam to spread out over a four-fold area, reducing exposure to one-quarter.

ty as the SID increased. The difference in density along a horizontal plane through the beam from the anode to the cathode side is due to the "heel effect" (see Chapter 17).

THE INVERSE SQUARE LAW

This relationship between distance and radiographic density follows the *inverse square law*, which may be stated as:

$$\frac{\text{Original density}}{\text{New density}} = \frac{(\text{New SID})^2}{(\text{Original SID})^2}$$

Let us apply this formula to the distance change illustrated in Figure 148 as an example. In this case, the original distance was 12 inches, and the new distance is 24 inches. Let us assign the original density a value of 1.0, and find how the new density would compare—The formula should be set up as follows:

$$\frac{1}{\text{New Density}} = \frac{(24)^2}{(12)^2}$$

and solving:

$$\frac{1}{X} = \frac{576}{144}$$

$$576X = 144$$

$$X = 144/576$$

$$X = 0.25$$

The new density will be 25 per cent, or one quarter, of the original. This agrees with the diagram in Figure 148, for there are four times as many squares across which the x-ray beam has spread. Each square must have one-fourth the original exposure.

Simple inverse square law problems can be solved mentally by simply applying the *name of the law* to the *proportional change in distance. Invert* the change, then square it. For example, if the distance is reduced to one-half the original, what would the resulting density be? Mentally invert one-half– this is two. Now square two. The radiograph will be four times darker if it is exposed at one-half the distance and no compensation is made. One third the distance results in nine times the exposure, tripling the distance results in one-ninth the exposure, and so on.

Try the following brief exercise, and check your answers from the Appendix.

EXERCISE: 19

Use the inverse square law to solve these problems:

	FROM	TO
1	40" SID	72" SID
	Density = 1	Density = _____
2.	60" SID	72" SID
	Density = 1	Density = _____
3.	50" SID	36" SID
	Density = 1	Density = _____
4.	72" SID	96" SID
	Density = 1	Density = _____

The inverse square law works because the x-ray beam *fans out* across greater areas as it travels, and to find an area, one must square the length of its sides. The following experiment and Figure 148 demonstrate the effect of increasing distance upon image density when all other factors are kept constant.

EXPERIMENT NO. 1–SID DENSITY RELATION

Purpose. To demonstrate the relation between source-image receptor distance and radiographic density.

Theory. Any change in SID influences the intensity of radiation. The intensity varies inversely as the square of the SID. Since changes in SID produce changes in intensity, radiographic density changes.

Procedure

1. The SID-density relation can be readily demonstrated by making a series of three posteroanterior radiographs of the hand using the following materials and exposure factors:

Materials	Film:	Screen-type, 8 x 10-inch
	Exposure holder:	8 x 10-inch
Factors	kVp:	50
	mA:	50
	Time:	1 sec.
	mAs:	50
Variable	Exposure No.	SID
Factors	1	25 inches
	2	36 inches
	3	48 inches

Comment. It may be observed that *as the SID increased, the radiographic density diminished* because the intensity of the x-radiation reaching the film diminished (Figure 150).

THE SQUARE LAW

Distance changes should usually be compensated for by using mAs, rather than kVp. Changes in distance alter the intensity of the x-ray beam–energy levels or penetrating ability are not affected. Adjusting the mAs restores the original intensity of the beam, without changing its quality. If kVp is used to compensate, the altered penetration of the beam will lead to different con-

Figure 150. Demonstration of effect of increasing SID on radiographic density on hand radiographs. Note the loss of density at increased distances: (A) 25 inches SID, (B) 36 inches SID, and (C) 48 inches SID, all other factors equal.

Figure 151. Demonstration of time-SID relation on hand radiographs, maintaining density by using the adjustment factors in Table XVII. Factors: (A) 25 inches SID with 25 mAs, (B) 36 inches SID with 50 mAs, and (C) 48 inches with 90 mAs, all other factors equal.

trast levels in the image, an undesirable side-effect.

Whereas the inverse square law is used to predict image density, the *Square Law* is used to compensate technique so that density is maintained when distance changes. The formula for the square law is

$$\frac{\text{Original mAs}}{\text{New mAs}} = \frac{(\text{Original SID})^2}{(\text{New SID})^2}$$

Simply stated, the change in technique should be equal to the square of the change in distance. If the distance were doubled, as illustrated in Figure 148 the technique change required to maintain density would be *2 squared* or 4 times the original.

Suppose 20 mAs had been used for the exposure taken at 12 inches in Figure 144. What new mAs would be required for an exposure taken at 24 inches? Using the formula:

$$\frac{20 \text{ mAs}}{X} = \frac{(12)^2}{(24)^2}$$

$$\frac{20 \text{ mAs}}{X} = \frac{144}{576}$$

$$144X = 20(256)$$

$$144X = 11,520$$

$$X = 11,520/144$$

$$x = 80$$

At 24 inches, 80 mAs would be required to maintain the original density level. Note

TABLE XVII
mAs Multiplying Factors for Use When SID Is Changed

Original SID	New SID								mAs Multiplying Factors
	20"	25"	30"	36"	40"	48"	60"	72"	
20"	1.00	1.56	2.25	3.22	4.00	5.76	9.00	12.96	
25"	.64	1.00	1.44	2.07	2.56	3.68	5.76	8.29	
30"	.44	.69	1.00	1.44	1.77	2.56	4.00	5.76	
36"	.31	.48	.69	1.00	1.23	1.77	2.77	4.00	
40"	.25	.39	.56	.81	1.00	1.44	2.25	3.24	
48"	.17	.27	.39	.59	.69	1.00	1.56	2.25	
60"	.11	.17	.25	.36	.44	.64	1.00	1.44	
72"	.08	.12	.17	.25	.31	.44	.69	1.00	
	mAs Multiplying Factors								

that this is four times the original mAs. Table XVII was derived using this formula. If the original mAs is unknown, a "1" may be placed in the formula, and the resulting number will be a *factor* by which mAs must be multiplied.

Experiment No. 2 and Figure 151 prove that the square law works in maintaining density. Note that, from exposure #1 to exposure #3, the distance is nearly doubled (from 25 inches to 48 inches), while the mAs was nearly quadrupled (from 25 mAs to 90 mAs). Inspection of the resulting radiographs in Figure 151 reveals a constant density level.

Following this experiment are three examples of applying the square law, one for an adjustment in exposure time, one for total mAs, and one for a mAs adjustment factor.

EXPERIMENT NO. 2 –TIME-SID DENSITY RELATION

Purpose. To demonstrate the interrelation of time of exposure and source-image dis-

tance to radiographic density when all other factors are constant.

Theory. The time required for a given radiographic density is directly proportional to the *square* of the SID when all other factors are constant.

Procedure

1. The time-SID relation may be demonstrated by making a series of three posteroanterior radiographs of the hand employing the following materials and exposure factors:

Materials	Film:	Screen-type, 8 x 10-inch		
	Exposure holder:	8 x 10-inch		
Factors	kVp:	50		
	mA:	50		
Variable	Exposure No.	SID	Time	mAs
Factors	1	25 inches	1/2 sec.	25
	2	36 inches	1 sec.	50
	3	48 inches	$1^{8/10}$ sec.	90

Comment. In comparing these radiographs, (Figure 151) it may be seen that the densities are approximately the same because suitable exposure time compensation has been made for each SID change in accordance with the square law. Since the SID has a material effect on radiographic density, it is recommended that once an SID is established for a given projection that it should be considered a constant. When some unusual need arises for varying the SID, the square formula should be used to equalize density.

EXAMPLE NO. 1–TIME AND SID

RULE. The exposure time required for a given radiographic density is directly proportional to the *square* of the SID when the remaining factors are constant. This rule may be expressed by the following formula for the purpose of solving the exposure problems:

$$\frac{\text{Original Time}}{\text{New Time}} = \frac{\text{Original SID}^2}{\text{New SID}^2}$$

Example. Assume that an exposure time of 10 seconds (T_1) and an SID of 30 inches (D_1) have been used, and it is desired to decrease the SID to 24 inches (D_2). What exposure time (T_2) would be required?

Solution. T_1, D_1, and D_2 are known; T_2 is unknown. The following working equation adapted from the above basic formula should be employed to solve the problem:

$$T2 = \frac{(T_1)(D_2)^2}{(D_1)^2}$$

$$T2 = \frac{10 \times 24^2}{30^2} = \frac{10 \times 4^2}{5^2} = 6.4 \text{ sec. Answer.}$$

EXAMPLE NO. 2–MAS AND SID

RULE. The mAs required to produce a given radiographic density is proportional to the *square* of the SID when the remaining factors are constant. This rule may be expressed by the following formula for the purpose of solving exposure problems:

$$\frac{\text{Original mAs}}{\text{New mAs}} = \frac{\text{Original SID}^2}{\text{New SID}^2}$$

Example. Assume that an exposure of 10 mAs (M_1) at an SID of 25 inches (D_1) is employed. The SID is increased to 60 inches (D_2). What mAs (M_2) must be employed to maintain the same radiographic density?

Solution. M_1, D_1, and D_2 are known; M_2 is unknown. The following working equation adapted from the above formula should be used to solve the problem:

$$M2 = \frac{M_1(D_2)^2}{(D_1)^2}$$

$$M2 = \frac{10 \times 60^2}{25^2} = \frac{36000}{625} = 57.6 \text{ mAs. Answer.}$$

To facilitate the mathematics involved, Table XVII may be employed to determine mAs values when common SID values are changed. For example, under the column headed "Original SID" find 25 inches. Find the vertical column headed by the new SID of 60 inches. Where these two columns intersect will be found the mAs multiplying factor 5.76. Multiply the original mAs of 10 by 5.76. The answer is 57.6 mAs.

EXAMPLE NO. 3–TECHNIQUE CHANGE FACTOR AND SID

RULE. The factor by which technique must be changed to maintain a given density is proportional to the *square* of the SID when all other factors are constant. This rule may be expressed by the formula:

$$\frac{1}{X} = \frac{\text{Original SID}^2}{\text{New SID}^2}$$

Example: Suppose the SID is increased from 40 inches to 60 inches. The technique chart lists a technique for 40 inches. What change would need to be made in the mAs from the chart to maintain adequate density at 60 inches SID?

$$\frac{1}{X} = \frac{40^2}{60^2}$$ Since the actual mAs is not given, place a 1 for "mAs_1" D_1 is 40 inches and D_2 is 60.

$$\frac{1}{X} = \frac{1600}{3600}$$ Square the distances

$$1600(X) = 3600$$ Cross-multiply.

$$X = \frac{3600}{1600}$$ Isolate X by dividing both sides of the equation by 1600.

$$X = 2.25$$ This is the *factor* by which mAs should be changed

The 40-inch technique should be increased 2.25 times to maintain density at 60 inches SID.

The solutions to square law problems are always the inverse of those for solving inverse square law problems. For example, if a distance change would result in twice as dark a film by the inverse square law, then the technique that would be required in order to maintain the original density at the new distance would be one-half the mAs. If the density change can be predicted, simply invert this change to find the technique adjustment.

Try the following exercise and check your answers from the Appendix. You will need to find square roots to solve for the distance in numbers 7 and 8. Calculators are allowed!

EXERCISE 20

Use the square law to solve these problems:

1. $\dfrac{5\text{ mAs}}{50\text{" SID}} = \dfrac{\rule{2cm}{0.4pt}\text{ mAs}}{60\text{" SID}}$

2. $\dfrac{2.5\text{ mAs}}{40\text{" SID}} = \dfrac{\rule{2cm}{0.4pt}\text{ mAs}}{72\text{" SID}}$

3. $\dfrac{2.5\text{ mAs}}{60\text{" SID}} = \dfrac{\rule{2cm}{0.4pt}\text{ mAs}}{20\text{" SID}}$

4. $\dfrac{12\text{ mAs}}{96\text{" SID}} = \dfrac{\rule{2cm}{0.4pt}\text{ mAs}}{30\text{" SID}}$

5. $\dfrac{25\text{ mAs}}{96\text{" SID}} = \dfrac{\rule{2cm}{0.4pt}\text{ mAs}}{40\text{" SID}}$

6. $\dfrac{40\text{ mAs}}{80\text{" SID}} = \dfrac{\rule{2cm}{0.4pt}\text{ mAs}}{36\text{" SID}}$

7. $\dfrac{180\text{ mAs}}{96\text{" SID}} = \dfrac{20\text{ mAs}}{\rule{2cm}{0.4pt}\text{ SID}}$

8. $\dfrac{45\text{ mAs}}{90\text{" SID}} = \dfrac{5\text{ mAs}}{\rule{2cm}{0.4pt}\text{ SID}}$

RULES OF THUMB FOR DISTANCE CHANGES

Although the inverse square law is important to understand, in practice radiographers rarely use a calculator or pencil to apply it accurately—Rather, when doing a mobile procedure at 60 inches SID, for example, they will likely make a mental estimate of the increase in technique required when compared to the usual 40-inch SID. This section provides some simple rules of thumb which, if committed to memory, will greatly improve your accuracy in making this kind of technique adjustment.

A handful of distances (30 inches, 40, 60, 72 and 96 inches), applies to more than 95 per cent of radiographic procedures. By taking the most commonly used 40 inches as a standard and comparing the others to it, rules of thumb are easily derived and learned.

It helps to think of distance changes in factors of two, that is, doublings and halvings. For example, the square law formula shows that if SID is increased from 40 inches to 80 inches (a doubling), the technique must be increased by 4 times in order to maintain density. However, by thinking of this quadrupling of the technique as *two doublings*, rules of thumb can be formulated for other distance changes:

Think of increasing the SID from 40 inches to 60 inches as going *half-way to doubling* the SID. That is, 60 inches is halfway from 40 to 80. Since 80 inches would require two doublings of technique, 60 inches will require one-half of that increase, or *one doubling*. For a 60-inch projection, double the mAs used at 40 inches.

In a similar manner, 30 inches can be considered as half-way to cutting 40 inches in half. A 20-inch distance would require $1/4$ of the overall technique, or two halvings. Thus, 30 inches requires only one halving of the 40-inch technique.

Table XVIII summarizes these rules of thumb for the most used distances. A column listing the actual solution based on the square law formula is provided as well so that you can see how close these rules of thumb are for accuracy. Keeping in mind that density must be changed by at least 30 per cent to see a visible difference, the rules of thumb are clearly accurate enough for practical use.

Radiographers performing mobile procedures must be especially wary of the fact

TABLE XVIII
Rules of Thumb for Distance Changes
Starting at 40 inches

New Distance	Technique Change Computed by the Square Law	Rule of Thumb Technique Change
30 inches	0.56	$1/2$
40 inches	1.0 (standard)	1
60 inches	2.25	2 x
72 inches	3.24	3 x
80 inches	4.0	4 x
96 inches	5.76	6 x

that only a 20 per cent change in SID will result in an unacceptable density level unless technique is adjusted. A classic example occurs when a radiographer who places the mobile unit at the foot of the patient's bed for an AP chest exposure asks another radiographer for a technique. If the advice-giver is used to placing the

mobile unit alongside the bed, he may be using as little as 55-60 inches SID. Using his technique at 72 inches (x-ray tube near the foot of the bed) will result in such a light exposure that a repeat will be needed. *A ten-inch difference in SID is always significant enough to require a technique adjustment.*

By far, the most useful of these rules of thumb will be those for 60 inches and 72 inches because these distances are frequently used both in mobile procedures and in the radiology department. For mobile procedures, the rules of thumb can be taken one step further to derive a technique for 50 inches SID:

Considering 50 as the half-way to 60, the technique would be increased half-way to doubling, or increased 50 per cent. By the square law formula, the needed increase is 1.57 times the original. The rule of thumb rounds it to 1.5 times. Radiographers assigned to mobile units should remember that *compared to the usual 40-inch technique, a 50-inch SID requires a 50 per cent increase in overall technique* (preferably using mAs), *a 60-inch distance requires a doubling, and a 72-inch distance requires a tripling.*

Since chest radiography is commonly performed with the 72-inch SID, it is well to emphasize that the 72-inch distance requires 3 times the 40-inch technique, and that a 40-inch distance requires $1/3$ of the 72-inch technique. This relationship is frequently encountered in performing upright or decubitus abdomen radiographs along with chest radiographs. Remember that the *relationship between a 40-inch SID and a 72-inch SID is a factor of 3.*

These rules of thumb can also be used to solve for density problems, if you remember to invert them (make fractions out of them). For example, if the distance is increased from 40 inches to 72 inches, and the technique is NOT compensated for this change, how dark will the radiograph be? Simply invert the factor for 72 inches from

Table XVIII. The answer is that the new radiograph will have $1/3$ the density of the original. A radiograph taken at 60 inches without compensating technique would be $1/2$ as dense as a 40-inch radiograph, and so on.

Complete the following exercise *mentally, using the rules of thumb*. Note that those starting at 60 inches or 30 inches can also be solved in your head, if you analyze the distance changes as doubling, halving, halfway to doubling, or half-way to halving. Check and review your answers using the Appendix.

EXERCISE #21

Use the technique rules of thumb to solve these problems:

	FROM	*To MAINTAIN DENSITY*
1	25 mAs	_____ mAs
	40" SID	72" SID
2	15 mAs	_____ mAs
	40" SID	60" SID
3	7.5 mAs	_____ mAs
	40" SID	80" SID
4	6 mAs	_____ mAs
	40" SID	96" SID
5	60 mAs	_____ mAs
	40" SID	20" SID
6	2.5 mAs	_____ mAs
	30" SID	60" SID
7	30 mAs	_____ mAs
	40" SID	30" SID
8	12.5 mAs	_____ mAs
	30" SID	45" SID

EFFECT ON CONTRAST

Although the intensity of both the secondary and the primary radiation in a beam changes as the inverse square of the distance changes made, they both change by the same proportion. Therefore, at any distance in the beam, the *ratio* of scattered x-rays to primary x-rays will remain the same. Since there is no change in the relative proportion of scatter in the beam, image contrast will not be affected (see Figure 151). Two adjacent densities may both be lighter or darker, but the ratio of difference between them will be unchanged.

Source-image receptor distance, as a controlling factor over density, is similar in its effects to mAs. Both simply control the intensity of the beam. Like mAs, very extreme changes in SID leading to a blank underexposed film or to an overexposed film will clearly destroy the contrast of the image. But within the diagnostic ranges of distances used in real practice, SID is not a consideration in controlling contrast.

SUMMARY

1. A longer SID reduces penumbra and therefore increases *sharpness* of recorded detail. Increasing the SID extends the SOD. Sharpness is *directly proportional to the SOD.*

2. A longer SID reduces the amount of image *magnification*. Magnification is *inversely proportional* to the SID.

3. Source-image distance is not directly related to alignment of the beam and part and does not affect shape *distortion*. Once shape distortion is present in the

image, the magnification effect of distance may make it more or less noticeable. But distance changes do not cause distortion.

4. Increasing source-image distance reduces image *density* by the inverse square law, because the area over which the x-rays are distributed spreads out with distance.

5. Regarding *technique*, the square law may be used to accurately compensate mAs values for changes in SID.

6. SID has no effect upon image *contrast* within typical diagnostic ranges, because the numbers of x-rays penetrating through the patient, interacting by Compton effect, and interacting by photoelectric effect, are all changed by the same proportion, so that the ratio between them is unaffected.

7. *Teleradiography* using an SID of 96 inches is recommended for routine chest radiography, to reduce magnification of the heart.

REVIEW QUESTIONS

1. Decreasing SID _____ penumbra. (Increases, decreases, or has no effect on)

2. Why would you intentionally use a short SID on such procedures as sternoclavicular joints or temporomandibular joints?

3. List the *three* image qualities which are affected by changes in SID.

4. Image density is related to changes in the SID by the _____ law.

5. If the density of one radiograph is 4 times greater than that of another, all other factors equal, the SID must have been changed to a factor of _____ the original.

6. A technique chart lists $1/20$ second for a procedure using 40 inches SID. At an SID of 80 inches, what new time would be required to maintain density?

7. As a rule, the _____ feasible SID should always be used.

8. Increasing SID _____ magnification. (Increases, decreases, or has no effect on)

9. Any change in distance of _____ per cent or greater will require an adjustment in technique.

10. What does "teleradiography" mean?

11. Changing from 72 inches SID to 40 inches SID, technique must be adjusted to _____ the original.

12. Image sharpness is directly proportional to which distance?

13. Image magnification is inversely proportional to which distance?

Chapter 19

OBJECT-IMAGE RECEPTOR DISTANCE

OBJECT-IMAGE RECEPTOR DISTANCE is a crucial factor in controlling radiographic image quality. Although it is primarily a geometric, *recognizability* factor, it affects most of the aspects of the radiograph, directly or indirectly, in dramatic fashion. When the object is placed directly upon the radiographic film, all of the image qualities are optimized. Relatively small changes, such as placing the film four inches away from the anatomy, result in large effects on density, contrast, sharpness, and magnification. Therefore, every effort should be made to minimize the OID on all radiographic procedures.

EFFECT ON SHARPNESS OF RECORDED DETAIL

When the object is at some distance from the film as shown in diagram, Figure 152, the sharpness is not as great as it is when the object is next to the film. *The larger the object-image distance, the greater the penumbra grows, and therefore the less the sharpness of recorded detail.* Image sharpness and OID are inversely proportional. The use of Bucky grids requires a slight increase in object-image distance, causing a small amount of image unsharpness to be introduced.

Example. The series of four posteroanterior radiographs of a hand, Figure 153, was made in which all factors were constant except the object-image distance. Radiograph A was made with the hand on the film; B, the OID was 2 inches; C, 6 inches; and D, 8 inches. Note that as the OID increased, the edges of the carpal and metacarpal bones can be seen to have become more blurred, thin joint spaces between the carpals are less distinct, and there is less detail visible within the bone marrow. Sharpness has been reduced,

resulting in a loss of information.

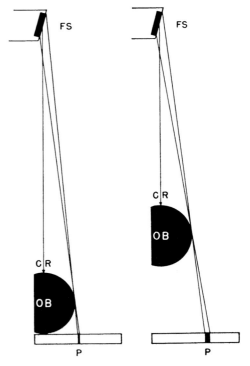

Figure 152. Diagram of effect of increasing OID. (*Right*) penumbra spreads at large OID, reducing sharpness.

Figure 153. Radiographs of hand demonstrating that OID increases (B through D), magnification and unsharpness at the edges of the bones become apparent. Factors: (A) no OID, (B) 2 inches OID, (C) 6 inches OID, (D) 8 inches OID.

EFFECT ON MAGNIFICATION

Magnification in the radiographic image is a normal occurrence. The degree of enlargement is a function of the source-image and object-image distance. *When the object is close to the film, enlargement is minimal.* When the center of the part is traversed by the central ray, normal magnification occurs. Whether the SID is great or small, the image will always be magnified when a large OID exists (Figure 154).

The use of a long SID in these situations serves only slightly to increase the sharpness of definition and decrease the image size. Therefore, the film should always be placed as near the object as possible.

The following example will illustrate the effects of simple magnification when the OID is varied.

Example. Two series of lateral radiographs of a dry skull, Figure 155, were made in which the source-image distance was varied as indicated on the radiographs. The dry skull was placed directly on the exposure holder in radiographs A-D, Top. Note that as the OID was increased, the images became smaller. Radiographs E-H, Bottom: the various source-image distances were the same as in Figure 155, Top, but the OID was increased to 4 inches in each case.

EFFECT ON SHAPE DISTORTION

As with SID, changes in OID do not affect shape distortion. Changes in OID only cause changes in magnification, as previously described.

Distortion will occur from improper beam-part-film alignment. Once distortion is created by these types of problems, a longer OID will make that distortion more apparent by magnifying it. But the shape, measured as the ratio of length to width, will not change. Changes in object-image distance do not *create* distortion.

FOCAL SPOTS

Figure 154. Diagram illustrating effect of increasing OID upon image magnification of the overall image. (B) both umbra and penumbra expand at greater OID.

EFFECT ON CONTRAST

The emission of scatter radiation and its influence on the image may be simulated radiographically by the use of paraffin—a material that generates large quantities of scatter radiation. A block of paraffin $2^{1}/_{2}$ x 6 x 10 inches may be used for this purpose.

Two principal conditions under which scatter radiation fog may be produced on film are illustrated by the series of diagrams and radiographs shown in Figures 156 and 157.

WHEN OBJECT IS NEAR FILM

When the emitter is placed on the film and a coin is mounted on its top (Figure 156-A), the radiograph will show the image of the coin to be fogged by the scatter radiation that undercuts the object. This diagram and radiographic example (Figure 157-A) demonstrate that images of objects in or on an emitter, located at a distance from the film will be fogged when the emitter is adjacent to the film.

WHEN OBJECT IS DISTANT

When the emitter together with the disc on its top is moved away from the film (Figure 156-B), the degree of fog in the

Figure 155. Radiographs of dry skull illustrating the interrelation of SID and OID in controlling magnification of the image. SID's are marked on each radiograph. The top series was taken with no OID, the bottom series with 4 inches OID. The least magnification is at (D) with 72 inches SID and no OID, the greatest magnification is at (E) with 20 inches SID and 4 inches OID.

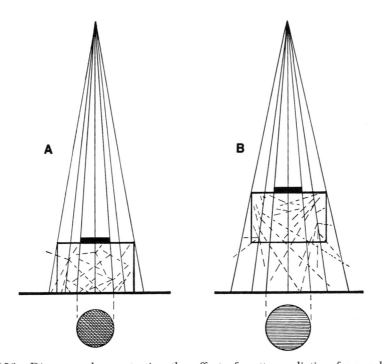

Figure 156. Diagrams demonstrating the effect of scatter radiation from a block of paraffin on the image of a coin: (A) When the coin is on top of the emitter, scatter edition from the paraffin fogs the coin image. (B) When the block and coin are moved away from the film, the fog density is reduced, because the scatter radiation is allowed to spread out (by the inverse square law).

Figure 157. Radiographs of a disc on a paraffin block demonstrating the effects diagrammed in Figure 156. (A) fogged image of disc, (B) reduction of fog due to placing the disc and paraffin block 5 inches off of the film.

image will be *less* than that shown in Radiograph (A) (Figure 157), since the scatter radiation reaching the film has been diminished by reason of its greater distance from its source. Therefore, *by increasing the distance between the emitter-disc combination and the film, the intensity of the scatter radiation reaching the film diminishes.*

Since the scattered photons spread out more as they move away from the object, they are less concentrated in any given area on the film (Figure 158). In fact, at a large OID, some scatter misses the film entirely. Primary photons which have penetrated the object are travelling in a nearly vertical direction and maintain the same concentration over a given area on the film that they would have had with no OID. This means that the *ratio* of scatter to primary photons striking a given area on the film is reduced. *With less fogging, image contrast is enhanced.*

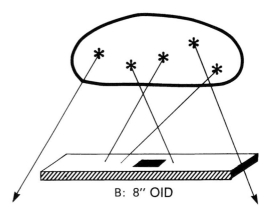

Figure 158. Diagram of effect of increasing OID (air gap technique) upon both density and contrast. As OID increases (B), scattered photons *miss* a given area (the black square) because of greater divergence. The scattered rays to the far sides completely miss the film. With the reduced concentration of scatter, contrast is improved, while density is reduced.

EFFECT ON DENSITY

The diagram in Figure 158 and the radiographs in Figure 157 demonstrate the effect of increasing the object-image distance on image density as well as contrast. *Since the scatter x-rays diverge more* before reaching the film, they are less concentrated in any given area of the film; consequently, *a loss in density occurs.* At significant object-image distances, an increase in mAs is required to maintain image density at a diagnostic level.

AIR GAP TECHNIQUE

Because of its contributory effect on image contrast, a large OID may be occasionally used to advantage in combatting image fog. A common application of this concept is found in chest radiography of very large patients. When an excessive amount of scatter fogging is present on the radiograph, a repeat exposure may be taken, with the patient placed six to eight inches away from the film. This procedure is called the *air gap technique* and is effective in restoring a portion of the desired image contrast.

But, the air gap technique creates problems with other image qualities which must be compensated for. First, since the anatomy will be magnified considerably, the largest practical SID should be used along with the high OID in order to compensate for some of the magnification. A minimum of 72 inches, and ideally 96 inches, SID are suggested. Sharpness of detail lost from the OID will also be partially restored in this manner. Second, the loss of image density from both the high OID and from the inverse square effect of an increased SID must be compensated for by an appropriate increase in mAs.

SUMMARY

1. Increasing the object-image receptor distance results in the growth of penumbra at the image edges and thus reduces *sharpness* of recorded detail. Sharpness is *inversely proportional* to the OID.
2. Increasing object-image distance also *magnifies* the image.
3. Increasing object-image distance has no direct effect upon shape *distortion* in the image. If distortion is already present from poor alignment of the beam and part, the magnifying effect of a larger OID may make it more noticeable. But a larger OID does not *cause* distortion.
4. Increasing the object-image distance reduces image *density,* because scattered radiation produced within the patient diverges more and loses intensity before reaching the film.
5. Increasing the object-image distance enhances image *contrast,* because scattered radiation reaching the film is reduced while the primary rays penetrating the patient remain at the same

intensity.

6. The *air gap* technique is recommended for very large patients, in order to restore some of the image contrast. However, magnification and unsharpness also result.

REVIEW QUESTIONS

1. Always use the _____ feasible OID.
2. The greater the OID, the _____ the image contrast.
3. The greater the OID , the _____ the image sharpness.
4. Explain *how* increased OID enhances image contrast.
5. List the three essential steps to the "air gap technique":
6. Which image quality is inversely proportional to the OID?

Chapter 20

DISTANCE RATIOS

The previous two chapters have discussed SID and OID separately, explaining the results in image qualities when one of these is changed and *all* other factors are kept equal. This approach works well when considering image *visibility* qualities such as density and contrast. But when examining the *geometric* qualities of sharpness and magnification, the SID, SOD and OID should be considered *in relation to each other*. For example, a proportionate change in the SID may completely offset the magnifying effects of a change in the OID.

Both sharpness and magnification are actually determined and controlled by *similar triangle geometry*, and can be calculated by forming *ratios* between the appropriate distances. Similar triangles are defined as triangles whose respective corners are of the same number of degrees. When a ratio is made between the same part of two similar triangles, it will always be equal to the ratio formed between any other part of the two triangles. For example, the ratio between the heights of the two triangles will always equal the ratio between their

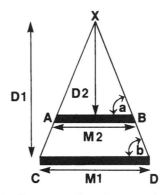

Figure 159. Diagram of similar triangle geometry for magnification: Triangles XAB and XCD are similar (angle a = angle b). AB represents an object or the aperture of a collimating device. CD represents the image or the field size at the film. The ratio D_1/D_2, or SID/SOD, will determine the factor of magnification (M_1/M_2).

bases. The geometry of the x-ray beam forms similar triangles between the tube, object and film, with the height of each triangle representing a distance–SID, SOD or OID. Certain ratios between these distances can be used to predict changes in both sharpness and magnification of the image.

MAGNIFICATION: THE SID/SOD RATIO

Figure 159 depicts the similar triangle geometry of *magnification*. Two similar triangles are formed, one by the SID and the film, the other by the SOD and the object, both sharing the apex "X' at the focal spot of the x-ray tube. *Magnification is simply defined as the ratio between the size of the image and the size of the object.* In Figure 159, the size of the image is represented by M_1, the base of triangle *XCD*, and the object is represented by M_2, the base of triangle *XAB*. The ratio between M_1 and M_2 should equal the ratio between the distances D_1 and D_2 (the heights of the triangles):

$$\frac{M_1}{M_2} = \frac{D_1}{D_2}$$

By definition, the ratio M_1/M_2 is the factor of magnification and may be abbreviated *M.* Since D_1 is the *SID* and D_2 is the *SOD,* these may be substituted and a formula for radiographic magnification derived as:

$$M = \frac{SID}{SOD}$$

Magnification is determined and controlled by the ratio SID/SOD. If the SID/SOD ratio is 2.0, this means that the projected image is magnified twice as large as the real object. If the ratio is 1.5, the image is half-again as large, or 50 per cent larger, and so on. *Magnification is directly proportional to the SID/SOD ratio.* Note that the *OID* is not used in calculating magnification. In Figure 155, the OID does not represent a triangle, but rather a trapezoid formed by the points *A, B, D and C.* It cannot be used for calculations. When the OID is given in a problem and the SOD is not, you must first subtract the OID from the SID to obtain the SOD, then work the formula.

Example No. 1

With an SID of 30 inches and the object placed 20 inches away from the film, how much will the image be magnified?

First, find the SOD as:
SID - OID = 30 - 20 = 10

$$\frac{SID}{SOD} = \frac{30}{10} = \frac{3}{1} = \quad \text{Magnification Factor of 3.0}$$

Solution: The image will be three times as big as the real object

Example No. 2

An image measures 8 inches across. A 30-inch SID was used along with an SOD of 20 inches. What is the size of the original object?

$$\frac{SID}{SOD} = \frac{30}{20} = \frac{3}{2} = \quad \text{Magnification Factor of 1.5}$$

Solution: The image size, given as 8 inches, is 1.5 times larger than the real object. Designating the real object as X then 8 = 1.5 times X:

$$1.5(X) = 8 \; and$$

$$X = \frac{8}{1.5} = 5.3 \text{ inches}$$

The real object is 5.3 inches in width.

Note that any change in SID, SOD, or OID will be exactly offset by a *proportionate* change in one of the other distances. For example, suppose that the OID and the SID are *both* doubled: As shown in Figure 156, this results in the SOD also being doubled, and the SID/SOD ratios are maintained equal, (40/38 = 20/19). Magnification will be identical as long as the distances are changed proportionately so that they offset each other.

Try the following exercise for practice, then check your answers in the Appendix.

EXERCISE 22

Magnification ratios are calculated identically for both the light field/x-ray field size and also for the magnification of an object being radiographed. For each of the following, three factors are given—solve for the fourth, using the ratio SID/SOD. Don't forget to subtract the OID when needed to get the SOD:

	Width of Distal End of Cone or Collimator	Width of X-Ray Field at Film	SID	SOD
1.	8 inches	_____	60 inches	30 inches
2.	6 inches	_____	60 inches	45 inches
3.	_____	10 inches	60 inches	20 inches
4.	1 inch	9 inches	72 inches	_____
5.	5 inches	15 inches	_____	60 inches

	Width of Light Field on Patient's Surface	Width of X-Ray Field at Film	SID	**O.I.D.**
6.	8 inches	_____	60 inches	40 inches
7.	10 inches	_____	24 inches	8 inches
8.	4 inches	5 inches	_____	6 inches
9.	_____	12 inches	96 inches	84 inches
10.	4 inches	6 inches	96 inches	_____

	Width of Actual Object	Width of Object's Image on Film	SID	SOD
11.	10 cm	_____	80 inches	20 inches
12.	6 cm	_____	100 inches	80 inches
13.	_____	24 cm	96 inches	72 inches
14.	8 cm	12 cm	60 inches	_____
15.	12 cm	18 cm	_____	60 inches

SHARPNESS: THE SOD/OID RATIO

The sharpness of recorded detail in the image is also determined by similar triangle geometry, but in this case a pair of triangles are formed by the penumbra diagram at each edge of the image as shown in Figure 160. Note that in Figure 160, triangle *XAB* and triangle *XCD* are inverted to each other with their common apex, *X*, being the edge of the projected object. The height of triangle *XAB* represents the *SOD*. Triangle *XCD* represents the *OID*. If the object were moved twice as far away from the film, triangle *XCD* would stretch twice as high, and the penumbra *CD* would spread exactly twice as much. Penumbra or blur is directly proportional to the OID.

THE "GEOMETRIC UNSHARPNESS" FORMULA

As demonstrated in the last chapter, image blur or unsharpness is directly proportional to the OID. In Chapter 16 we learned that blur is also directly proportional to the size of the focal spot. In Chapter 18 we learned that blur is *inversely proportional* to the SOD. All three of these relationships can be mathematically expressed by the *geometric unsharpness formula* used in many textbooks:

$$\text{Unsharpness} = \frac{\text{FS X OID}}{\text{SOD}}$$

Theoretically, one can calculate the actual size of penumbral spread due to geometrical penumbra in millimeters, given the focal spot size in mm and the two distances. For example, if the OID is 10 cm and the SOD is 40 cm, how much geometrical penumbra would be produced by an 0.5mm focal spot? The calculation would be 0.5 X 10/40 = 5/40 = 0.125 mm of penumbral spread. Unfortunately, the actual *total penumbra* produced in an image includes *absorption penumbra* which must be added to the *geometrical penumbra*. This is explained fully in Chapter 24. Therefore, the geometrical penumbra formula is of limited practical application. It is useful in theoretically comparing the *relative* unsharpness between different techniques using varied distance and focal spot combinations.

SHARPNESS OF RECORDED DETAIL

"Geometrical sharpness" may be mathematically expressed by simply inverting the above unsharpness formula. It would then state:

$$\text{Sharpness} = \frac{\text{SOD}}{\text{FS X OID}}$$

Theoretical calculations can also be made for *relative* sharpness values. For example, two techniques are compared, *A* using an 0.5 mm focal spot, 40 cm SOD and 10 cm OID, and *B* using an 0.4 mm focal spot, 50 cm SOD and 25 cm OID. Which produces a sharper image?

Figure 160. Diagram showing a doubling of SID, SOD and OID. As long as the ratios between these distances are maintained, there is no change in sharpness nor in magnification: Relative Sharpness (SOD/OID) = 38/2 = 76/4 = 19. Magnification (SID/SOD) = 40/38 = 80/76 = 1.05.

$A = 40/0.5 \text{ X } 10 = 40/5 =$

8 (relative sharpness value)

$B = 50/0.4 \text{ X } 25 = 50/10 =$

5 (relative sharpness value)

Solution: A is sharper than B

(8/5 = 1.6 times or 60 per cent sharper)

More importantly, though, this formula may serve to remind us that sharpness is directly proportional to SOD, and inversely proportional to FS and OID. In Figure 160, the OID was doubled, which would normally double the blur and cut sharpness to one-half. However, the SID was also doubled in Figure 160, and this resulted in twice the SOD. On the left, the SOD/OID ratio is 38"/2" = 19. On the right, the SOD/OID ratio is 76"/4" = 19. The distances, having been changed proportionately, offset each other exactly, and result in the same ratio. The sharpness is therefore mainlined equal, and so is the magnification, as you can see in Figure 160. As long as the SOD/OID ratio is maintained, no geometrical changes will be noted in the image.

VISIBILITY FUNCTIONS

Distance ratios are not directly related to the visibility functions in the image.

Since increases in SID and increases in OID both decrease image density, the loss of density is exaggerated when both are increased. Since SID has no effect upon image contrast, and increasing OID enhances contrast, increasing both will result in a net increase in contrast.

MACRORADIOGRAPHY (MAGNIFICATION TECHNIQUE)

As discussed in Chapter Nineteen, in most radiographic practice the object-image distance (OID) should be kept as small as possible in order to minimize magnification and preserve sharpness in the image. There are some applications, most notably for angiography and mammography, in which a magnified image is desired as a way of enhancing its visibility. For example, cerebral angiography is commonly performed with an intentional OID of 8 to 10 inches. With the usual 40-inch SID, the SID/SOD ratio will be 1.25 to 1.33 achieving 25 to 35 per cent magnification of the vessels of the brain. For the 8-inch OID, the formula would be:

$$\frac{\text{SID}}{\text{OID}} = \frac{40}{32} = 1.25 \text{ magnification factor}$$

(1.25 - 1) x 100 = 25 per cent magnification

In this case, the loss of image *sharpness* caused by the high OID must be compensated for with some factor other than distance. Focal spot size is ideal, since it affects only sharpness. *Microfocus* x-ray tubes, with focal spots from 0.1 to 0.3 millimeters in size are therefore used. With the smaller focal spot, sharpness of recorded detail is restored to the normal level even though the image is magnified. The smallest available focal spot should always be used when performing magnification technique. This method is called *macroradiography*, meaning "big radiography."

SUMMARY

1. The SID/SOD ratio is the primary controlling factor over *magnification.* Magnification is *directly proportional* to the SID/SOD ratio.
2. The SOD/OID ratio is the primary controlling factor over *sharpness of recorded detail.* Image sharpness is *directly proportional* to the SOD/OID ratio.
3. A *relative geometric sharpness value* may be calculated with the formula S = SOD/FS X OID.
4. *Geometric unsharpness* may be calculated with the formula U = FS X OID/SOD.
5. Distance ratios are not related to shape distortion, density or contrast in the image. When determining density or contrast changes, SID and OID should each be considered separately.
6. In *Macroradiography*, fractionally small focal spots are employed to restore most of the sharpness which is lost by using an air gap OID.

REVIEW QUESTIONS

1. Aside from the effects of focal spot, the sharpness of an image is *directly* proportional to the ratio of the _____ _____ distance divided by the _____ _____ distance.
2. If the SID is 40 inches and the SOD is 20 inches, the projected image of the object will be magnified by a factor of _____.
3. An original technique is used with an SID of 40" and an OID of 2 inches. If the *OID* were increased from 2 inches to 3 inches, what new SID would be required in order to *completely* eliminate the blurring effects of the OID change.
4. An original magnification ratio is 50 per cent. If the *SID AND OID* were *both* tripled the new magnification ratio will be _____.
5. What are the two essential steps to performing macroradiography (magnification technique)?

Chapter 21

BEAM-PART-FILM ALIGNMENT

THE ORIENTATION of the central ray of the x-ray beam, the anatomy being radiographed, and the film, in relation to each other, their shapes, angles and centering are all alignment factors which relate to positioning in controlling the geometrical integrity of the recorded image. Blanket statements such as "Angling the x-ray beam *always* causes shape distortion" are misleading. The effects of beam-part-film alignment on the image are complex and must be discussed on a case-by-case basis for the sake of accuracy.

OFF-CENTERING VERSUS ANGLING

Off-centering of either the central ray or the part in relation to each other places the part in the diverging peripheral rays of the beam. These peripheral rays angle away from the central ray. The further they are from the central ray, the more angled they are from it. Therefore, off-centering has identical effects to angling the beam or part (Figure 161). Although the following demonstrations are all produced by angulation, equivalent effects are caused by off-centering.

EFFECT ON SHAPE DISTORTION

The traditional rule of keeping the part parallel to the film and the central ray perpendicular to both the part and the film effectively minimizes shape distortion in the image. But, this ideal situation is possible in not more than 70 per cent of the radi-

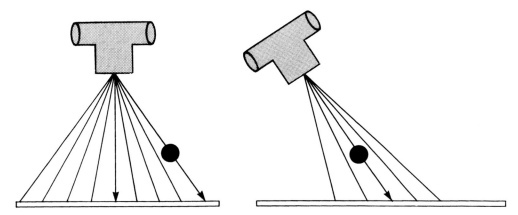

Figure 161. Diagram showing how off-centering the x-ray beam has an equivalent effect of angling the beam, since off-centering places the object in diverging rays.

ographs commonly taken. The remainder of cases consist of anatomy which cannot be placed parallel to the film or the necessity of angles to desuperimpose overlying structures. In these cases, shape distortion must be minimized and keeping the beam perpendicular to the film or part is not always applicable in doing so. There are four major factors which affect shape distortion in the image: (1) The shape and thickness of the object being radiographed, (2) the centering of the central ray with respect to the object, (3) the angle formed between the central ray and the long axis of the object, and (4) the angle formed between the long axis of the object and the film. All of these must be understood in controlling distortion.

SHAPE OF THE ANATOMICAL PART

The shape of the anatomical part or object being radiographed affects the degree to which its image is distorted by changes in beam-part-film alignment. Objects that are spherical or cubical in shape distort under more circumstances than do flat, wedge-shaped or tubular objects. Further, when the x-ray beam is angled, spherical or cubical objects which have no distinct long axis will be more distorted than flatter objects whose long axis parallels the film. Examples of anatomical parts which are spherical or cubical include the cranium, the femoral condyles, the heads of the femur and humerus, the vertebrae and the tarsal bones.

Objects which are flat, such as the sternum and scapulae, wedge-shaped, such as the sacrum and anterior teeth, or tubular, such as the shafts of the long bones and the ureters, may not distort significantly with tube angles as long as their long axis is maintained parallel to the plane of the film. Thus, the shape of an object has a direct bearing upon the occurrence of visible shape distortion when the beam is angled or off-centered.

Figure 162. Diagram demonstrating that angling or off-centering the x-ray beam against a thin, flat object may not cause visible shape distortion if the object is kept parallel to the film, since the ratios of SID/SOD are maintained. Only relatively thick objects exhibit noticeable shape distortion.

OBJECTS WITH
A DISTINCT LONG AXIS

When a relatively flat, wedge-shaped or tubular object is kept parallel to the film, angulation of the central ray may not lead to appreciable shape distortion (Figure 162). This is because at *any* given ray in the beam, the angle will have caused SOD to increase by the same proportion as the SID. The SID/SOD ratio is therefore unchanged across the beam of x-rays and there is no distortion.

When a flat, wedge-shaped or tubular object is tilted in relation to the film, *foreshortening* distortion will occur (Figure 163). The image recorded is shorter in the axis of the tilt than the real object is. This can cause misleading information on the radiograph. (Since a spherical or cubical object has no identifiable long axis, its orientation in relation to the film is of no consequence.)

If a flat, wedge-shaped or tubular object is tilted in relation to the film, and the central ray is angled to place it perpendicular to the long axis of the object (Figure 164), *elongation* distortion occurs in the axis of the

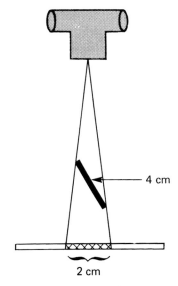

Figure 163. Diagram of foreshortening distortion caused by tilting the object while the beam and film are kept perpendicular.

tilt. Again, misinformation is recorded on the radiograph.

Ceiszynski's Law of Isometry

Since tilted objects present distortion regardless of whether the central ray is

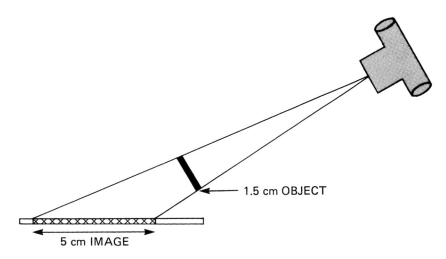

Figure 164. Diagram of elongation distortion caused when the beam is directed perpendicular to an object that is tilted in relation to the film.

placed perpendicular to the film or perpendicular to the object (foreshortening on the one hand and elongation on the other), the minimal distortion must be achieved at some angle between these two extremes. *Ceiszynski's Law of Isometry* states that an *isometric* angle, equal to one-half of the angle formed between the object and the film, will eliminate or minimize distortion. A classical example of the use of isometric angles is found in radiography of the AP sacrum. The sacrum is a fairly flat wedge-shaped object. Note that although the normal sacrum lies at an angle of 30-35 degrees from the film when a patient is lying supine, positioning atlases recommend the use of a 15-degree cephalic angle of the central ray, one-half of the anatomical angle, for the AP projection (Figure 165). This angle minimizes shape distortion of the sacrum.

Figure 167 demonstrates these various

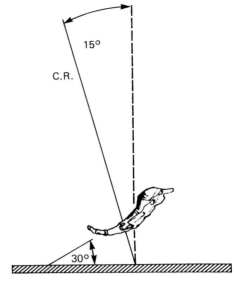

Figure 165. Ceiszynski's law of isometry applied to the AP sacrum projection: To minimize shape distortion of an object that cannot be placed parallel to the film, angle the beam one-half of the part/film angle. The sacrum lies at a 30-degree angle, the CR should be angled 15 degrees.

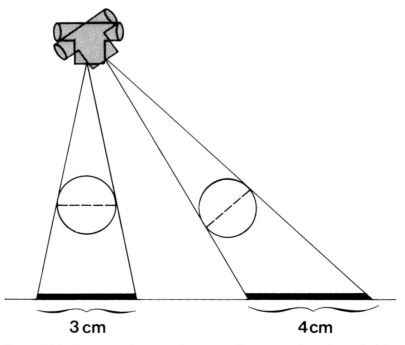

Figure 166. Diagram showing elongation distortion of a spherical object when the x-ray beam is angled or off-centered.

Figure 167. Radiographs demonstrating various cases of shape distortion: (A) flat coin parallel to film with beam perpendicular to both showing no distortion, (B) coin tilted and beam perpendicular to film showing foreshortening, (C) coin tilted and beam perpendicular to *coin* showing elongation, (D) coin angled 45 degrees to film, beam angled isometrically at 22.5 degrees showing no distortion, (E) coin parallel to film and beam angled 30 degrees to both showing no noticeable distortion because coin is flat and thin, (F) spherical head of femur in normal projection, and (G) angulation of beam 30 degrees showing elongation distortion of femoral head.

effects radiographically, using a coin for a flat object.

OBJECTS WITHOUT A DISTINCT LONG AXIS

Angling (or off-centering) the central ray distorts spherical or cubical objects. This occurs because, since they have no true long axis, the x-ray beam sees an artificial axis which is always perpendicular to itself. Thus, when the beam is angled, the same effects occur as if if a linear object were tilted to the film and distortion occurs (Figure 166). These effects on actual radiographs are shown in Figure 167.

In the case of off-centering objects in the beam, using shorter source-image distances may indirectly lead to exaggerated distortion problems as follows: When a shorter SID is used, the radiographer must often open the collimator or otherwise increase the field size to avoid cutting off anatomy of interest. In doing so, objects that are placed at a given distance away from the central ray will be recorded on the film by more peripheral beams that are more angled from the central ray (Figure 168). In effect, these objects have been angled against more, and if they are relatively thick objects they will be distorted in shape more (Figure 169). Therefore, off-centering of objects in the x-ray beam causes more severe distortion problems at short distances than at long distances.

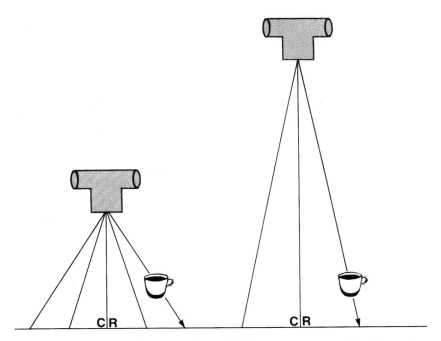

Figure 168. Diagram illustrating how SID becomes a controlling factor (but not a causing factor) when shape distortion is already occurring due to off-centering: By increasing the SID (*right*) the object is projected by more vertical beams, thus reducing shape distortion.

EFFECT ON DENSITY

Angling the central ray, part, or film does not directly affect image density. However, angling the C.R. *without* compensating the tube-to-tabletop distance results in an increased SID. The longer SID then leads to a loss of density, as described in Chapter 18. The distance change, not the angle itself, causes the density loss. To compensate for this reduction in density, use the rule of thumb: *One inch less tube-to-tabletop distance for every 5 degrees of CR angle.* It is not necessary to apply this rule at tube angles of 15 degrees or less, since the density loss at these angles is negligible. This rule serves to maintain an actual SID of 40 inches.

Tilting or angling the part may result in an effective increase or decrease in part thickness as measured through the central ray location. This will change image density accordingly. The change in density is due to the effectively changed part thickness and not to the angle itself.

EFFECTS ON OTHER QUALITIES

All of the preceding diagrams on distortion demonstrate the effects of alignment changes caused in *one* axis only–the axis of the angle or off-centering shift. In the opposite axis, across or perpendicular to the angle or off-centering shift, no change

Figure 169. Radiographs of several mugs demonstrating the contributing effects of SID when distortion is already present. Note the centering of the darker area within each cup: (*left*) Using 30 inches SID, peripheral cups are distorted, while (*right*) using 72 inches SID this effect is diminished. Also, note that the cup centered in the CR is not distorted at either distance, because it is not in a diverging beam.

occurs. This may be documented by comparing the crosswise *width* of the sphere in Figure 167F-G, which does not change even though elongation distortion is occurring. Since magnification is defined as an increase in the *total* image size across *both* axes, it may be said that beam-part-film alignment does not affect magnification.

Misalignment can also be seen in these same radiographs to not affect sharpness of detail at image edges. Neither magnification nor sharpness are affected by alignment changes, because the ratio of the SID/SOD remains equal in all of the rays across an angled or off-centered beam.

Any SID increase resulting from CR angles is accompanied by an equivalent SID increase, so that the ratio between them is unchanged (Figure 162). As described in Chapter 20, as long as this ratio remains equal and the focal spot is not changed, no change in sharpness or magnification will occur.

Alignment of the beam, part and film is strictly geometrical in nature and has no effect upon the ratio of scatter radiation produced within the patient or upon the penetration characteristics of the beam. It cannot, therefore, have any relationship to image contrast.

SUMMARY

1. *Distortion* of the shape of an image is absent when the x-ray beam, part and film are centered, the part is parallel to the film and the beam is perpendicular to the film.

2. *Off-centering* of either the central ray or the part results in the same effects as angling the beam.

3. Angling or off-centering the beam against spherical or cubical objects causes *elongation* distortion.
4. When a relatively flat, tubular or wedgelike object is tilted in relation to the beam and film, *foreshortening* distortion occurs.
5. If the beam *and* object with a long axis are equally angled to the film, *elongation* distortion occurs.
6. When a flat or linear object cannot be made to parallel the film plane, an *isometric angle* of the central ray of the beam, one-half of the object-to-film angle, should be used to minimize distortion.
7. If a relatively flat, wedge-shaped or tubular object is kept *parallel* to the film,

angling the beam may not result in visible distortion of its shape.
8. Angulation of the beam or part does not directly affect radiographic *density*. However, effective patient thickness, and distances if uncompensated for, may be changed in the course of angling the beam or part. These changes may then affect image density.
9. To compensate for distance changes from beam angulation so that density may be maintained, use the rule of thumb *one inch for every five degrees* in adjusting tube-to-tabletop distance.
10. Angulation of the beam or part has no effect upon image *contrast, magnification* or *sharpness of detail.*

REVIEW QUESTIONS

1. As long as the body part is placed parallel to the film, the central ray should always be _____ to the film to minimize shape distortion.
2. Why is off-centering of the central ray similar in its effects to angling the x-ray beam?
3. Why do positioning atlases suggest a 15-degree cephalic angle for the AP sacrum projection, when the average sacrum lies at 30-35 degrees from the plane of the film?
4. Which of the following would distort *most* in shape with a 35-degree angle of the central ray: the head of the femur, the shaft of the femur, or the sternum?
5. If a flat object is angled in relation to the film, and the x-ray beam is angled to place the central ray perpendicular to the object, what type of image distortion occurs?
6. The distorting effects of off-centering

an object within the x-ray beam are indirectly worsened if a _____ target-film distance is used.
7. If you angle the x-ray beam 20 degrees, the tube-to-tabletop distance must be changed from 40 inches to _____ inches in order to maintain a 40-inch SID and avoid loss of image density.
8. If the x-ray beam is angled 35 degrees, and the tabletop-tube distance is left at 40 inches, an increase in mAs will be required to maintain image density, NOT because of the angle itself, but because of:
9. List the four aspects of beam-part-film alignment which affect image shape distortion:
10. Why will the cranium distort more with an angled x-ray beam than the head of a femur, even though both are spherical in shape?
11. State Ceiszynski's Law of Isometry:

Chapter 22

GEOMETRIC FUNCTIONS OF POSITIONING

POSITIONING, at its most fundamental level, is a geometrical factor affecting the recognizability of the image details. Every specific position has as its purpose one of the following objectives:

1. To increase sharpness of recorded detail by placing the anatomy of interest closer to the film.

2. To reduce magnification by placing the anatomy of interest closer to the film.

3. To minimize distortion of the shape of the anatomy of interest by optimizing the alignment of the anatomy with the x-ray beam and the film.

4. To increase the visibility of the anatomy of interest by desuperimposing other overlying, contrasty anatomical structures which are not of interest and, therefore, represent *noise* in the image.

PROJECTION ROUTINES

The diagnostic radiograph is dependent upon proper positioning of the patient before exposure. This is facilitated by the use of standard projections. Such projections produce images that reveal the maximum amount of diagnostic information with a minimum of distortion. An accurate idea of the anatomic arrangement of the internal structures with relation to some external landmark aids materially in positioning the patient. A convenient method is to visualize the part as though it were transparent, so that the usual structures which appear on the radiograph may be identified in relation to an external land-mark. The relation of the central ray to the part to be examined, and to the film, must be carefully considered in each projection. Imperfect centering of the part on the film and alignment of the tube to the part are the causes of image distortion. The requirements of radiography are such that slight differences in position do not necessarily rule out the diagnostic value of the radiograph. A certain degree of latitude in routine may be permissible, because the radiologist ordinarily can make satisfactory adjustment by reason of his experience and knowledge. However, in order to secure reliable diagnostic results, it is best to conform to a procedure which is precise and accurate.

To derive the maximum information concerning the size and shape of body parts and foreign objects in relation to their position in the body, projections should be made from different directions. The need for multiple views is clearly demonstrated in Figures 170 and 171.

In routine radiography, two views, each at right angles to the other, are made as shown in Figure 170, wherein posteroanterior and lateral views of the femur are illustrated.

These radiographs demonstrate the value of two opposing projections. In radiograph A, a portion of the image appears abnormal. When viewed at right angles, it may be seen in radiograph B that the ends of the bone are not united but are quite distant to each other, yet their ends were projected so that their images were superim-

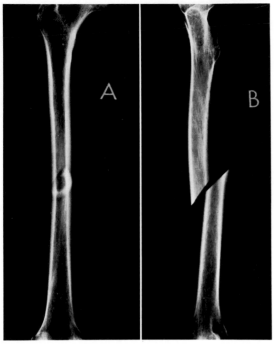

Figure 170. Radiographs of a dry femur, (A) in AP and (B) in lateral projections emphasizing the importance of a second projection at right angles to determine misalignment of a fracture.

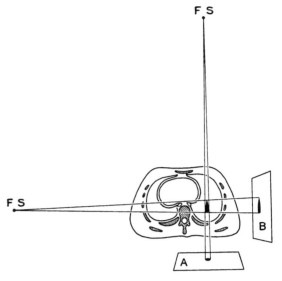

Figure 171. Diagram illustrating the need for two projections to determine the true nature of a foreign body, in this case a bullet which appears only as a circular density on the AP projection.

posed.

To determine the nature of a foreign body, two views are also necessary, Figure

171. In this diagram an anteroposterior radiograph would show a foreign body as a circular object (image A). Another, when viewed at right angles to the original projection (image B) would show by its shape that the foreign body was a bullet.

SUMMARY

1. Radiographic *positioning* is essentially a geometrical factor designed to increase sharpness of recorded detail, minimize magnification, minimize shape distortion or desuperimpose overlying structures.

2. *Standardized* projections, including at least two views at right angles to each other, are necessary for complete diagnosis.

REVIEW QUESTIONS

1. When the contrasty spine is obscuring the gall bladder because of the particular position used, and if interest is only in the gall bladder, the spine then is considered as what type of undesirable image quality?

2. Explain why two views must be taken at right angles to each other as standard radiographic procedure, and give an example:

3. State the four objectives of positioning:

Chapter 23

MOTION

MOTION OF A BODY part being examined directly influences sharpness of recorded image detail. Motion may be voluntary on the part of the patient, or may be involuntary. The only means for controlling the effects of motion are (1) patient cooperation, (2) immobilization of the part being examined, and (3) short exposures.

Voluntary motion may take several forms. The noncooperative child who needs restraint is common. The patient who does not understand the manner in which he is to cooperate is usually the fearful one. A satisfactory explanation of the procedure usually suffices to create confidence. When in doubt, immobilize the part and use short exposures.

Involuntary motion is normally associated with the physiologic activity of the body tissue. Respiration produces movement of the thorax and its contents so that short exposures are mandatory (Figure 172). The normal adult respiratory rate is 16 to 18 respirations per minute; in some pulmonary or cardiac lesions, the rate may be greater; in the newborn, it may be 30 to 40 per minute. Respiration also influences in some degree the viscera adjacent to the diaphragms.

Movement of the heart and great vessels is an important factor in radiography of the chest. The pulsation of the arterial system in all parts of the body at the rate of about 5 to 8 meters per second creates various

Figure 172. Radiographs of the PA chest demonstrating blurring of pulmonary and mediastinal anatomy due to movement (A) compared to a properly exposed film (B).

287

degrees of movement in the tissues they supply.

Esophageal peristalsis begins about 1 second after the initial swallowing act. The rate of travel is not the same at all levels. In the first 7 to 8 centimeters of its course, the rate is rapid (1 second); in the next 7 centimeters, the rate is 1 to 2 seconds; and in the lower segment, the rate is about 3 seconds. Solid or semisolid food takes between 6 and 7 seconds to pass from the mouth to the stomach. When liquids are ingested, the rate is relatively more rapid. Movement of the gastrointestinal tract requires proper use of exposure time to avoid unsharpness in the image. Motion of the stomach exhibits great individual variations. In some stomachs, the peristaltic wave travels rapidly and lasts 10 to 15 seconds. In others, the wave may occupy as much as 30 seconds to move from its origin

to the pylorus. The slower waves, however, are more common. Peristalsis in the small intestine is about 10 centimeters per second; the colonic rate is very slow.

The gallbladder exhibits rhythmic contractions that may last 5 to 30 minutes. Contractions also occur in the common bile duct.

In the urinary tract, peristaltic waves begin at the kidney and extend to the urinary bladder at the rate of 20 to 30 millimeters per second or 3 to 6 contractions per minute.

To summarize, there are four general categories of motion: (1) peristalsis, (2) heart motion, (3) breathing motion, and (4) voluntary or involuntary movement of the body itself or its limbs. The effects of the first three are localized to specific areas on the final image. Body movement certainly has the greatest effect on the overall image.

EFFECT ON SHARPNESS OF RECORDED DETAIL

The influence of motion in producing image unsharpness is diagrammatically shown in Figure 173. In this illustration, the object moved during the exposure resulting in unsharpness in the margins of the image. A typical radiographic example of patient movement is shown in a radiograph of the hand (Figure 174-B). Note the blurring of all image details and the double edges.

Immobilization

Immobilization is imperative in radiography, for differential diagnoses depend upon the visualization of sharp, undistorted images. Movement should be practically eliminated during the exposure in order to avoid blurring of details in the image.

Composing the Patient

The responsibility of keeping the part immobile is the job of the radiographer, not the patient, for movement may occur consciously or unconsciously. Respiration and body tremor are physical conditions that are important enough to warrant close attention. To some patients, the mere fact it is necessary to lie on a table for an x-ray examination is perturbing. Some may show signs of trembling. A few words of assurance will help to restore peace of mind. Too much cannot be left to the patient in the matter of keeping still during the exposure because most patients are not familiar with the requirements for making a radiograph. Frequently, they are nervous and afraid; so it is the job of the radiogra-

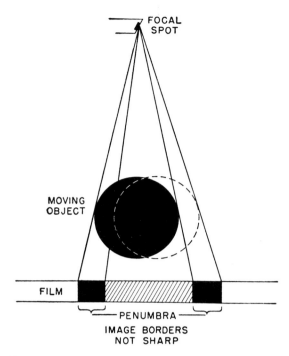

FOCAL SPOT

MOVING OBJECT

FILM

PENUMBRA

IMAGE BORDERS NOT SHARP

Figure 173. Diagram illustrating the influence of motion in producing image unsharpness.

not end there, however, for much of his success is dependent upon the closeness and the firmness with which the part is juxtaposed to the filmholder and the method of immobilization used. Even with the short exposures now possible, immobilization is necessary. There is no usable exposure so short as to fail to record uncontrollable or involuntary tremor of the area under examination. Proper immobilization assures comparison of symmetrical parts, for it also serves to prevent involuntary rotation of the part. The tube carriage always should be locked in position, because its vibration is a common cause for blurred radiographs.

Immobilization Methods

There are a number of good methods for immobilizing the body part: sandbags, compression bands, cones, and special clamps, etc. Many of these devices for immobilization are found in the modern laboratory. An important aspect of immobilization is compression of tissues, particularly in the abdomen. By displacing some of the tissues, less scatter radiation is produced and better contrast attained.

pher to put the patient at ease—so that he will be comfortable, mentally and physically. When the patient is passive and relaxed as a result of his comfort, he will be most cooperative. The radiographer's task does

EFFECT ON CONTRAST

Motion of the x-ray tube, patient or film during the exposure causes extraneous densities from other structures to be superimposed over the anatomy of interest. If this overlapping of adjacent densities is severe, the differences between them becomes less distinct and image contrast is reduced. If the motion is slight, the loss of contrast only occurs in the peripheral portions of each density area (tissue type) but is nonetheless sufficiently destructive to image quality to render it unacceptable.

Note in Figure 172 that in radiograph A where motion blurring occurred, the contrast in the peripheral portions of the heart shadow against the density level of the surrounding lung tissues is not as great as it is in radiograph B, where no motion occurred.

Motion is the only variable which may affect image contrast *without* doing so through the mechanism of scattered radiation proportions in the remnant beam. Motion is not related in any way with the production of scatter radiation. But since sufficient levels of blurring will lead to excessive overlapping and superimposition of image densities, these densities tend to cancel each other out and contrast may be lost.

The hand radiographs in Figure 174 demonstrate how the effect of motion on contrast is dependent on the severity of the motion. Radiograph B shows the effect of moderate motion when compared to the sharp radiograph A. While B is obviously blurred, any change in overall image contrast is arguable. In radiograph C there is severe motion and a gross loss of contrast is apparent when compared to A: The finger bones are a "washed out" darker gray, while the tissues of the palm are a "washed out" very light gray.

The mechanism by which this superimposition process can result in reduced contrast is fully described in the next chapter. Breathing, heart motion and peristaltic motion are usually *not* sufficient to affect overall image contrast, but whole body motion can certainly destroy it. Although it should not be considered as a *controlling* factor over image contrast, *motion generally reduces contrast* in the image.

EFFECT ON DENSITY

Since motion causes adjacent densities on the radiograph to overlap each other, there is clearly an effected change in the density of some small, *confined* areas of the radiograph. However, in discussing radiographic density, we normally refer to the *overall* density of the radiograph, or, in other words, the average density. Further, the overlapping of densities may not alter the overall average density of the image. For example, the mixing of a white area over a black area will result in a medium-gray density. It is not then said that the black area became *more white* and that the white, area became *more black* but simply that a new density has been created in place of the two originals, namely, the gray. The new gray density has exactly the same *average* density measurement as the average density between the original black and white.

The effects of motion on density are at best completely unpredictable and at worst nonexistent. Therefore, *motion should not be considered to be a controlling factor over image density.* To confirm this fact, observe Figure 172 once again and note the similar densities present in both radiographs despite the presence of motion in one.

EFFECT ON OTHER QUALITIES

There is a very common misconception that motion causes shape distortion in an image. True elongation or foreshortening of an image are caused only by alignment changes as discussed in Chapter 21. When motion occurs, new images are actually created in the radiograph by the interaction between the anatomy present and the motion itself. The most common of these new images are the familiar *streaks* seen in the image when doing linear tomography or when the tube, patient or film is moved in one direction during the exposure. The streaks and other similar artifacts are *false*

Figure 174. Radiographs of the hand showing (A) a sharp and high contrast image, (B) a blurred image due to motion, but still possessing high contrast in some areas, and (C) a severely blurred image showing the destruction of contrast as well as sharpness.

images, not distorted images.

These *false images, created by the geometrical interaction between the anatomy present and the movement of the tube, part or film, may be categorized as image noise.* Noise is any unwanted and deleterious information in the image which impedes the visibility of the desirable information. Any false image is a form of noise.

When motion is very slight, the shape of the image will be still recognizable although the edges are blurred. Again, this is a blurred image, not a distorted one. True distortion only occurs from changes in beam-part-film alignment.

For the same reasons, it may be said that *motion has no direct relationship to image magnification.* If motion results in an average distance from the film which is greater than normal, magnification may be present. But, in this case the change in distance, not the motion itself, causes the magnification.

SUMMARY

1. Motion destroys *sharpness* of image detail by expanding penumbra at image edges. It is the most destructive factor affecting image sharpness.
2. Severe motion can destroy image *contrast* by superimposing the various densities.
3. Motion has no direct relation to *overall* image *density.*
4. Motion does not cause *magnification* nor shape *distortion* of the gross image.
5. Motion does create *noise* in the form of *false images* on the radiograph.

REVIEW QUESTIONS

1. Motion has the *most* detrimental effect upon which image quality:
2. List two internal body functions which may result in involuntary blurring of the radiograph, even though the breath was properly held:
3. Explain why excessive motion can reduce image contrast:
4. Sometimes the relationship between the movement of the x-ray tube during tomography and the shape of the anatomy *produces* streaks or other images on the radiograph which do not represent any real anatomical structure. Such images are classified as:
5. Name the three methods of reducing the probability of motion leading to visible blur on the radiograph:

Part IV

COMPREHENSIVE TECHNIQUE

Chapter 24

ANALYZING THE RADIOGRAPHIC IMAGE

We have now covered some twenty types of variables which affect the quality of the radiographic image prior to processing it. We have described how each variable affects the six primary radiographic qualities: Density, contrast, noise, sharpness of recorded detail, magnification and distortion. This material is frequently taught in reverse order, taking each image quality and then listing all of the variables that affect it. By using this approach in this chapter, it will serve as a comprehensive review.

We have been further limited by treating each quality and each variable one at a time. In reality, several of the image qualities and the variables affecting them are intimately related to each other in rather complex ways. The overall ability of an imaging system to bring out the maximum number of details in an image, or the most visible information, is called its *resolution*. Resolution determines the overall quality of the image. The ways in which image qualities interrelate to produce a highly resolved image will be discussed later in this chapter.

The ability to critique the technical quality of finished radiographs is essential for radiographers to keep patient dose due to repeated exposures at a minimum. This ability will also be discussed.

VISIBILITY FUNCTIONS

The visibility of a radiographic image depends upon three things only–its density, its contrast and the presence of any noise. These qualities were defined and illustrated in Chapter Three. We shall briefly review the variables affecting each.

DENSITY

Milliamperage

Milliamperage is directly proportional to image density. For example, doubling the mA from 100 to 200 will double the apparent darkness of the radiograph, if all other factors are kept constant and no compensations are made. During the exposure, x-rays are emitted from the tube at twice the *rate*, and the x-ray beam is therefore twice as *intense*.

Exposure Time

Exposure time is also directly proportional to density. If no compensation is made, increasing the time from $1/20$ second to $1/10$ second, or from 0.35 to 0.7 second, will double the density.

Milliampere-Seconds (mAs)

The total mAs is the product of mA and exposure time. It controls the total density resulting on the film in a directly proportional fashion. Doubling the mAs doubles the density. To see a visible difference in image density, mAs must be altered by at least $1/3$ or 30 per cent.

In producing a total mAs value, mA and exposure time are inversely proportional to each other. A doubling of the mA may be compensated for by halving the exposure time to achieve the original density. *The total mAs is the prime factor for controlling image density*, because it does not directly affect other image qualities.

Kilovoltage-Peak

Kilovoltage-peak directly affects image density. However, this relationship is *exponential* rather than *proportional*. That is, a small increase in kVp results in a large increase in image density. The relationship follows the *15 per cent rule*: A 15 per cent increase in kVp causes twice as dark a radiograph (100 per cent darker). A 15 per cent decrease in kVp results in an image one-half as dark.

Two useful correlaries follow: An 8 per cent increase in kVp increases density by one-half or 50 per cent, and a 5 per cent change in kVp is the minimum required to see a visible difference in image density.

The 15 per cent rule should be used when compensating for mAs changes. To maintain the original density when the mAs is doubled, reduce kVp by 15 per cent. Kilovoltage can be used for density compensations, but is not recommended as a control for density. *Optimum kVp*, however, is essential to allow the production of adequate density: kVp affects density because it controls the *proportion* of the original x-rays which are able to penetrate through the body and reach the film. Adequate density cannot be produced without sufficient penetration.

Machine Phase and Rectification

The type of electrical generators and rectifiers used in x-ray equipment affects the output intensity of the x-ray beam, as well as its average energy, and directly bears upon the resulting density of the image. Operated at the same mAs, three-phase equipment produces twice the density when compared to single-phase machines.

Constant potential generators such as battery-powered mobile units, and high-frequency generators can be equal to or somewhat higher than three-phase units in their efficiency. They often require less kVp to obtain the same density levels. Half-rectified units require four times the mAs used on a three-phase unit in order to achieve adequate density.

Protective Filtration

Excessive filtration in the x-ray beam can lead to a visible reduction in image density, due to its absorption of x-rays. However, the removal of filtration (or a small increase in it) will not visibly affect the density of radiographs in daily practice, because the body of the patient will absorb nearly all of what the filtration "missed."

Compensating Filtration

Compensating filters, such as wedges and troughs, are specifically designed to even out the density on radiographs of anatomy with irregular thickness or absorption characteristics. These filters are as much as five times thicker than protective filtration, and thus result in visible density effects. If they were inappropriately used on regular anatomy, the thicker end of the filter would result in less image density. They can be used to advantage on irregular anatomy, however, to produce more consistent densities across the radiograph.

Field Size Limitation

Collimation of the field size to smaller, confined areas results in a loss of image density. Density may drop by one-third to one-half, depending on how drastic the change is, and should be compensated for by a corresponding increase in mAs. The loss in density is brought about because less tissue is exposed, producing less scatter radiation. Even though the intensity of primary radiation is maintained, the reduction in scatter radiation results in a lower total exposure to the film, and a visible drop in density.

Patient Status and Contrast Agents

Larger body part thicknesses result in a loss of image density, simply because more radiation is absorbed within the patient and less reaches the film. The *four-centimeter rule* should be used to compensate for deviations in patient thickness from the average of 22 cm measured anterior-to-posterior and 30 cm laterally. For every increase of 4 cm, mAs should be doubled. For patients who are thinner than average, cut mAs in half for every 4 cm.

The radiographer must be observant of body habitus, anthropological factors and condition in deriving appropriate techniques to maintain density. Large muscular patients require a much greater increase in technique than hypersthenic patients. Fluid distention requires more technique than obesity. Brachiocephalic skulls often require more technique than average. Expiration chest radiographs require more exposure than the normal inspiratory views.

The main technique consideration when contrast agents are introduced into body cavities is to obtain the optimum kVp to achieve penetration of some of the x-rays through the contrast bolus. Iodine compounds require at least 80 kVp, while solid-column barium studies require over 100 kVp with a corresponding reduction in mAs, and air-contrast barium studies about 90 kVp. These compensations are necessary to "see through" the contrast bolus to obtain maximum information, and the bolus should thus appear as a very light gray rather than blank white. Blank areas on the radiograph contain *no* information and are diagnostically useless.

Pathology and Casts

Additive diseases which increase the bone or fluid component of tissue require increases in technique, typically from one-third to one-half again as much. Destructive diseases which reduce bone or fluid content, or which increase gas or fat content, necessitate a technique reduction. Recommendations for specific diseases are presented in Chapter 11. Failure to make these compensations will result in densities that are either too light or too dark.

Casts and splints will result in inadequate image density unless technique is increased to compensate for them. Plaster casts require from 2 to 4 times the average technique, while half-casts, wood splints and similar devices require a 50 per cent increase. Specific recommendations are given in Chapter 11. Using the 15 per cent rule, kVp may be used to make these types of technique adjustments.

Extraneous Fog

Scattered radiation, from whatever source, always increases overall image density, and can thus contribute to overexposure. Since fog density is always destructive to the image, field size limitation, optimum kVp, grids, leaded masking sheets, and other methods must be used to control it.

Fogging of the radiograph can also occur from accidental exposure to light, heat or chemical fumes. All fog results in undesirable, darker density.

Grids

The use of grids always lightens the radiographic density unless compensated for. The higher the grid ratio, the more severe the loss of image density. The recommended compensation is an increase in mAs from 2 to 5 times that of a nongrid, tabletop technique, depending on grid ratio. Chapter 13 lists specific recommendations.

Misuse of grids can lead to grid cut-off, an unacceptable loss of density over particular regions of the radiograph. Causes of grid cut-off include off-angling, off-centering, SID outside of the grid radius and grids placed upside-down.

Intensifying Screens

The use of intensifying screens always enhances radiographic density and allows the reduction of patient exposure by compensated techniques. If technique is not compensated, then the higher the speed of the screen, the darker the resulting image density. Special gradient screens can be used to even out the density for radiographs of body parts with irregular thicknesses.

State-of-the-art radiology departments currently use 400-speed "regular" rare earth screens. "Medium" rare earth screens and "High-speed" calcium tungstate screens are typically 200 to 250 speed, and require about double the mAs from the 400-speed screen. "Extremity" screen cassettes usually require 6 times the technique

for a "regular" screen, or 3 times the technique for a "medium" screen, to maintain density. There are many variations in screen speeds, types and brands. Specific compensating factors and special circumstances are described in Chapter Fourteen.

Films

The higher the speed of radiographic film, the darker the image density will be for a given exposure level. Faster films allow lower mAs values in obtaining the same density. Films are designed according to the types of screens or exposure holders used with them, and the type of film must be appropriately matched according to manufacturer specifications, or a light density will result.

Anode Heel Effect

The anode heel effect results in a slight loss of density toward the end of the film nearest the x-ray tube anode. This is used to advantage for wedge-shaped anatomy by placing the thinnest anatomy toward the anode, but is detrimental to radiographs of regular anatomy.

Source-Image Receptor Distance (SID)

Image density is inversely related to distances in an exponential fashion. Small changes in distance cause substantial changes in density. The greater the SID (the distance from the x-ray source to the image receptor), the less the density. This relationship follows the *inverse square law* described in Chapter 18. Density will be inversely proportional to the square of the change in distance. For example, doubling the distance results in one-fourth the image density.

To prevent such dramatic changes in

density, the *square law for technique* must be applied: Adjust the mAs according to the square of the distance change. For example, if the distance is doubled, the mAs should be quadrupled to maintain density.

Distance changes should be compensated with mAs rather than with kVp. Distance and mAs both affect the x-ray beam intensity without changing its quality (energy). An adjustment in kVp would unnecessarily change other image qualities besides density.

Object-Image Receptor Distance (OID)

Dramatic changes in object-image receptor distance can cause visible differences in image density. The larger the OID, the less the resulting density. When the air-gap technique is used, or whenever the OID cannot be minimized, an increase in mAs from one-third to one-half is required to maintain adequate density.

Processing

If an exposed radiographic film is developed for too long, at too high a temperature, or in chemicals that are too concentrated, it will turn out dark. Details of these relationships are explained in Chapter Thirty-Seven.

CONTRAST AND GRAY SCALE

Kilovoltage-Peak

Kilovoltage-Peak (kVp) should be considered as the prime factor for controlling radiographic image contrast and gray scale. It does so both through its effect upon x-ray beam *penetration* and upon the *proportion of scatter radiation reaching the film*. At higher kVp levels, more different types of tissue are penetrated by the x-ray beam and recorded as shades of gray. With more shades of gray present in the image, there is a smaller degree of difference from one shade to the next, therefore, contrast decreases. When long gray scale is desired, high kVp should be used. When high contrast is desired, low kVp should be used. Optimum kVp is the minimum kVp which still penetrates *all* tissues of interest. At this level, both contrast and gray scale will be balanced.

In addition to its penetration effects, high kVp also results in a loss of most photoelectric interactions in the tissues. The remaining image is then controlled mostly by penetrating rays and scattered rays. Also, more scatter radiation reaches the film because it is produced with higher energy and in a more forward direction. Image fog becomes more visible, and contributes to the reduction of apparent contrast.

Machine Phase

Three-phase and high-frequency generators produce a higher average x-ray beam energy. Penetration is enhanced, slightly lengthening the gray scale and slightly reducing the contrast in the resulting image.

Field Size Limitation

When the field size is collimated to a smaller area, image contrast is enhanced. Less exposed tissue is available to produce scatter radiation, but the primary beam concentration is unaffected. With a reduction in the proportion of fog in the image, contrast will increase.

Patient Status and Contrast Agents

With thicker patients, more exposed tissue is available to produce scatter radiation. Even as the primary beam is attenuated by the tissue mass, scatter increases, fogging the film and reducing contrast. Technique must be increased to maintain density, so the only ways to counter this fog are to use grids, collimate the field size, and if possible for chest radiographs use the air-gap technique.

Contrast agents are designed to enhance subject contrast by exaggerating differences in penetration through different tissues. Positive contrast agents absorb radiation, but should not stop *all* of the beam. Therefore, optimum kVp must be used for these agents to obtain partial penetration through them and maximize radiographic information. Negative agents are highly radiolucent and generally require a decrease in kVp to optimize both density and contrast levels in the image.

Pathology and Casts

Muscular or fluid-distended tissues produce much more fog than fatty tissues, and air produces almost no fog. Plaster casts produce additional scatter, especially when wet. The Radiographer should be aware of these effects in evaluating each patient.

Extraneous Fog

Anything that reduces the occurrence of photoelectric interactions in the patient, or that increases the occurrence of Compton scattering interactions, will result in more visible fog in the image, as explained in Chapters 4 and 12. Fog may also be caused from light, heat, chemical fumes or over-processing. Fogging destroys image contrast.

An important and interesting point is that *fog also destroys gray scale.* When all of the shades of gray are darkened by a blanket density, there will be a net loss in the number of shades present, because extremely light shades will no longer be present and shades that should have been dark gray will be black.

Grids

Grids were developed for the express purpose of restoring image contrast when larger body parts are radiographed. The large amounts of exposed tissue result in more scatter radiation produced. Grids eliminate much of this scattered radiation before it reaches the film, as described in Chapter 13. The higher the grid ratio, the more effective it is in "cleaning up" scatter, and the higher the resulting image contrast.

Intensifying Screens

Because of their magnifying effect on film exposure, the use of intensifying screens results in much higher image contrast than direct exposure techniques, as described in Chapter 14. Generally, high-speed screens produce somewhat higher contrast in the image than slow-speed screens, however, this is not *always* the case. Screens were developed to enhance density, and any effect they have on image contrast is a side-effect. Therefore, they are not of primary concern when regarding image contrast.

Radiographic Film

Generally, higher-speed films also produce higher image contrast. Film can be chemically treated to produce either longer gray scale or higher contrast, according to the needs of the diagnostician. The recommendations of manufacturers should be strictly followed when matching films and screens to obtain a desired image quality.

Object-Image Receptor Distance (OID)

When the OID is increased, leaving a gap between the body and the film, scattered radiation produced within the tissues and emitted at random angles is allowed to diverge more before reaching the film, in accordance with the inverse square law. The divergence of the primary beam, however, is unaffected by a change in OID. Hence, the concentration of scattered rays is reduced while the primary beam remains at the same intensity. A smaller proportion of the resulting image will be composed of fog, and contrast will increase. The intentional use of a large OID for the purpose of enhancing contrast is called the *air gap technique*.

Motion

Motion should not be considered as a *controlling* factor for image contrast. If it is severe enough, however, it can reduce contrast because of the superimposition of different densities across the image. This process is explained later in this chapter.

Processing

There are optimum times, temperatures and chemical concentrations for processing radiographic film, as described in Chapter Thirty-Seven. Although slight increases in any of these may increase contrast, excessive development time, temperature or chemical action will fog the film and destroy contrast as a rule.

NOISE

Milliampere-Seconds (mAs)

Insufficient mAs leaves such a light exposure reaching the film that the uneven distribution of x-rays within the beam becomes visible on the finished image. The resulting blotchy or freckled appearance in the image is called *quantum mottle*, and is a form of image noise because it interferes with the visibility of details.

Kilovoltage-Peak

Because of the loss of photoelectric interactions at high kVp levels, the remaining image is composed only of penetrating rays and scattered rays. Further, a higher proportion of those scattered rays that are produced will reach the film, because they have more energy and are emitted in a more forward direction. Fog in the image becomes more apparent. A high proportion of fog interferes with the visibility of image details. Therefore, high kVp may be considered as a contributor to image noise.

Field Size

Larger field sizes increase the amount of exposed tissue producing scatter radiation. The scatter creates noise in the image in the form of fog. This noise is reduced by limiting field size to the anatomy of interest.

Patient Status and Pathology

Large patients also increase the amount of exposed tissue creating scatter radiation, causing more noise in the form of image fog.

Artifacts and Casts

Artifacts include any object or substance inadvertently left within the passage of the x-ray beam which impedes visibility of image details. A few examples are objects or clothing left on the patient, removable devices on the patient's person such as dentures, objects left on the x-ray table or film, particles of dirt or paper inside intensifying screens, and contrast agents soaked into positioning sponges from previous spills. Casts and splints also interfere with the image quality, and constitute noise, even though they may not be removable.

Extraneous Fog

Fog on the radiograph, whatever the source, constitutes noise since it reduces visibility of details.

Grid Lines

Grid cut-off may be considered an extreme case of artifacts occluding the image. But stationary grids such as those taped to cassettes during mobile procedures will result in grid lines even when they are used properly. On close inspection, one can see the clear white lines where grid strips absorbed radiation, reducing the amount of information reaching the film. Grid lines interfere with details and are a form of noise.

Intensifying Screens and Film

The use of extremely high speed intensifying screens can lead to very low mAs values. As previously explained, this will lead to quantum mottle, a form of noise. Clumping of crystals in the manufacture of emulsions for screens or for radiographic film can cause a mottled appearance in the finished radiograph that is unrelated to the x-ray beam itself. This type of image noise is referred to as screen mottle or as film mottle, respectively.

Motion

In addition to its blurring effects, motion of the patient, the x-ray tube or the film during exposure can cause the production of false images such as streaks, described in Chapter Twenty-Three. False images can obscure the anatomy of interest, and are a form of image noise.

GEOMETRICAL INTEGRITY (RECOGNIZABILITY)

The geometrical functions of an image are those qualities which allow correct recognition of the object it represents. There are three such functions fully defined and explained in Chapter Three: Sharpness of recorded detail, magnification and shape distortion. The variables determining the integrity of the image by affecting these three qualities will be reviewed:

SHARPNESS OF RECORDED DETAIL

Focal Spot Size

The size of the focal spot should be considered as the primary control for sharpness of recorded detail in the image, for two reasons: (1) It is the only variable that *exclusively* affects sharpness, without affecting any other image characteristic, (2) It is readily manipulated by the radiographer. The smaller the focal spot, the sharper the recorded detail. The relationship is inversely proportional: If the focal spot size is reduced to one-half the original, sharpness of detail doubles.

Radiographers should be conscientious enough to utilize the small focal spot whenever high detail resolution is of essence, (for example, whenever "extremity" cassettes are used). The large focal spot must be employed whenever high techniques might overheat the x-ray tube.

Anode Bevel

Through the line-focus principle described in Chapter Seventeen, steeper anode bevels (at a smaller angle from vertical) result in smaller projected focal spot sizes, and therefore contribute to sharpness of recorded detail.

Source-Image Receptor Distance (SID)

SID is directly proportional to the sharpness of recorded detail produced in the image. If the distance is doubled, the sharpness is doubled, provided all other factors are equal. SID should not, however, be considered as a primary control for sharpness, because it affects other image qualities as well, and because it cannot always be easily modified.

Object-Image Receptor Distance (OID)

When the distance from the object to the image receptor is increased, sharpness of recorded detail is reduced. If all other factors are kept equal, the sharpness is inversely proportional to the OID. When OID is doubled, sharpness is cut to one-half due to a doubling of the penumbra. The OID should always be kept at a minimum.

SOD/OID Ratio

The ratio of SOD to OID is directly proportional to sharpness of recorded detail, as discussed in Chapter Twenty. If both the SID and the OID are doubled, the SOD will also be doubled. The SOD/OID ratio will therefore be unchanged, and image sharpness will remain equal.

Positioning

If the body is positioned so that the anatomy of interest is further from the film than necessary, sharpness of recorded detail is diminished. This effect is due to a change in the OID where the "object" is restricted to the specific anatomy of interest. Radiographers must utilize those positions which place the anatomy as close as possible to the image receptor.

Motion and Exposure Time

Motion blurs the image and is therefore the prime enemy of sharpness of recorded detail. Radiographers must use communication skills, immobilization and short exposure times to reduce the probability of motion occurring.

Long exposure times are not the *direct cause* of motion. But in chest radiography, for example, heart motion is unavoidable, and can only be eliminated radiographically by the use of very short exposure times. In addition, the longer the time, the greater the chance for peristaltic motion, breathing motion or movement of the patient to occur. Therefore, exposure time should be considered as a *contributing factor* of motion during radiographic procedures. Generally, the shorter the exposure time, the sharper the recorded detail.

Intensifying Screens

The use of an intensifying screen always results in less sharpness of detail than the use of direct exposure holders, because light from a screen diffuses prior to reaching the film. When changing from one screen speed to a higher speed, image sharpness *may* be compromised depending on the manufacturing method by which the higher speed was achieved. If a thicker emulsion or larger crystals were used, sharpness will be reduced. If chemical differences were used, sharpness may be unaffected, or even enhanced if the resulting emulsion layer is thinner. As a general rule, the higher the speed, the less the sharpness.

Image Receptor Systems

Usually, the higher the speed of a radiographic film, the lower the sharpness of recorded detail. As with screens, chemical changes will not affect sharpness. But most speed differences in films are due to crystal size or emulsion thickness. Any increase in these will reduce sharpness.

Duplitized film is less sharp than single-emulsion film, because of the parallax effect of viewing two images in two separate emulsions.

Single-screen cassettes result in better sharpness of detail than double-screen cassettes, due to the elimination of the crossover effect described in Chapter Fourteen.

MAGNIFICATION

Source-Image Receptor Distance (SID)

The SID is inversely related to magnification, but not proportional to it. A longer SID projects the image of the object with more parallel beams, and results in less magnification. The reduction in magnification, however, is relatively small compared to the change made in the SID. The longest feasible SID should always be used to minimize image magnification.

Object-Image Receptor Distance (OID)

The OID is directly related to magnification, but again, is not proportional to it. The greater the OID, the greater the magnification. If the OID is doubled, the image size will not double, but it will increase (by about 30 per cent). The OID should always be minimized to control magnification.

SID/SOD Ratio

The SID/SOD ratio should be considered as the primary controlling factor for magnification of the image size. The SID/SOD ratio is directly proportional to the magnification factor.

For example, a 20-inch SID and a 15-inch SOD yields a magnification factor of $20/15 = 1.25$ or 25 per cent magnification. Doubling the SID to 40 inches without changing the object-film distance results in an SOD of 35 inches, and the magnification factor becomes $40/35 = 1.14$ or 14 per cent magnification.

To minimize magnification of the image, the SID/SOD ratio should always be kept as low as possible. This is accomplished by long SID's and short OID's.

Positioning

Since positioning of the patient may place the anatomy of interest nearer to or further from the film, effectively changing the OID it can result in unnecessary magnification of the anatomy of interest. To minimize magnification, radiographic positioning should always be done with an eye to placing the anatomy of interest as close to the film as possible.

SHAPE DISTORTION

Beam-Part-Film Alignment and Positioning

The *only* variable which affects shape distortion in radiography is beam-part-film alignment. Nonetheless, this variable has several aspects including positioning of the patient, the actual shape of the anatomy of interest, centering of the central ray, angulation of the x-ray beam, and proper placement of the film holder or image receptor. Beam-part-film alignment is the controlling factor for distortion.

If the anatomy of interest is thick and spherical or cubical in general shape, any distortion of it will be exacerbated. If it is thin and flat, linear, tubular, or wedge-shaped, with a distinct long axis, then distortion effects will not be as severe.

When the long axis of an object is angled in relation to the film, while the beam is perpendicular to the film, foreshortening distortion will occur.

When the object and the film are parallel to each other, any angling of the x-ray beam so that it is not perpendicular to them will cause elongation distortion. However, when the object is angled in relation to the film, distortion is minimized by using Ceiszynski's law of isometry: Angle the central ray one-half of the angle formed between the object and the film.

Off-centering of the central ray from the anatomy of interest causes distortion effects similar to angulation. Positioning must be performed with an eye to maintaining a perpendicular beam-film relationship and a parallel part-film relationship whenever possible.

RESOLUTION

In evaluating the overall quality of any image, the concept of resolution is of essence. A dictionary may define optical resolution as the "ability to distinguish the individual parts of an object or closely adjacent images," as being separate from each other. On a radiograph, in order for two small, closely adjacent details to be recog-

nized as distinct and separate from each other, density and contrast must be optimal, sharpness of recorded detail must be high, and magnification, distortion, and noise must be minimal. *All of the image qualities affect resolution.*

To fully understand resolution, these six qualities must be considered collectively, in

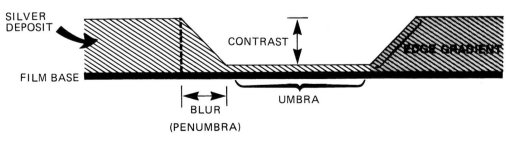

Figure 175. Density trace diagram. Image *contrast* is indicated by differences in the vertical depth of the silver deposit on the film, comparing the middle of the image to the background deposit. The *edge gradient* is the slope in the silver deposit at the edges of the image. Penumbra or blur is indicated by the *horizontal* spread of the edge gradient.

relation to each other, rather than individually. A helpful aid in studying these interrelationships is the density trace diagram.

DENSITY TRACE DIAGRAMS

Density trace diagrams are simple diagrams of a physical "cross-section" of the radiographic film emulsion after development. They demonstrate the thickness of metallic silver deposit remaining on different areas of the film. Where the thickness

of the silver is great, the film would appear dark, thinner regions would appear gray, and areas with little or no silver thickness would appear nearly clear or "white."

Contrast can be defined as the ratio between two adjacent densities. This difference is shown on a density trace as the *vertical* distance through which the image edge drops (Figure 175). This contrast measurement must be taken at the center of the image, as compared to the density outside the image.

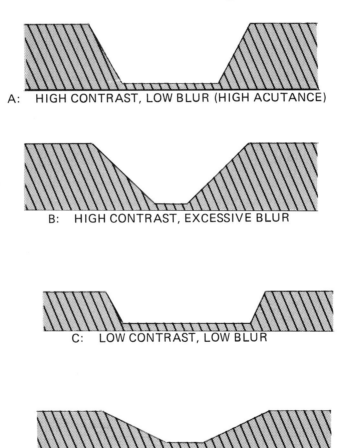

A: HIGH CONTRAST, LOW BLUR (HIGH ACUTANCE)

B: HIGH CONTRAST, EXCESSIVE BLUR

C: LOW CONTRAST, LOW BLUR

D: LOW CONTRAST, EXCESSIVE BLUR

Figure 176. Density trace diagrams for various contrast and sharpness levels. (A) is the best resolved image, with high contrast (vertical density drop) and high sharpness (steep edge gradients). (B) shows increased blur, but still has high contrast. (C) shows a loss of visibility low contrast, but has sharp edges. (D) is the poorest image, with both low contrast and excessive blur.

One can see that the density at the edge of a radiographic image does not drop straight down. Rather, it drops more or less gradually, forming a slope of decreasing silver deposit on the film. This slope is called the *edge gradient*, Figure 175. The edge gradient can be measured by dividing the height of the slope by its width. For example, if the silver deposit drops 10 microns over a horizontal distance of 2 microns, the edge gradient is $10/2 = 5$ (A in Figure 176). If it takes 4 microns of horizontal distance for the silver deposit to drop 10 microns, the edge gradient is $10/4 = 2.5$ (B in Figure 176). A high edge gradient indicates a steep slope, a low edge gradient indicates a gradual slope.

The abruptness of the edge of a radiographic image is called its *acutance*, how *acutely* it drops off. Acutance is closely related to the sharpness of recorded detail. A steep edge gradient indicates high acutance, and results in a high level of image sharpness.

Sharpness is defined in terms of the *horizontal* distance through which the edge gradient passes. More precisely, the horizontal measurement of the edge gradient represents penumbra or blur from *un*sharpness, Figure 175.

At this point, one can readily see that contrast and sharpness are closely related to each other, because they both affect the slope of the edge gradient. In other words, contrast and sharpness are both essential to the *resolution* of image detail. Resolution of detail depends upon both sharpness and contrast.

Nonetheless, contrast and sharpness are different image qualities, and they must not be confused, even though they are related. Figure 176 illustrates the traces for various images with different contrast and blur levels. High contrast images can still have poor resolution if edges are blurred (Figure 176-B). Low contrast images can be sharp in spite of poor visibility (Figure 176-C).

Image resolution may be measured with the unit *line pairs per millimeter*, using a test template as shown in Figure 36, Chapter Three. Exposure of this device records alternating black- and white lines on the film so that it can be visually determined which ones can be distinguished from each other, as shown in Figure 132, Chapter 16. The smaller the lines resolved, the more of them would fit into one millimeter. This measurement is called *spatial frequency*, the number of details that fit into a given *space* of one millimeter and still be visibly distinct. Spatial frequency depends on both contrast and sharpness. It is a direct measurement of overall image resolution that the radiograph can achieve.

MODULATION TRANSFER FUNCTION

Physicists use a complex measurement of the total resolution capacity of an imaging system called *modulation transfer function* or *MTF*. A full discussion of MTF is not necessary for radiographers, but it is worth noting that MTF is very similar to density trace diagrams. If one were to expose a resolution test template (Figure 36), the density trace diagram for the resulting silver deposits on the film would be essentially identical to an MTF graph. A high MTF indicates that the imaging system produces high resolution, and therefore provides images with maximum diagnostic information. A low MTF indicates poor overall image quality.

GEOMETRICAL PENUMBRA

X-rays can be emitted at various angles and from different points within the area of the focal spot, and yet record the same edge of an object on the film. This means that the same edge of the object will actually be recorded several times in various different locations on the film, Figure 177. This "spreading" of the edge constitutes blur or *penumbra,* and is fully explained in Chapter 16 (see Figure 134).

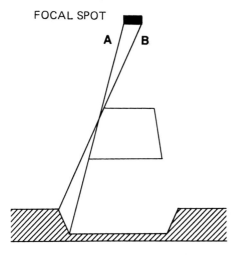

FOCAL SPOT

A   B

Figure 177. Density trace diagram illustrating geometrical penumbra. The extent of penumbra is represented by the horizontal spread of the edge gradient slopes.

In Figure 177, between "A" and "B" absorption of the x-ray beam is *partial,* increasing toward the object. Hence, "penumbra" may be thought of as a *partial absorption* process (bearing in mind that "partial" refers to a portion of the total amount of x-rays which the object in question is capable of absorbing, not to a portion of the total x-ray beam).

Motion and Parallax Blur

Motion blur and parallax blur (from double-coated film) are actually both superimposition processes which result in *horizontal* spreading of the edge (Figure 178). Motion should not be considered to affect image contrast unless it is so severe that this horizontal spreading crosses the middle of the image, effectively reducing the vertical component of the density trace at mid-image (Figure 178-B).

ABSORPTION PENUMBRA

"Absorption unsharpness" or "absorption penumbra" is a blurring of the edge of an image due to the relationship between the shape of the object being radiographed and the diverging x-ray beam. Suppose that several objects having different shapes, but made out of the same, homogeneous material, are to be radiographed:

The "ideal" shape for an object to be radiographed would be a trapezoid whose slanted sides coincide exactly with the angles of the diverging x-rays (Figure 179-A). All portions of the x-ray beam striking such an object will be attenuated by the same thickness of material. The density trace diagram in Figure 179 shows that there will be no blur due to absorption unsharpness at the edge of the image produced. Note that the black silver deposit on the film drops off straight down at the edge of this image. The image of the trapezoid is as "white" just inside the edge as it is in the middle. This "sudden" change in density at the edge of the image represents a sharp edge with no blur.

Imaging a *cube* of the same material (Figure 179-B) yields different results: Note that the lateral diverging x-rays pass through only a small thickness of material at the upper corners of the cube. Little absorption occurs, and the density trace shows a reduced but still dark deposit of silver. As inner beams pass through thicker portions, the density trace drops until the full thickness of the cube is reached at the lower corners (dashed line). On observing this image, the density would gradually

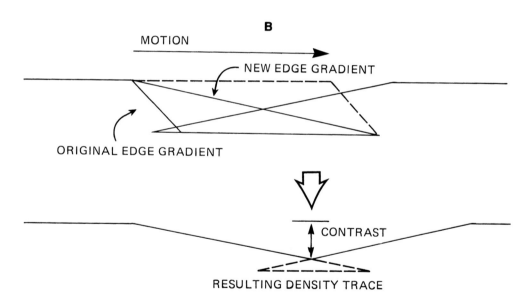

Figure 178. Density trace diagrams showing the effects of motion on image sharpness and contrast. Slight motion (A) increases the horizontal spread of the edge gradient, reducing sharpness, but contrast at the middle of the image is unchanged. With *severe* motion (B), the edge gradients may begin to overlap, causing a loss of contrast.

change from dark to light as one scans across its edge. This effect is identical to geometrical blurring, even though it is caused by a different process.

Worse yet is the spherical object (Figure 179-C), whose full thickness is found only at the center. The density trace shows that the drop in density is very gradual and the edges of the image very indistinct.

Referring to Figure 179, note that all three objects are of the same thickness in the center, and should have identical absorption and identical contrast at this point. Indeed, the density traces have dropped the same vertical distance in the center of each image.

TOTAL PENUMBRA

A representation of total blur or penumbra may be obtained by combining the diagram for geometrical blur with that for absorption blur (Figure 180), using a cube or a spherical object. In this case, all beams are not absorbed at the inside penumbral line, but rather at the (dashed) absorption line. Within the penumbral (solid) lines, absorption varies primarily because the beams originate at different points within the focal spot. Within the dashed lines, absorption continues to vary, but strictly because of changing object thickness. *Total penumbra is comprised of geometrical penumbra plus absorption penumbra.*

MAGNIFICATION, DISTORTION AND NOISE

Magnification or distortion of an image does not cause any change in edge gradient. The slope of the edge will drop at the same rate. (Many of the same variables that create magnification also cause unsharpness, and it is easy to mistake the two as being directly related to each other, but they are not. If the magnification of an image is accompanied by increased blur, that is, if the expansion of the umbra is accompanied by an expansion of the penumbra, then adjacent details may overlap and image resolution will be lost. But, this loss of resolution is due to the *blurring,* which does affect the slope of the edge gradient, *not* to the magnification. Desirable magnification techniques, such as those used in angiography, can be employed without a loss of sharpness.)

Clearly, the enlargement of any image makes it more visible overall, but results in an inaccurate representation of its true size. The value of magnification depends on

Figure 179. Density trace diagrams for absorption penumbra, using objects of equal width but different shapes. The trapezoid object (A) will produce *geometrical* penumbra as shown in Figure 177, but will have no *absorption* penumbra as shown here. The square object (B) absorbs most radiation at the thickest portion of its projected edge, causing a penumbral edge gradient. For a spherical object (C) the edge gradient (penumbra) extends to the middle of the image. This represents the most severe absorption penumbra.

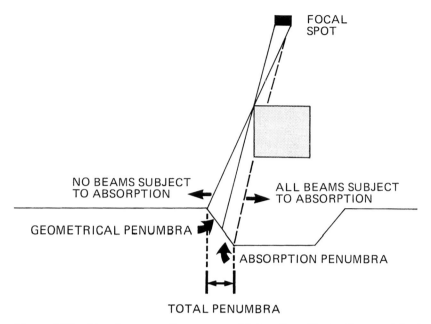

FOCAL SPOT

NO BEAMS SUBJECT TO ABSORPTION

ALL BEAMS SUBJECT TO ABSORPTION

GEOMETRICAL PENUMBRA

ABSORPTION PENUMBRA

TOTAL PENUMBRA

Figure 180. Density trace diagram combining the effects of geometrical penumbra and absorption penumbra in producing the total penumbra or total amount of blurring at the edge of the image.

whether the diagnostic emphasis is on measurement or simple detection.

Noise, such as an artifact or fog, superimposes and obscures the visibility of the anatomy of interest. This does not change the slope of the edge gradient, but since details are obscured, overall image resolution is lost. The effects of scatter radiation are thoroughly discussed in Chapter 12.

CRITIQUING AND REPEATING RADIOGRAPHS

Radiographers must develop, primarily through experience, the ability to accurately assess the technical qualities of the finished radiograph–its density level, contrast, gray scale, noise level, sharpness of recorded detail, and any magnification or distortion present. This ability is *essential* to the control of unnecessary repeated exposures to the patient. A review of the radiographs used throughout this book, particularly in Chapter 3, should help.

The single greatest technical cause for repeated exposures is improper density levels. Exposed radiographs that are either too light or too dark account for *73 per cent* of all repeats in radiology departments without quality control programs, and for *33 per cent* of all repeats in departments with quality control (see Table XXVIII, Chap. 30).

The following exercise is designed to help the student develop an ability to visually estimate the needed adjustment in overall technique when repeating an exposure that turned out too light or too dark. In each of two series of radiographs (Figures 181 and 182), a radiograph with optimum density level is first shown for

Figure 181. Chest radiographs: Estimate density change needed. Answers in Appendix II.

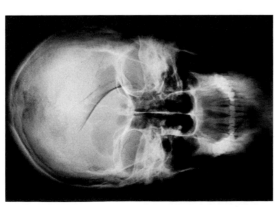

Figure 182. Skull radiogrpahs: Estimate density change needed. Answers in Appendix II.

comparison. The following numbered radiographs were taken at precisely selected techniques at rounded out values, such as double the original mAs or one-third the original mAs. For each of the numbered radiographs, estimate the *overall technique change* required to restore density to the optimum level. All answers are in factors of 2, 3 or 4. Check your answers using the Appendix.

EXERCISE 23:
CRITIQUING RADIOGRAPHIC DENSITY

A: For the series of chest radiographs in Figure 181, compare each of the *numbered* radiographs to the *optimum* radiograph first shown. List the *factor* to which the density for each numbered radiograph should be changed to restore it to optimum density. The correct answer will be *4X, 3X, 2X, 1/2, 1/3 or 1/4*.

B: For the series of skull radiographs in Figure 182, compare each of the *numbered* radiographs to the *optimum* radiograph first shown. List the *factor* to which the density for each numbered radiograph should be changed to restore it to optimum density. The correct answer will be *4X, 3X, 2X, 1/2, 1/3 or 1/4*.

SUMMARY

1. Image *density* is affected by mAs, kVp, machine phase, filtration, field size, patient condition and casts, contrast agents, fog, grids, screen/film combinations, the anode heel effect, SID, OID, and processing.

2. Image *contrast* and gray scale are affected by kVp, machine phase, field size, patient condition and contrast agents, fog, grids, screens and film, motion and processing.

3. Image *noise* can be caused by insufficient mAs, excessive kVp, excessive field size, large patients, fog, grids, screens and film, motion, and artifacts.

4. *Sharpness of recorded* image *detail* is affected by focal spot size and the anode bevel angle, SOD, OID, SOD/OID ratio, positioning, motion, and image receptor systems.

5. *Magnification* of the image is affected by SID, SOD, the SID/SOD ratio and positioning.

6. *Distortion* of the image shape is affected by beam-part-film alignment, which includes angling and centering considerations, and positioning.

7. Image *resolution* depends upon *both* contrast and sharpness of recorded detail. A loss of either one of these qualities makes it more difficult to distinguish adjacent details. Resolution is determined by the *edge gradient* of the image, and can be measured by modulation transfer function (MTF) or by spatial frequency in line pairs per millimeter (LP/mm).

8. The *total penumbra* or total *blur* in an image is the sum of geometrical penumbra plus absorption penumbra.

9. One of the most fundamental skills for the radiographer is the ability to analyze proper image density to determine if a repeated exposure is indicated. Improper density can account for $1/3$ to $3/4$ of all necessitated repeats. This skill must be developed by practice.

REVIEW QUESTIONS

1. What variable is the primary *control* for image density?
2. What variable is the primary *control* for image contrast?
3. What variable is the primary *control* for sharpness of recorded detail?
4. What variable is the primary *control* for image magnification?
5. What variable is the primary *control* for distortion of image shape?
6. What effect do additive diseases or casts generally have upon image density?
7. What effect does the anode heel effect have upon image density?
8. What variable is the primary *control* for image gray scale?
9. What form of noise destroys *both* image contrast and gray scale?
10. How can stationary grids contribute to image noise, even if they are properly aligned ?
11. Artifacts should be classified in the hierarchy of image qualities as _____.
12. Name *two* types of mottle that high-speed receptor systems might lead to:

13. Streaks caused by motion or by tomography should not be considered as distorted images but rather as _____ images, a form of image noise.
14. Positioning can be *indirectly* related to both sharpness and magnification because it can alter the _____ distance to the anatomy of interest.
15. As demonstrated with density trace diagrams, what *two* image qualities combine to determine image resolution (the ability to distinguish adjacent details as being separate)?
16. As demonstrated by density trace diagrams, what *two* types of penumbra combine to form the total penumbra of an image?
17. The quantitative measurement of the total resolution of an imaging system used by physicists is called:
18. Even for departments with quality control programs, one-third of all repeated exposures is caused by improper image _____.
19. What is the only shape of object that would produce *no* absorption penumbra when projected by an x-ray beam?

As a general review of the variables that affect each image quality, complete the following EXERCISE 24, and check your answers from the Appendix.

EXERCISE 24

Directions: For each technique change listed at the left, indicate the effect it will have upon each image quality by placing a plus sign in the box if it increases the image quality, a minus sign if it decreases it, or a zero if it is not a *direct* cause of changes in the image quality. Assume that all factors are maintained equal except the listed change. For example, when the x-ray beam is angled, assume that the SID is maintained equal through compensating tube-to-tabletop distance.

	Density	Contrast	Sharpness	Magnification	Distortion
Increase mA					
Increase Exp. Time					
Increase kVp					
Increase Filtration					
From 1-Phase to to 3-Phase or HFG					
Increase Field Size					
Increase Motion					
Increase Patient Size					
Increase Grid Ratio					
Increase Screen Speed					
Increase Size of Focal Spot					
Increase SID					
Increase OID					
Misalign or Misangle Beam					

Chapter 25

SIMPLIFYING AND STANDARDIZING TECHNIQUE

THE FUNDAMENTALS of exposure are easy to understand and there seems to be no reason why they should be made complicated. It must be realized that the radiologist is not so much interested in the occasional "beautiful" radiograph–or poor one–as he is with *uniform* radiographic quality. Such uniformity from day to day and year to year can only be achieved through complete control and standardization of exposure and processing procedures. The *appearance* of the radiographic images should always be fairly consistent. The busy radiologist should not be obliged to interpret radiographs made with a particular projection in which the image of a body part is seldom twice alike. The apparatus, x-ray tube, x-ray film, and processing chemicals have been scientifically designed so that radiographic standardization may be more readily employed to produce radiographs from which the radiologist can make competent interpretations.

The common lack of unanimity on the subject of radiographic exposure is aptly demonstrated by the numerous recipes advanced in the form of complicated exposure tables. The lack of systematic and workable exposure method becomes readily apparent when it is necessary to train a student in radiographic exposure.

Standardized projections of an anatomic part portray the structures always in the same manner. It has been demonstrated repeatedly that an essential point in the radiographic diagnosis often appears in an inconspicuous portion of the image. Therefore, a systematic analysis and evaluation of the *entire* image should always be made. This requires that the entire image should be diagnostically informative and that translucent silver deposits representative of the anatomic structures always be produced.

RADIOGRAPHIC QUALITY

Radiographic quality should be evaluated along realistic lines rather than upon the emotional response of the individual observer to the image. Quality results when sound judgment is employed in the selection of the exposure factors and in the manner in which the exposed x-ray film is processed. Also, there should exist a balance in compromise between the exposure factors employed, the clinical situation as it is presented to the radiographer, and the objective of the examination–the diagnosis.

When a radiologist views a good radiograph, he is not particularly interested in how it was produced. But, if the quality is not what he should reasonably expect, then the *practical* reasons for failure should be recognized and investigated.

CRITERIA

The following criteria for attaining satisfactory radiographic quality may serve as a guide to better radiography.

1. All image densities should be translucent when viewed before a conventional x-ray illuminator.

2. All portions of the image should have silver deposit. Areas devoid of silver deposit are diagnostically useless. Excessive silver deposits should be avoided for they obscure detail and also are diagnostically useless.

3. The part examined should be fully penetrated.

4. The *basic mAs* factor should be selected so as to provide the best overall radiographic density for the patient whose measurement is within the *average* thickness range.

5. Contrast and gray scale should be balanced such that differentiation between densities or details can be readily made.

6. Image details should not be obscured by scatter radiation or chemical fog.

7. Maximum sharpness and true shape and size of the image should be consistent with the clinical needs of the examination.

EVOLVING THE EXPOSURE SYSTEM

The foregoing chapters have described in detail the functions of x-ray exposure factors. From this material may be summarized essential features that can serve as a basis for formulating a standardized exposure system. The ideal should establish all factors as constants with the exception of one to be employed as a variable. Hence, kilovoltage should be regarded as the factor of penetration, exposure latitude and radiographic contrast; milliampere-seconds as the factor of radiographic density; and the focal spot size, SID, SOD and OID as geometric factors influencing image sharpness, shape, and size. Thus, standardization of radiography resolves itself into three phases.

1. **Standardization of Exposure Factors.** The reduction of all exposure factors in a given projection to constants with the exception of one variable (mAs).

2. **Standardization of Projections.** A standard method for positioning the patient and projection of the central ray for a given procedure.

3. **Standardization of the Processing Procedure.** The reduction of time and temperature values to constants so that changes in radiographic density can more properly be attributed to exposure.

OPTIMUM (FIXED) KILOVOLTAGE TECHNIQUE

The bulk of modern radiography is expeditious effort. A standardized system for selecting and applying exposure factors therefore becomes a necessity. Such a system, however, must produce consistently good radiographic quality. The optimum kilovoltage technique satisfies these requirements. This technique was evolved to eliminate many complexities in the application of exposure factors and reduce them to simplicities. Specifically, it is based upon standardization of the processing procedure and the reduction of exposure factors to constants with the exception of one variable. The technic is based on the following general principles. By trial, a fixed or optimum kilovoltage is established for an average tissue thickness range and for a given projection. Once it has been found that the kilovoltage selected produces the most desirable amount of penetration and contrast for the given human part, irrespective of size, it is established as a constant. A basic mAs value is then decided upon that will produce the required amount of radiographic density within the average range. When a patient is classified as outside the average thickness range—smaller or larger—the basic mAs value is adjusted. All other factors, including processing, are constants.

TECHNIQUE

In working out an optimum kilovoltage technique, each projection must be considered individually. It must be understood that for a given thickness of a particular body part, the wave length of the x-rays employed to penetrate the tissues must be adequate or, in other words, *optimum*. The amount and kind of tissue—the relation of bone to soft tissue—and its penetrability by x-radiation must be evaluated. Measurement of the part must be made along the course traversed through the tissues by the central ray, and the average range of measurements verified by checking many individuals. On the basis of this information, a kilovoltage is selected that will thoroughly penetrate the part, irrespective of size, and produce a satisfactory contrast. Once established as optimum for the projection, it should not be changed unless the conditions under which the kVp was established are changed.

With the kVp fixed, a basic mAs or density value must be established for the average thickness range of the part. In deriving mAs values for thicknesses outside the average range or for variations in the physiologic or pathologic state of the tissues, a rule of thumb for density changes by mAs is employed. The source-image distance

need seldom be changed and may, in most cases, be considered a constant.

When the wave length is optimum, a lower mAs value is usually more adequate for the exposure than that habitually employed for the same purpose with the lower kilovoltages. Less mAs, of course, permits a greater number of radiographs to be made in a given projection before the limit of radiation safety is reached. The overall radiographic density produced by this method is uniform from case to case—a point of considerable diagnostic value because any differences from the normal density may then be attributed to abnormal changes within the tissues. Duplication of results is easy to attain in followup cases. The technique may be employed with any type of rectified or self- rectified apparatus. Whatever the type of generator, the only variable factor to adjust is the mAs; all other factors are constant.

Role of Thickness Ranges

Average thickness ranges are actually guides for establishing basic mAs values for various projections since approximately 85 per cent of all patients fall within these ranges. However, thickness ranges have been established for a number of projections shown in Table VII, Chapter 10. The approximate frequency in percentage with which these thicknesses appear is also listed.

Illustrated in Figures 183-184 are groups of unretouched radiographs in which, for the respective projections the exposure factors were identical since the thicknesses of the parts in each case were within the average range. Note the uniformity in density and contrast manifested in each group.

An overview of the optimum kVp determined for each type of anatomical part and procedure is presented in Table IV,

Figure 183. Radiographs of AP lumbar vertebrae of various patients made using a standardized technique chart.

Figure 184. Radiographs of lateral knee of various patients made using a standardized technique chart.

Chapter 6. Only in the most extreme cases of departure from the average would a kVp other than those listed in Table IV be necessary. Variable mAs, primarily through the use of exposure time, should be used to adjust for most changes in thickness.

OPTIMUM MILLIAMPERAGE

There are only three considerations in selecting an mA station: How short exposure times it will allow the technologist to use to reduce the probability of patient motion, how small a focal spot it will allow the technologist to use to obtain the sharpest geometric detail, and the heat generated at the surface of the anode which may cause anode damage.

First, it must be determined whether the small focal spot size is necessary. If so, this will narrow the choices of mA stations to a range from 10 to 300 mA. At the large focal spot size, mA stations from 200 up to as much as 1200 may be available. Milliamperage stations in the small focal spot range do not usually present overheating problems at the anode, precisely because they are limited to 300 mA or less. An overload condition can occur at these stations if the small focal spot is imprudently used on procedures requiring high kVp levels. The more common problem with overheating occurs at the large focal spot when milliamperage stations above 600 mA are used. Therefore, the maximum mA stations for general use should be considered as 200 or 300 at the small focal spot (depending on the equipment) and 600 mA at the large focal spot.

For a given procedure, the mA station should be standardized at one of these maximum levels in order to achieve the shortest possible exposure times in obtaining the needed total mAs values. But, mA settings above 600 should not generally be used, except in special procedures where the time factor becomes critical. Having optimized both kVp and milliamperage, the short exposure times achieved will minimize the probability of motion unsharpness. This method also reduces the number of exposure variables changed during the procedure to one, which is simpler and narrows the probability of mathematical technique errors. The ability to obtain an exact mAs is not a serious problem, because any desired mAs can be very nearly obtained at any mA station with the times available, with few exceptions. As a rule, then, once it is decided which focal spot to use for a given procedure, the maximum mA station available at that focal spot size should be used so that minimum times can be achieved for "manual" technique..

Secondly, eliminating mA as a density control during a procedure reduces the number of factors that the technologist must consider when setting technique, making it easier to deal with and reducing the probability of error.

CONTROLLING DENSITY WITH EXPOSURE TIME

It is confusing indeed when a technologist looks up a technique on a chart for the second or third view in a procedure and finds a different kVp, a different mA station, and a different time setting from the previous view. It turns out that the smallest density adjustments practical can nearly always be achieved by a change in exposure time. Thus, changing kVp or mA amounts to unnecessary work when done within a procedure from one view to the next.

SELECTION OF BASIC mAs

The mAs factor is the most reliable factor for regulating the *amount* of overall silver (density) in the image. There should be a satisfactory range of densities for interpretations of all portions of the image. The mAs can become a constant within certain limitations for a given projection. A *basic* mAs value can be established for any average thickness range of a part, provided it is established for an adult person.

Thickness Only a Guide

The thickness of any part serves only as a guide which the radiographer can use to expose the normal part and in determining what mAs will compensate for abnormal tissue changes. Obviously, if the part is normal and is in the average thickness range, the basic mAs can be employed. Knowledge of the structural makeup of the area is necessary when the kilovoltage has been fixed as a constant for the projection. The part should also be judged from a physiologic and pathologic standpoint as to whether it is reasonably normal. For the *small* part, the basic mAs value is halved; for the *average* part, the basic mAs value is employed; and for the *large* part, the basic mAs value is doubled. By means of these modifications, the radiographic density obtained will be approximately correct. If not, a slight increase or decrease in the mAs value in exposing a second film should provide the most desirable density. However, it will be found that a "remake" is seldom required.

OVEREXPOSURE

To the trained eye, the overexposed radiograph is easily identifiable. One type of overexposure exhibits an over-all grayness with low contrast. Another type of overexposure produces such a great density of the thinner portions of the part radiographed that they are obliterated. Regardless of how it is developed, an over-

exposed film lacks the requisites of ideal radiographic quality–proper radiographic density and contrast–as one or the other is invariably sacrificed. If the kilovoltage is correct, overexposure due to the mAs factor may usually be corrected by making another radiograph with one-half the original mAs ($^{1}/_{2}$X). Very frequently, the density of this second radiograph is satisfactory or is so near in quality that if a third radiograph is made, only a minor adjustment of the mAs is needed to secure the most desirable quality.

Example. Two anteroposterior screen-grid radiographs of the lumbar vertebrae, Figure 185, were made with 70 kVp and a 36-inch SID. The first radiograph (A) was made with a trial exposure of 200 mAs. The density was excessive. Applying the rule of thumb for density, the second radiograph (B) was made with 100 mAs. The density was reduced, which yielded a satisfactory image density.

Figure 185. Screen radiographs of lumbar vertebrae demonstrating the effect of halving the mAs in correcting for a very dark image.

UNDEREXPOSURE

A radiograph is underexposed when important details are lacking because of inadequate radiographic density. Details of thin structures may be visible but those representing the heavier parts will be absent. When the kilovoltage is of a value to secure proper penetration of the part yet the mAs is insufficient to secure proper density, the radiograph will reveal very faint detail in image areas corresponding to the greater tissue densities. It may be presumed, therefore, that the kilovoltage is satisfactory for the part and that detail may be better visualized if more silver were deposited on the film. To achieve this result, the first step in correction is to *double* the mAs. Usually the density will then be satisfactory. However, a further small adjustment in the mAs may be made, if necessary, to provide a more satisfactory image.

Example. Two lateral screen-grid radiographs of the thoracolumbar vertebrae, Figure 186, were made employing 85 kVp, 36-inch SID; 100 mAs and 200 mAs; thickness 32 cm. The first radiograph (A) made with 100 mAs was obviously underex-

posed. By doubling the mAs value to 200 in making the second radiograph (B), a satisfactory overall density was obtained.

Figure 186. Screen radiographs of the lateral thoracolumbar vertebrae demonstrating the effect of doubling the mAs in correcting for a very light image.

VARIABLE KILOVOLTAGE TECHNIQUE

Technique systems using various approaches to varying the kVp have been developed over the years. Many of these are actually hybrid systems, using both variable mAs and variable kVp, a practice difficult to rationalize. A few have proven to work with good reliability in controlling image density, and will be discussed briefly.

Probably the most common variable kVp system consists of using a "base" kVp of 40, to which an additional value equal to two times the measured part thickness is added. For example, for a cervical spine measuring 14 centimeters in thickness, the kVp would be:

$$40 + (2 \times 14) = 68 \text{ kVp}$$

A proper mAs value must still be established for each general body area, such as lower extremity, upper extremity, abdomen, chest and head. Let us suppose

that the determined mAs value for chest radiographs is 10 mAs. The average chest measures 22 centimeters in PA projection and 30 centimeters in lateral projection. The derived techniques would then be:

PA: $40 + (2 \times 22) =$ 84 kVp at 10 mAs
LAT: $40 + (2 \times 30) =$ 100 kVp at 10 mAs

Varying the kVp in this manner would cause a change in image contrast between the two views, with the lateral view presenting lower contrast than the PA view. For many procedures, the changes in kVp from one view to another would not be extreme enough to appreciably alter image contrast, but as the above example shows, this is not always the case, since a change of 16 kVp will result in a visible difference in image contrast. Typically, this discrepancy is adjusted for by using a new mAs value, resulting in a hybrid approach to technique.

Variable kVp systems are workable from the standpoint of controlling image density, and are indeed impressive in their accuracy for this. But they fundamentally ignore the fact that kVp affects other image qualities. Worse, the use of variable kVp may frequently lead to reductions in kVp for thinner patients that result in inadequate penetration for the tissue. Optimum kVp is essential for proper penetration and radiographic demonstration of each body part, in accordance with the proportions of different types of tissue that create subject contrast for the image. While kVp can be safely increased above the optimum level to a certain extent, reductions in kVp can prove disastrous to image quality. The use of fixed kVp and variable mAs, on the other hand, has the following advantages:

1. Changes in mAs made within the reasonable ranges of daily practice, affect *only* image density.

2. mAs is *directly* proportional to image density, while kVp is not. This allows more accurate prediction of densities that will result from adjustments made in technique.

3. Because mAs is directly proportional to image density, the entire proportional anatomy system presented in Chapter 26 can be applied with ease. Variable mAs is compatible with the proportional anatomy approach.

4. Since variable mAs is predicated upon fixed, optimum kVp, adequate penetration of anatomy is assured with high reliability.

5. Because mAs adjustments are easier to calculate than kVp changes in their effect on image density, less errors are likely to be made, and less repeats taken.

For all of these reasons, *only a fixed kVp approach, using optimum kVp techniques, can be recommended.*

SUMMARY

1. *Uniformity* and *consistency* in image qualities between the radiographs of a given procedure are essential to accurate diagnosis.

2. The use of an *optimum kilovoltage* level for each procedure will eliminate variations in image contrast and make technique manipulation more accurate and simple.

3. The use of *optimum milliamperage* for a given focal spot size within a procedure will improve the accuracy of density control, simplify technique, and reduce the probability of patient motion.

4. In most cases, a *halving* of the *mAs* will correct for a light exposure, and a *doubling of the mAs* will correct for a dark exposure.

5. Three factors should be standardized in a radiology department: (1) exposure factors, (2) projection routines and (3) processing procedures.

REVIEW QUESTIONS

1. Define "optimum mA":
2. Name two advantages to standardizing an optimum kVp on all techniques used within a procedure:
3. Name the three areas in which radiographic procedures should be standardized within a radiology department:

4. If an x-ray machine is properly calibrated, the most accurate and reliable technique factor to vary in compensating for different thicknesses of patients is:
5. In most cases, a very light or dark radiograph can be corrected by adjusting the mAs by a factor of _____.

Chapter 26

TECHNIQUE BY PROPORTIONAL ANATOMY

MANY WORKABLE TIPS or "tricks of the trade" regarding technique are passed from one radiographer to another, whereby a technique for a certain body part may be derived from a known technique for another body part. A central pattern emerges from these which is based on the logical premise that the body parts can indeed be proportionately related for the average body habitus. A close examination of any good technique chart will reveal the same pattern of *total techniques* (that is, mA-time-kVp combinations) when the 15 per cent rule is used to adjust for kVp differences and total resulting mAs values are compared. For example, the techniques listed below from a typical technique chart are all roughly equal in terms of *total technique*:

AP Lumbar Spine = 300 mA, $^1/5$ sec., 80 kVp
AP Abdomen = 200 mA, $^3/10$ sec., 78 kVp
AP Pelvis = 300 mA, $^1/10$ sec., 92 kVp
Townes Skull = 200 mA, $^1/5$ sec., 86 kVp

To become comfortable with the concept of "total technique" as the above example illustrates, the student must completely familiarize himself with the 15 per cent rule. The exercises in Chapter Six are recommended for this purpose. In the tables that follow, *total technique* levels and adjustments are stated according to the proportional change they would normally cause in the final density of the image. *These tables do not recommend whether to change kVp or mAs specifically, they only list the desired end result in overall technique.*

The radiographer must then decide whether to use kVp or mAs to make the adjustment. If kVp is used, it must be done according to the 15 per cent rule. Some examples are given in the following table:

To change total technique by a factor of	Adjust the kVp up or down by
2	15%
3	22%
4	30%
50% up or 30% down ($^1/2$ up or $^1/3$ down)	8%

In making this decision, *the rules of optimum kVp for each body part must not be broken. The kVp used should never be less than the optimum amount listed for each body part as given in Table IV, Chapter Six.* For example, Table XX states that a knee technique may be derived by doubling an ankle technique. However, simply doubling the mAs to accomplish this might violate the optimum kVp recommendation in Table IV, which lists 70 kVp as optimum for the knee, and 64 kVp for the ankle. By the 15 per cent rule, one can surmise that a 6-kVp increase in this range will increase density by about one-half or 50 per cent, and thus takes us half-way to the desired total doubling. An increase in mAs of 50 per cent, added to the 6-kVp increase, will result in an overall doubling of *total technique*.

The entire proportional anatomy system can be adapted to the variable kVp approach by applying the 15 per cent rule. Many technologists increase about 8 kVp when changing from an AP foot technique to a lateral foot technique, leaving the original mAs. This agrees perfectly with Table XX, which recommends a doubling of the AP foot technique to derive a lateral foot technique. Fifteen per cent of 60 kVp is 9 kVp. Hence, the popular 8-kVp increase approximates an overall doubling of *total technique.*

A second important consideration is the minimum change in overall technique required to see a visible difference in image density. It will be recalled that changes of less than 30 per cent in *total technique* are unlikely to cause a visible difference in the image. When using kVp adjustments, any change of less than 5 per cent will not be visible.

Finally, one must bear in mind that the following tables are applicable only to *average, adult patients.* In assessing a patient to derive an appropriate technique, the radiographer must consider the *shape* of the patient as well as his habitus and size. No amount of instruction can compensate for carelessness in doing so. Figure 187 illustrates how body torso shape, in cross section, deviates from that of the average adult (c) for premature babies, healthy infants and fluid-distended hypersthenic patients.

The average adult torso is oval in shape, measuring 22 cm in AP by 30 cm laterally. Table XX recommends 4 times the AP technique for lateral projections of all torso anatomy, including the chest and the abdomen. (Note that this also agrees with the 4-centimeter rule, since two doublings would be required where the anatomy is 8 centimeters thicker.) This very workable rule of thumb fails, however, for very young children or for fluid-distended abdomens.

Healthy newborn infants have a rounder torso, (Figure 187-B), so there is less difference in technique from the AP projection to the lateral projection. A good rule of thumb for infants (less than one year old) is to double the AP technique for the lateral view. An increase of about 8 kVp will accomplish the overall doubling. This will work for both chest and abdomen radiography. Experienced radiographers know that the same technique can be used for both the AP and the lateral views on premature babies in intensive care that are well below normal birth weight. These babies have torsos that are nearly circular in cross-section, so there is little difference in thickness from any angle, Figure 187-A.

Some hypersthenic patients, particularly those with fluid distention of the abdomen, have a very round torso shape, Figure 187-D. After increasing the AP technique from average for the added thickness, the radiographer may find himself using the same technique for a lateral projection.

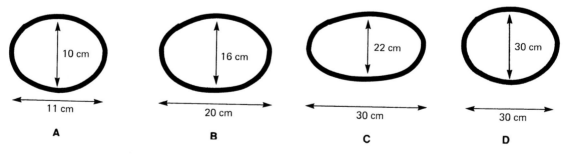

Figure 187. Cross-sectional diagrams of body torso shapes and dimensions (not to scale) of (A) premature infant presenting an essentially round torso; (B) helathy baby with more oval shaped torso, requiring a doubling of the AP technique for lateral projections; (C) average adult measuring 8 cm more laterally than in AP projection, requiring almost two doublings of technique from AP to lateral; and (D) fluid-distended hypersthenic adult, with AP and lateral techniques roughly equal.

Radiographers who are observant of body shape as well as body habitus and thickness will have lower repeat rates and save unnecessary patient exposure.

USEFULNESS OF THE PROPORTIONAL ANATOMY SYSTEM

Having reviewed the foregoing considerations, Tables XIX and XX can be applied to daily radiography practice in estimating techniques. It is recommended that both of these closely related tables be memorized. At a glance, this will seem overwhelming to the student, but rest assured that many of the factors listed are duplicated several times, and that the commitment of these rules of thumb to memory will be well worth the effort because they are so useful in daily practice.

Figure 188 demonstrates a series of radiographs which were taken using the proportional anatomy system to derive techniques. The AP lumbar spine projection (A) was exposed using 30 mAs and 80 kVp on a three-phase machine with 200-speed "medium" rare earth intensifying screens. This patient measured average dimensions, 22 cm in AP and 30 cm in lateral. The lateral lumbar spine (B) was taken with 120 mAs at 80 kVp, four times the mAs used for the AP projection in (A) and maintaining optimum kVp for the series. The lateral view of the lumbosacral junction (C) utilized the same 120 mAs as in (B), but with kilovoltage increased to 90 in order to penetrate the additional iliac bones which are superimposed over the spine at this level.

Radiograph (D) is a PA skull projection taken with 20 mAs at 80 kVp. Note that this technique is precisely 2/3 of the lumbar spine in (A). Derived by proportional anatomy using Table XX, the Townes view of the skull would be equivalent in technique to the average AP abdomen or lumbar spine, and the PA skull would be 2/3 the mAs used for the Townes view, i.e., 2/3

the AP lumbar spine technique.

Radiograph (E) is an AP projection of the cervical spine taken with 12 mAs and 76 kVp. By Table XX, this view would require one-half the technique for the PA skull in (D). Note that the mAs is cut almost to one-half, but that the kVp has also been reduced by 4, making an overall reduction in *total technique* of slightly less than one-half the PA skull.

Radiograph (F) is a PA wrist projection taken with 6.4 mAs at 58 kVp. Derived by proportional anatomy from the AP cervical spine in Table XX, this adjustment is made in several steps as follows:

Cervical Spine to Knee:
Minus 8 kVp = 10 mAs @ 68 kVp

Knee to Ankle:
$1/2$ (using 15% kVp) = 10 mAs @ 58 kVp
*200-Speed "Medium" Rare Earth Screen to
75-Speed "Extremity Cassette" (See Chapter 14):
Slightly less than 3 X technique = 28 mAs @ 58 kVp

Ankle to AP Foot or AP Elbow:
$1/2$ = 14 mAs @ 58 kVp

AP Elbow to PA Wrist:
$1/2$.... = 7 mAs @ 58 kVp

Using the proportional anatomy system, the derived technique is only 14 per cent off from the actual technique used. Remembering that a 30 per cent change is required to see a visible difference, this calculation is close indeed.

The lateral wrist (G) was exposed using 13 mAs and 58 kVp, double the mAs from the PA projection as recommended by Table XX. All of these views were exposed using the same x-ray machine, and illustrate the practical value of the proportional

TABLE XIX
Proportional Anatomy Groupings

Group 1: (Reference: AP Abdomen, Average 22 cm)

Technique: 3-phase equipment, 400-speed screens:
15 mAs, 80 kVp
If single-phase OR 200-speed screens:
30 mAs, 80 kVp

AP Abdomen
AP Pelvis
AP Lumbar Spine
AP Dorsal Spine
AP Hip
Lat Hip
Townes (Grashey) View, Skull

Group 2: (Reference: AP Cervical Spine, Average 13 cm)

Technique: 3-phase equipment, 400-speed screens:
5 mAs, 76 kVp
If single-phase OR 200-speed screens:
10 mAs, 76 kVp

AP Cervical Spine
All Cervical Spine Views (if at same distance and grid)
Open-Mouth Odontoid (George View)
AP Shoulder
AP Clavicle
AP Femur
Lat Femur
AP or PA Chest (grid)
Lateral Skull
AP Sacrum/Coccyx

Group 3: Solid Column Barium Studies (Reference: AP Views)

Technique: 3-phase equipment, 400-speed screens:
4 mAs, 110 kVp
If single-phase OR 200-speed screens: 8 mAs, 110 kVp

Upper G.I., AP
Barium Enema (solid column), AP

Group 4: Extremity Groupings, Using "Extremity" Cassettes

Subgroup	Technique using 75-speed screens
1. AP Foot AP Elbow	} 3-phase: 5 mAs, 64 kVp 1-phase: 10 mAs, 64 kVp

TABLE XIX (*Continued*)

Group 4 (Continued):

Subgroup	Technique using 75-speed screens
2. Lat Foot AP Ankle Lat Ankle AP Humerus	} 3-phase: 10 mAs, 64 kVp 1-phase: 20 mAs, 64 kVp
3. AP Leg Lat Leg Lat Humerus	} 3-phase: 10 mAs, 68 kVp 1-phase: 20 mAs, 68 kVp

anatomy system.

Technique derivation by proportional anatomy has proven to be extremely useful in at least three types of situations: (1) Complete technique charts and other radiographers are not always available when performing mobile radiography. If the radiographer does not have a written or memorized technique for a knee, for example, but does have one for an ankle, a good knee technique can be derived from the ankle technique. (2) When asking another radiographer for recommended techniques for a particular procedure, one would only have to ask for and remember a single technique. For example, having been given a technique for the PA view of the skull, one can then derive techniques for the remaining views. (3) In devising a new technique chart "from scratch," perhaps for a newly installed x-ray machine, many techniques can be derived from just a few proven exposures. In the next chapter, the derivation of an *entire technique chart* using this approach is demonstrated. If a handful of proven exposures are used to cross-check the development of the techniques, an entire chart can be derived with remarkable accuracy. Naturally, such a chart would need refinement in use, but the proportional anatomy system provides the radiographer a systematic starting point that is helpful indeed.

PROPORTIONAL ANATOMY GROUPINGS

Table XIX presents groupings of anatomy which share roughly equivalent technique requirements. Approximately the same technique can be used for all projections listed within a group. Groups 1 and 2 cover over fifteen projections that can be taken with just two memorized techniques! It is this simplification that makes the system worth memorizing.

For example, Group 1 shows that the same technique can be used for an AP abdomen, a lateral hip, an AP dorsal spine and a Townes view of the skull *on a patient of average habitus.* The radiographer may wish to slightly decrease this technique for the AP dorsal spine, or slightly increase it for the lateral hip view, but for an average patient, these techniques are so close that one "rounded" technique will produce adequate density for all of them. Naturally,

adjustments must be made for patients that are not average and situations that are not normal.

For each grouping, an actual technique is listed for the "reference" anatomy, assuming that three-phase equipment with 400 speed "rare earth regular" screens are used. If the machine is single-phase, *or* if the screens are 200-speed "rare earth medium" or "high-speed" calcium tungstate, then the mAs must be doubled. All possible variations on technique cannot be listed here, but those two listed should cover the most common circumstances. Group 4 lists three subgroupings of extremities which share equivalent techniques. Again, two variations on technique are given for each group assuming the 75-speed "extremity cassettes" (or "slow-speed" calcium tungstate screens) are used.

TECHNIQUE DERIVATIONS BY PROPORTIONAL ANATOMY

Table XX lists a series of comparisons of total technique according to average body parts, so that a given technique may be derived from any one of several other known techniques. Of course, not every possible derivation can be listed, nor every projection. But, the list is quite comprehensive and unlisted techniques can be extrapolated from those listed in many cases.

Many of these rules of thumb can be proven out before actually trying them by simply observing good radiographs. For example, examine the cervical spine on a lateral view of the skull. You will see that the lateral skull technique is ideal for demonstrating the cervical spine. Examine the clavicles on a radiograph of the cervical spine, or the pelvis on an abdomen view.

Two precautions bear mention: First, Table XX does *not* indicate adjustments for changes other than anatomy, such as changes in screens, grids or distances. These adjustments must be made *in addition* to the rules of thumb presented here. For example, a lateral cervical spine is equivalent in technique to the AP cervical spine. But since the lateral is normally taken upright using a 72-inch SID, the mAs must then be tripled as described in Chapter Eighteen to adjust for the increase in distance from the 40-inch AP projection. If the upright cassette holder has no grid, an additional compensation must be made.

Second, note that oblique projections of the torso are broken down into 30-degree and 45-degree obliques. There is great variation in the amount of obliquity used in practice. Very shallow obliques of torso anatomy require no increase in technique from the AP projections. Many oblique views are close to 30 degrees and require a 50 per cent increase in technique. But, the oblique lumbar spine, for example, must be taken at a true 45-degree angle to properly demonstrate the anatomy of interest, and this steep oblique will require a doubling of the mAs when compared to the AP view.

Five *key derivation references* are listed, below. These might be thought of as the five most important derivations to memorize, because they allow one to "jump" between very different portions of the body and still arrive at an estimated technique. The first takes us from a distal lower extremity or an upper extremity to the knee, the second from the knee to the neck, the third and fourth from the neck to the skull, and the fifth from the skull to the torso:

KEY DERIVATION REFERENCES

1. AP Knee = 2 X AP Ankle OR 2 X AP Humerus
2. AP Cervical Spine = AP Knee + 8 kVp
3. Lat Skull = AP Cervical Spine
4. Townes (Grashey) Skull = 3 X Lat Skull

5. *Average* AP Abdomen = Townes (Grashey) Skull

Memorize these five relationships first, then review Table XX.

TABLE XX
Technique by Proportional Anatomy

A. TRUNK:

AP Abdomen
AP Pelvis
AP Hip
Lat Hip } all are roughly equal to each other and equivalent to a Townes (Grashey) Skull
AP Lumbar Spine
AP Dorsal spine

30° Obliques on All Above = $1\frac{1}{2}$ x AP
45° Obliques on All Above = 2 x AP (average thickness increase is about 4 cm)
Laterals on All Above = 4 x AP (average thickness increase is about 8 cm)
All Barium Studies = about $\frac{1}{4}$ mAs and up about 30 per cent kVp

B. SKULL:

PA/Caldwell = $\frac{2}{3}$ Abdomen, = $\frac{2}{3}$ Townes, = 2 x Lateral, = 2 x C-Spine
Lateral = $\frac{1}{2}$ PA, = C-Spine, = Shoulder = Femur = PA or AP grid Chest
Lateral Sinus = $\frac{1}{3}$ PA
Townes = $1\frac{1}{2}$ x PA, = 3 x Lateral, = AP Abdomen
Submentovertex = Townes ($1\frac{1}{2}$ x PA)
Waters = PA + 4-6 kVp
Mandibles, Mastoids, etc. = roughly $\frac{1}{3}$ PA

TABLE XX (Continued)

C. *CHEST:*

PA CXR = AP Shoulder, = Cervical Spine, 0R = AP Knee + 10 kVp IF BOTH are done non-grid or both in the bucky (if one is grid and one non-grid, technique must be adjusted by a factor of 4)

Lateral = 4 x PA (the common "double mAs and up 10 kVp" is equivalent to two doublings, or 4X)

D. *PEDIATRICS:*

Skull: Newborn = $^1/_4$ Adult
1 Year = $^1/_2$ Adult
5 Years = $^3/_4$ Adult

Torso: Newborn = $^1/_4$ Adult
1 Year = $^1/_2$ Adult
5 Years = $^3/_4$ Adult

Extremities: Newborn= $^1/_6$ Adult
2 Years = $^1/_4$ Adult
8 Years = $^1/_2$ Adult
12 Years = $^3/_4$ Adult

E. *EXTREMITIES, ETC.:*

Cervical Spine: AP = AP Shoulder grid, = Lateral Skull, = $^1/_2$ PA Skull, = Femur
Obliques
Lateral* } all equal to AP
Odontoid
*If lateral is done at 72" FFD, but non-grid, technique will equal AP at 40" grid. Otherwise, adjustment must be made for distance or grid changes.

Femur = $^2/_3$ AP Abdomen, = 2 x Knee grid, = Shoulder, = Cervical Spine
Lateral = AP

Knee = 2 x Ankle, = PA Chest - 10 kVp if BOTH are grid or both are non-grid,
= AP Shoulder - 8 kVp or AP C-Spine - 8 kVp if grid
Lateral = AP

Leg = $^1/_2$-way between AP Ankle and AP Knee
Lateral = AP

Ankle = 2 x AP Foot, = $^1/_2$ AP Knee, = Lateral Foot
Lateral = AP

Foot = $^1/_2$ AP Ankle (usually down 8 kVp, NOT less mAs), = $^1/_4$ AP Knee, = AP Elbow
Lateral Foot = 2 x AP, = Ankle

Shoulder = C-Spine, = Knee + 8 kVp, = $^1/_2$ PA Skull, = PA Chest IF grid, = Lat Skull, = Femur

Humerus = $^1/_2$ way between elbow and shoulder
Lateral = AP + 6 kVp

Elbow = 2 x Wrist, = $^2/_3$ Humerus, = AP Foot
Lateral = AP + 4 kVp

Forearm = $^1/_2$ way between wrist and elbow

Wrist = $^1/_2$ Elbow, = $^1/_2$ Foot, = 1.5 x Hand (usually up 8 kVp, not mAs)
0blique = $1^1/_2$ x PA
Lateral = 2 x PA

TABLE XX (Continued)

E. EXTREMITIES, ETC.: (Continued)

         Hand = $1/3$ Elbow, = $2/3$ Wrist
                   Oblique = $1^1/2$ x PA
                   Lateral = 2 x PA

         Digit = PA Hand

F. CASTS AND SPLINTS:

         Plaster Casts: Dry plaster, small extremity = 2 x non-cast technique
                         Wet plaster, small extremity, OR   } 3 x non-cast
                         Dry plaster, large extremity (femur)
                         Wet plaster, large extremity (femur) = 4 x non-cast

         1" Wood Splint, two $1/2$-inch wood splints, or plaster half-cast = $1^1/2$ x non-cast technique
         Pure Fiberglass cast or Air Splint = No Change in Technique
         Fiberglass-Plaster Cast = $1^1/2$ x non-cast technique
         Wet Fiberglass Cast = $1^1/2$ x non-cast technique

APPLYING THE SYSTEM

For practice, try the following EXERCISE 25 to help in your memorization of proportional anatomy relationships. Check your answers from the Appendix.

EXERCISE 25:
PROPORTIONAL ANATOMY PRACTICE

For each of the following relationships of anatomy, write the proportional change in *total* technique required:
1. PA Skull to Townes Skull: _____
2. Lateral Facial Bones to PA Facial Bones: _____
3. AP Cervical Spine to Oblique Cervical Spine: _____
4. Barium Enema AP View to Sigmoid (35-degree angled) View: _____
5. PA Chest to Lateral Chest: _____
6. Townes Skull to AP Abdomen: _____
7. PA Wrist to AP Elbow: _____
8. AP Knee to AP Shoulder: _____
9. AP Leg to AP Leg With Dry Plaster Cast: _____
10. PA Adult Skull to AP Infant (2-week old) Skull: _____
11. AP Foot to Lateral Foot: _____
12. AP Ankle to Lateral Ankle: _____

Figure 188. Demonstration of usefulness of proportional anatomy derivations on average patient in producing balanced densities. Techniques: (A) AP lumbar spine with 30 mAs at 80 kVp, (B) lateral lumbar spine with 120 mAs at 80 kVp (4 X AP), (C) lateral L5-S1 spot with 120 mAs at 90 kVp, (D) PA

skull with 20 mAs at 80 kVp ($^{2}/_{3}$ the mAs in *A* for AP lumbar/abdomen or Townes skull), (E) AP cervical spine with 12 mAs at 76 kVp (approximately 1/2 the PA skull in *D* and equal to a lateral skull), (F) PA wrist with 6.4 mAs at 58 kVp using extremity cassette tabletop, and (G) lateral wrist with 13.2 mAs at 58 kVp (double the PA wrist).

SUMMARY

1. Using the proportional anatomy system, *groupings of anatomical parts* that require approximately the same *total radiographic technique* can be made, helping to simplify techniques.
2. Using the proportional anatomy system, *techniques can be derived* from one body part to another with fair accuracy.
3. *Optimum kVp* guidelines must never be neglected in deriving techniques by proportional anatomy. This means that the radiographer must be adept at using the 15 per cent rule in making adjustments.
4. No system can compensate for neglecting proper *evaluation of patient shape and habitus*, the radiographer's responsibility.
5. The proportional anatomy system must be used in conjunction with all of the technique guidelines presented in this text for changes in *distance, screen speed, grids*, and other variables.

REVIEW QUESTIONS

1. Compared to average adults, the torso of an infant requires _____ (more, less or equal) adjustment in technique from a frontal (AP) to a lateral view.
2. Changes in total technique for proportional anatomy adjustments may be made in mAs, kVp or both?

For the following, what is the proportional change in *total technique* required:

3. AP Pelvis to AP Lumbar Spine: _____
4. Lumbar Spine Oblique View to Lateral View: _____
5. AP Ankle to AP Knee: _____
6. Upper G.I. AP View to Lateral View: _____
7. PA Wrist to Lateral Wrist: _____
8. AP Foot to AP Ankle: _____
9. Lateral Leg to Lateral Leg With One-Piece 3/4-inch Wood Splint: _____
10. AP Adult Humerus to Infant (2-week old) AP Humerus: _____
11. PA Esophagus (with barium) to 15-degree Anterior Oblique: _____
12. AP Shoulder to AP Cervical Spine: _____
13. PA Skull to Lateral Skull: _____
14. Townes Skull to Submentovertex Skull: _____

Chapter 27

TECHNIQUE CHARTS

EVERY RADIOLOGY DEPARTMENT should develop technique charts for each machine. The use of technique charts has its limits. Whether using computer-generated charts, technique computers, the bit system, or homemade charts, no written device can replace the need for the technologist's assessment of each individual patient and situation. Nonetheless, the technique chart has been proven to reduce repeat rates considerably and to be indispensable as a starting point and a reference. Radiographers who are critical of the use of charts simply never learned how to construct and use them properly. It would be unprofessional to ignore something that has been scientifically, objectively demonstrated to reduce patient radiation exposure, as well as help control costs for the radiology department.

Table VII in Chapter 10 presents the results of thousands of measurements taken on adult patients, and states the average range of thickness for each body part. For most distal extremities and skulls, more than 90 per cent of adult patients fall within the average range of thickness. For these radiographic procedures, a single technique can be written on the technique chart. The radiographer must always be observant and capable of adjusting the "average" technique upward or downward for uncommon circumstances, but space on a written chart need not be committed to such rare adjustments. The "extremities" section of the technique chart in Table XXI demonstrates this format, with a single technique for each anatomical part.

Another look at Table VII shows that the abdominal (lumbar) region is the most variable area of the body for thickness. Even for abdominal procedures, a single technique would work for more than two-thirds (69 per cent) of adult patients. (This certainly remains a high enough factor of reliability to substantiate the value of a technique chart, even if only one technique were listed for each procedure.) To adapt for this level of variation, the torso section of a technique chart should be broken down into columns according to measured thickness as illustrated in Table XXI. Note that the technique changes listed there follow the *four centimeter rule*, doubling for each increase in thickness of four centimeters, and cut to one-half for equal reductions in thickness.

The chart in Table XXI is written for three-phase equipment, using 10:1 grids, and 400-speed screens. Variations in equipment and calibration may require the entire chart to be adjusted up or down by a certain ratio for it to be useful. If the *entire* chart is adjusted consistently, it should be more than 85 per cent accurate. Change ONLY mAs values, not kVp.

- For single-phase equipment, double all mAs values
- For rare earth "medium"-speed or for "high"-speed calcium tungstate screens, double the techniques listed, (except those marked EXTREMITY CAS)

- For other screen conversions, see Chapter 14, TABLES XV and XVI.

This chart, while it may be of practical use, is primarily presented to illustrate the concepts taught in Chapters 25, 26, and 27. Take special note of the format: The torso section is organized according to variable part thicknesses, with an average cm measurement given for reference. The extremities section lists a single mAs value, with adjustments described at the top for patients which are smaller than average or larger than average. "Small," "Average," and "Large" mAs columns could be used as an alternative, but generally measurements are not needed here. The extremities section also has an additional column just to illustrate how both the mA and the exposure time can be listed in one column, as an option to listing the total mAs. Overall it is concise and yet it covers nearly every procedure including pediatric procedures in just three pages.

This is a variable mAs, fixed kVp chart, as recommended in Chapters 6 and 25. Torso measurements are organized into 2-cm columns as discussed in this chapter. And, you will note that if you take both the kVp and the mAs values into consideration as a "total technique," it very closely follows the proportional anatomy rules of thumb presented in Chapter 26. Careful analysis of this chart in reference to the concepts in these chapters will prove a valuable learning experience.

The use of calipers as explained in Chapter 10 to measure the part thickness is a must for torso radiography and for pediatric radiography. Radiographers can become adept at estimating body part thicknesses after acquiring considerable experience, and only require calipers for exceptional cases. The student must not take this practice in the wrong vein—the less

the experience, the greater the need for the calipers. One should only engage in such a practice *after fully establishing their accuracy over the course of many months.* This is done by persistent practice, by estimating the thickness of each patient and then checking *with the calipers* to see how accurate the estimate was. For more rare procedures, or whenever there is any doubt at all regarding patient thickness and appropriate technique, *calipers and technique charts should be used in conjunction.*

It should be noted that the foregoing is a philosophical statement, and not a legal one. Some states require the use of both calipers and technique charts *by law.* Such requirements are not unreasonable, since the objective data obtained from taking actual measurements will be more reliable than any estimation, assuming that the calipers are used properly. This practice should reduce repeat rates and enhance professionalism.

DEVELOPING CHARTS

The proper construction and use of technique charts *must* include the following:

1. A quality control program for calibration of machines and monitoring of processing conditions.

2. Input from all radiographers using a given machine as the chart is developed and corrected.

3. Strict enforcement by administrative technologists that no individual radiographer be allowed to alter the chart in any way once it has been developed and tested. Radiographers who continually cross out and rewrite techniques are usually radiographers who use incorrect distances, incorrect screens or film, or incorrect positioning. The next radiographer to use the room may use the right distance, screen, film, and position, and have to repeat radiographs

TABLE XXI

TORSO / SKULL CHART

ABBREVIATIONS: GD = Grid
NG = Non-Grid

Total MAS by PART SIZE

PROCEDURE	Notes	VIEW	kVp	Ave CM	-6cm	-4cm	-2cm	AVE	+2cm	+4cm	+6cm	+8cm	+10cm
GRID CHEST	72"	PA/AP	106	22	1	1.3	2	2.5	3.7	5	7	10	14
		LAT	116	30	2	2.5	3.7	5	7	10	14	20	26
NON-GRID CHEST	72"	AP	80	22	1	1.3	2	2.5	3.7	5	7	10	14
		LAT	90	30	2	2.5	3.7	5	7	10	14	20	26
SUPINE CHEST 40" NG		AP	80	22	0.6	1	1.4	1.8	2.7	3.6	5.5	7	10
RIBS / Sternum	72"	AP↑Diap	60	22	8	10	15	20	30	40	60	80	120
		OBL↑Dia	64	24	11	15	22	30	45	60	90	120	170
	72"	AP↓Diap	76	22	22	30	45	60	90	120	180	240	340
ABDOMEN / IVP	GD	AP/PA	80	22	6.2	8	11	15	22	30	45	60	90
		30°OBL	80	24	8	11	15	22	30	45	66	90	130
PELVIS / HIP	GD	AP	80	22	6.2	8	11	15	22	30	45	60	90
HIP (Unil or Groin)	GRID	LAT	80	22	6.2	8	11	15	22	30	45	60	90
SACRUM	AP / Coccyx All		74	20	6.2	8	11	15	22	30	45	60	90
	GD	LAT	80	28	11	15	22	30	45	60	90	120	170
LUMBAR SPINE	GD	AP	80	22	6.2	8	11	15	22	30	45	60	90
		45°OBL	80	26	11	15	22	30	45	60	90	120	170
		LAT	80	30	22	30	45	60	90	120	180	240	340
		L5/S1 SP	*90	30	22	30	45	60	90	120	180	240	340
THORACIC SPINE	GD	AP	80	22	5	7	10	13	19	26	38	52	76
	Breathing LAT		64	30	25 mA / 2.5 s		25 mA / 4 sec		50 mA / 4 s		100 mA /4 s		
TWINING C/T	GD	LAT	76	28	10	14	20	28	38	56	78	108	150
CERVICAL SPINE	40" GD	AP/Odon	76	13	2	2.5	3.7	5	7	10	15	20	30
	72"GD	OBL/LAT	76	13	6.2	8	11	15	22	30	45	60	90
	72"NG	OBL/LAT	76	13	2	2.5	3.7	5	7	10	15	20	30
SKULL	GD	PA/Cald	80	19	4	5	7	10	15	20	30	40	60
		LAT	76	15	2	2.5	3.7	5	7	10	15	20	30
		Townes	80	22	6.2	8	11	15	22	30	45	60	90
SINUSES / FACIAL BONES	GD	PA/Cald	75	19	4	5	7	10	15	20	30	40	60
		Waters	80	20	4	5	7	10	15	20	30	40	60
		Lat	75	15	1.5	2	3	3.8	5.6	7.6	11	15	22
AIR CONTRAST U.G.I. / B.E.	GD	AP/PA	90	22	1.8	2.4	3.2	4	6	8	12	16	24
		OBL/SIG	90	24	3	4	5	6	10	14	20	28	40
		LAT	90	30	6	10	12	16	24	32	48	64	96
SOLID-COLUMN U.G.I. / B.E.	GD	AP/PA	110	22	1.8	2.4	3.2	4	6	8	12	16	24
		OBL/SIG	110	24	3	4	5	6	10	14	20	28	40
		LAT	110	30	6	10	12	16	24	32	48	64	96

TABLE XXI *(Continued)*

ABBREVIATIONS: GD =Grid, NG =Non-Grid, SFS =Small Focal Spot, EXTCAS =Extremity Cassette, REG =Regular Cassette, PIGOST = Pig-O-Stat$_{TM}$

EXTREMITY CHART

PROCEDURE	Notes	VIEW	kVp	mAs
HAND		PA /All Fingers	54	2.2
	SFS	OBL	54	2.5
	EXTCAS	Fanned Lat	54	4.5
WRIST		PA	60	2.2
	SFS	OBL	60	3.3
	EXTCAS	LAT	60	4.5
FOREARM	SFS	AP	64	2.2
	EXTCAS	LAT	64	4.5
ELBOW		AP	64	3
	SFS	OBL	64	4
	EXTCAS	LAT	64	6
HUMERUS	SFS	AP	72	2.2
	EXTCAS	LAT	72	3.6
TOES	SFS/EXT	All	60	2.2
FOOT		AP	64	2.5
	SFS	OBL	64	3.3
	EXTCAS	LAT	64	5
CALCANEUS	SFS	PD	68	7
	EXTCAS	LAT	68	3.6
ANKLE	SFS	AP/OBL	64	5
	EXTCAS	LAT	64	5
LEG	SFS	AP	68	5
	EXTCAS	LAT	68	5
TABLETOP KNEE	EXTCAS	AP	70	5
		LAT	70	5
TBLTOP KNEE REG		All	70	0.8
BUCKY KNEE	GD	AP/OBL	70	5
		LAT	70	5
FEMUR	GD	AP / LAT	76	12
HIP	GRID	FRG/GROIN	80	14
SHOULDER	GD	AP/Transax	76	6
		Transthoracic	90	15
CLAVICLE	GD	AP/PA	74	6
SCAPULA	GD	AP	74	6
		LAT	74	10

FACIAL CHART

PROCEDURE	Notes	VIEW	kVp	mAs
MANDIBLE	GD	PA	76	8
		OBL LAT	66	8
		NON-GRID OBL LAT	60	5
ORBIT Rheese	GD	PA OBL	76	5
SINUSES	GD	SMV	80	15
ZYG. ARCH	EXTCAS	SMV	62	2
NASAL BONE	EXTCAS	LAT	54	2

PEDIATRIC CHART

PROCEDURE	Notes	VIEW	kVp	mAs
"PREMIE" CHEST	40" NG	AP	54	0.6
		LAT	54	0.6
INFANT CHEST	40" NG	AP	60	1
		LAT	68	1
2-YEAR CHEST	72" PIGOST	PA	66	1.5
		LAT	76	1.5
6-YEAR CHEST	72" NG	PA	70	2
		LAT	80	3
ABDOMEN / IVP / PELVIS SPINES		INFANT NG	62	1.5
		2-YEAR GD	68	4
		6-YEAR GD	74	8
CERVIC. SP	2-YEAR	All	64	2
SKULL (PA/AP)		INFANT NG	62	1.5
		2-YEAR GD	68	3.5
		6-YEAR GD	74	5
UPPER EXTREMITY		INFANT EXTCAS	54	0.5
		2-YEAR EXTCAS	58	0.7
		6-YEAR EXTCAS	62	2
LOWER EXTREMITY		INFANT EXTCAS	58	0.5
		2-YEAR EXTCAS	62	1
		6-YEAR EXTCAS	66	2

because of the rewritten techniques.

4. Encouragement by administrative technologists that all radiographers use the system.

5. Periodic checks and updates of all technique charts using the same system of input by which they were originally developed. *Periodic* here means perhaps every 6 months.

Suppose you are in charge of a newly constructed radiology department and must devise some charts from scratch. Using the rules of thumb and relationships discussed in Chapter 5, 6, 7, 10, 25, and 26, you can write a reasonably accurate preliminary technique chart completely from just one test film on a phantom (or patient, if necessary). To demonstrate, try the following Exercise #26. Answers and explanations for Exercise #26 are found in Appendix II.

Once the correct mAs is determined, it then becomes the basic value to be employed for all thicknesses in the average thickness range established for the projection.

Example 1. In posteroanterior adult chest screen radiography, the average thickness range may be considered to be 20 to 24 centimeters. As shown in Table VII, this range of measurements represents those of about 82 per cent of patients. In this projection the basic mAs should be established for a normal healthy adult measuring 22 cm. (the middle thickness in the range). Projections that have relatively little variation from the average thickness range, such as a posteroanterior view of the chest, require refinement in application of the mAs values to those thicknesses in excess of or less than the average. A typical example of a standardized posteroanterior technique is shown in the unretouched radiographs, Figure 189. It is interesting to statistically evaluate in Table XXII the physical char-

acteristics of the patient's whose radiographs are shown in Figure 189.

Radiation that completely penetrates the part and produces a consistently uniform density and contrast is most important in applying a standardized technic. It becomes readily apparent that the characteristics of height, weight, or sex cannot per se be employed to determine the x-ray absorbing properties of the tissues being exposed.

Thickness Greater than Average

When a chest measurement is slightly greater than average, the only change that need be made in the factors is in the mAs. The increased thickness of the 26- and 27-centimeter chest only requires *more* radiation of the quality as produced with 80 kVp on chests within the average range. The kilovoltage is held constant since it has been predetermined that 80 kVp provides the necessary quality of radiation to penetrate any size adult chest within a reasonable range in the posteroanterior direction, using *nongrid* exposure.

Smaller Thicknesses

To balance the densities for the 18- and 19-centimeter chests, $1/2X$ mAs may be used. For chests that are 14 centimeters, $1/4X$ mAs may be employed. For infants (less than 10 centimeters) $1/4X$ mAs may be employed, but the kilovoltage should be reduced from 80 to 70 to provide the increase in contrast that may be needed for the chests of these young subjects. It should be pointed out that only *one exposure factor should be changed at a time* when any exposure technique is to be altered. Changing two factors at a time introduces too many variables that are difficult to control.

EXERCISE #26
CONSTRUCTING A MANUAL TECHNIQUE CHART

INSTRUCTIONS: Assuming that the listed technique was good, complete the rest of the chart using proportional anatomy and the 4 cm rule of thumb.

Procedure	Projection	kVp	Ave CM	MAS						
Lumbar Spine	AP	80	22	18 cm	20 cm	**22 cm** **16**	24 cm	26 cm	28 cm	30 cm
	Oblique	80	26	22 cm	24 cm	**26 cm**	28 cm	30 cm	32 cm	34 cm
	Lateral	80	30	26 cm	28 cm	**30 cm**	32 cm	34 cm	36 cm	38 cm
Skull	PA	76	19	15 cm	17 cm	**19 cm**	21 cm			
	Lateral	76	15	11 cm	13 cm	**15 cm**	17 cm			
Shoulder	AP	76	14	10 cm	12 cm	**14 cm**	16 cm			
Knee	AP	70	12	8 cm	10 cm	**12 cm**	14 cm			

Other Formats for Technique Charts: Referring to the completed mAs chart for a wrist series fill in the variable time chart and variable kVp chart:

Procedure	KVP	mAs for each view		
WRIST	60	PA	OBL	LAT
		5	7.5	10

VARIABLE KVP CHART

Procedure	mAs	kVp for each view		
WRIST	5	PA	OBL	LAT

VARIABLE TIME CHART

Procedure	KVP	mA	Time for ea. view		
WRIST	60	200	PA	OBL	LAT

Figure 189. Standardized chest techniques for various patients using a technique chart. Note consistency of results.

FORMATS FOR TECHNIQUE CHARTS

Formats for making a technique chart are as varied as the individuals who use them. Charts can be made using index card boxes with a card for each procedure, using a drawing of the body in frontal and lateral views with the techniques written near each part indicated, using a loose-leaf "flip chart," or using a table or grid lined out on paper.

Some useful observations may be made, however, which apply to any chart: First, standardizing the optimum kVp and mA for a given procedure, as discussed in Chapter 25, is necessary for building a chart. A table only accommodates two variables, one for the rows, one for the columns. One of these variables must be body part thickness, usually listed at the tops of the columns. The rows can then be used for exposure time or total mAs, but not for all three technique factors (kVp, mA, and time). Second, optional notes must be condensed so that the chart does not become cumbersome. For example, use one column for notes such as "extremity cassette," "bucky," "small focal spot," etc. And third, the chart must be broken down for different body part thicknesses on *any torso anatomy*, such as lumbar spines, barium enemas and chests. It is suggested that a new column be made for every change of 2 *centimeters* in part thickness, as shown in Table XXI.

Table XXI presents a sample completed technique chart using these concepts. Also examine this chart for comparison with the proportional anatomy rules of thumb listed in Chapter 26. A blank chart is found in Appendix I, which may be useful for you to copy.

TABLE XXII

List of Physical Characteristics of the Patients Whose Radiographs Appear in Figure 195

Radio-graph	Thick-ness (CM)	Sex	Age (Years)	Height (Inches)	Weight (Lbs.)
A	17	F	20	65	105
B	18	F	24	63	110
C	19	F	29	60	101
D	20	F	22	63	107
E	21	M	61	67	135
F	22	F	21	58	132
G	23	F	24	60	123
H	24	M	60	68	165
I	25	M	34	63	130
J	26	M	60	67	173
K	27	M	55	67	199
L	28	M	36	70	206
M	29	M	60	69	193

Finally, note that no chart attached to a wall will help you on a *mobile* procedure! *Every radiographer should carry a "portable" technique reference* in the form of a telephone/address booklet or a similar pocket-sized book. Simply list procedures alphabetically, and make a note of techniques that work as you learn them from experience. Mobile equipment often requires techniques that are very different from those used in the department. If it works, write it down!

TABLE XXIII

Bucky Automatic Exposure Control Guide

Based on: Three Phase Generator (12:1 Grid: A 200 Speed Film/Screen Combination)

ANATOMY	Projection	kVp	Dist	MILLIAMPERAGE		Backup mAs	Detector Selection	Master Density Selection	FOCAL SPOT	
				Suggested	Selected				Small	Large
SKULL	All	80	40"	200		100		(N) Normal	✓	
	Basilar (SMV)	86	40"	200		100		N	✓	
SINUSES	All (cone)	80	40"	200		160		N	✓	
	SMV (cone)	86	40"	200		160		N	✓	
FACIAL BONES	All (cone)	80	40"	200		100		N	✓	
OPTIC FORAMEN	Rhese (cone)	80	40"	200		100		N	✓	
NASAL BONES	Waters (cone)	80	40"	200		100		N	✓	
	PA Caldwell (cone)	80	40"	200		100		N	✓	
MANDIBLE	PA (cone)	80	40"	200		50		N	✓	
	Lat (cone)	70	40"	200		50		N	✓	
MASTOIDS	All (cone)	76	40"	200		100		N	✓	
CERVICAL SPINE	AP	76	40"	200		50		N	✓	
	Odontoid	80	40"	200		50		N	✓	
	Lat - Obl	76	72"	200		50		N	✓	
THORACIC SPINE	AP	80	40"	500		100		N		✓
	Lat - Obl	76	40"	50		100		N	✓	
LUMBAR SPINE	AP	80	40"	500		150		N		✓
	Lat - Obl	90	40"	500		150		N		✓
	Lat L5, S1 (cone)	100	40"	500		150		N		✓
PELVIS - HIP	AP	80	40"	500		100		N		✓
RIBS	AP AD	76	40"	600		100	or	N		✓
	Obl AD	76	40"	600		100		N		✓
	AP BD	80	40"	600		100		N		✓
	Obl BD	80	40"	600		100		N		✓
ABDOMEN - IVP	AP	80	40"	600		160		N		✓
KIDNEY	AP (cone)	80	40"	600		160		N		✓
ABDOMEN - IVP	Obl	80	40"	600		200		N		✓
	Lat	90	40"	600		200		N		✓
IVP HIGH CONTRAST	AP	70	40"	600 to 1,000		200		N		✓
	Cone AP	70	40"			200		N		✓
GALL BLADDER	PA	80	40"	600		200		N		✓
	Obl	80	40"	600		200		N		✓
GALL BLADDER HIGH CONTRAST	PA	65	40"	600		200		N		✓
	Obl	65	40"	600		200		N		✓
GI — STOMACH COLON	PA - AP	120	40"	400		100		N		✓
	Obl	120	40"	400		100		N		✓
	Lat	120	40"	400		100		N		✓
ESOPHAGUS	AP	110	40"	400		100		N		✓
	Lat	110	40"	400		100		N		✓
SHOULDER CLAVICLE SCAPULA HUMERUS	AP	76	40"	200		40		N	✓	
	Trans Thoracic	90	40"	600		180		N		✓
FEMUR	AP	80	40"	100		40		N	✓	
	Lat	80	40"	100		40		N	✓	
KNEE	All Views	70	40"	100		40		N	✓	
CHEST	PA	125	72"	400 to 500		50		N		✓
	Lat	125	72"			64		N		✓
HIGH KVP CHEST	PA	140	72"	400		20		N		✓
	Lat	140	72"	400		50		N		✓
	RAO	140	72"	400		50		N		✓
	LAO	140	72"	400		50		N		✓

from "How to Prepare an X-Ray Technique Chart" by the General Electric Company, 1981. Permission given.

AUTOMATIC EXPOSURE TECHNIQUE CHARTS

The use of automatic exposure controls (phototimers) does *not* preclude the need for technique charts! For each projection and anatomical part, optimum kVp must be listed for adequate penetration, the correct configuration of the photocells (which ones to activate) must be given, the density control setting must be specified, and the recommended back-up time stated. An optimum mA should also be stated, high enough to minimize motion, but not so high that exposure times are reduced beyond the response time for the detectors,

as discussed in Chapter 28. Additional notes may needed.

Table XXIII is a sample technique chart written for an automatic exposure unit. Note that in addition to the above mentioned factors, columns are also provided for focal spot size and distance. The *minimum* information for such a chart would included kVp, back-up time or back-up mAs, detector configuration, and density control setting for each projection. Measurement of the patient is not required for automatic exposures.

SUMMARY

1. *Technique charts* should be used in every radiology department. They have been scientifically proven to reduce *patient exposure.*
2. The *proper use* of charts includes initial and ongoing input from the staff radiographers as a group, strict enforcement by administrative technologists and quality control of equipment and processing.
3. A first draft of a complete technique chart may be developed from only one or two test exposures using the guidelines and methods found in preceding chapters. Only minor adjustments to such a chart would be needed in use.

The *development* of technique should be a *systematic* approach, not a trial-and-error approach.
4. *Calipers* must be used by radiographers to measure patients so that technique charts are utilized properly. This is required by law in some states.
5. Technique charts with *measurement columns* (for torso anatomy) should be organized with a technique listed for every change in part thickness of 2 cm.
6. Every radiographer should carry a *pocket-book technique chart* for personal reference.
7. Technique charts are also necessary for *automatic exposure controls.*

REVIEW QUESTIONS

1. Describe two reasons why a radiographer might claim that a certain technique chart "does not work" when in fact there is nothing wrong with the chart itself:
2. What is the *most important* reason for

utilizing technique charts instead of relying on intuition or memory?
3. Describe three of the things that an administrative technologist must have done in a department in order to ensure the reliability and proper use of tech-

nique charts:

4. It is recommended that technique charts for torso anatomy be organized into columns for every _____-c.m. change in part thickness.

5. What device must be used by radiographers to measure patients so that technique charts are utilized properly.

6. Why should pocket-book charts be kept by radiographers?

7. What three items must an automatic exposure control technique chart include *which are different from manual technique charts?*

8. Below is an incomplete technique chart which has one average technique listed. Assuming that the listed technique is good, complete the rest of the chart:

PROCEDURE	PROJ	kVp	AVE CM				mAs			
				18cm	20cm	22cm	24cm	26cm	28cm	30cm
	AP/OBL	110	22			8				
Barium	35°			22cm	24cm	26cm	28cm	30cm	32cm	34cm
Enema	Sigmoid	110	26							
	Lateral			26cm	28cm	30cm	32cm	34cm	36cm	38cm
	Rectum	110	30							

9. Below is a variable mAs technique chart for a wrist series. In the second chart, given the set mAs as indicated, convert the chart into a variable kVp chart, listing the appropriate kVp for each view:

PROCEDURE	kVp	mAs FOR EACH VIEW		
		PA	OBL	LAT
Wrist	56	5	7.5	10

PROCEDURE	kVp	mAs FOR EACH VIEW		
		PA	OBL	LAT
Wrist	5			

10. Referring to the original variable mAs technique chart for the wrist in #9 above, complete the following exposure time chart *using fractions,* (not decimals) which will result in the correct total mAs values:

PROCEDURE	kVp	mA	EXP. TIME FOR EACH VIEW		
			PA	OBL	LAT
Wrist	56	200			

Chapter 28

AUTOMATIC EXPOSURE CONTROLS

AUTOMATIC EXPOSURE CONTROLS or *phototimers* were developed for the purpose of achieving more consistent film densities, reducing repeat rates, and ultimately reducing patient dose. All automatic exposure control devices work on the same physical principles, based upon the ability of radiation detection devices to convert radiant energy into an electrical current.

The two most commonly used types of detectors are the ion chamber and the photomultiplier tube. The ion chamber induces an electrical current when gas atoms are ionized by the impinging radiation, freeing electrons from the gas atoms. These electrons are then attracted to and strike a positively charged anode plate. Continuing to be attracted toward the positive terminal within a circuit, the electrons flow out of the anode plate and down a wire, thus becoming an electrical

Figure 190. Diagram of basic AEC circuit. Remnant radiation penetrating through patient ionizes atoms within the detector cell (A), creating an electrical charge that is stored within the capacitor (B). The thyratron (C) releases the charge on the capacitor when a preset amount is reached, and can be adjusted by the density control. When the electrical charge is released, it flows to a relay which pulls a switch (D) open, thus terminating the exposure.

current.

The photomultiplier tube is similar but adds an additional step in the process: It uses a fluorescent screen to convert imping-ing x-rays into light. The light then strikes a photocathode which induces an electrical current from the light energy. In either case, the induced electrical current can be used to charge an electromagnet which pulls the main exposure switch open and terminates the exposure.

As remnant radiation from the patient reaches the detectors, the electrical charge induced by them is stored in an electrical capacitor. A device called a *thyristor* sets a maximum charge which the capacitor may hold. When the charge on the capacitor reaches this maximum level, the thyristor allows it to be discharged through the cir-cuit (Figure 190) and the exposure is termi-nated. The thyristor is preset by a service specialist to always produce the desired density level on the radiographs taken according to the film-screen system being used. If film or screen type is changed, the thyristor must be readjusted.

When a patient is turned sideways, or when larger patients are radiographed, more radiation is absorbed in their bodies so that there is less remnant radiation per second striking the detectors. Hence, it takes a longer time for the capacitor to reach its maximum electrical charge and the exposure time is automatically length-ened until proper film density is achieved.

It should be emphasized that automatic exposure controls only control the *exposure time*, and consequently the total mAs. *Optimum kVp and optimum mA must be man-ually set by the radiographer when using the AEC*, in accordance with all of the princi-ples discussed in Chapters 5 and 6. If the kVp used is less than optimum for the par-ticular anatomy of interest, this anatomy will be underpenetrated. Assuming that the anatomy is properly positioned over the activated photocells, the sensors will detect a reduction in exposure rate, and the automatic control will allow a longer expo-sure time to try to compensate.

As explained in Chapter 6, *no amount of mAs will compensate for inadequate penetration.* The radiograph will therefore come out slightly too light in spite of the automatic compensation. Even if the "density con-trol" knob is adjusted to darken the overall image, with insufficient penetration the mAs required will be excessive, and result in unnecessary patient exposure. This is a particularly insidious problem, because the radiographer is not aware (at least until after the fact) of the final mAs value. Such a practice is both uninformed and unpro-fessional. The radiographer must know by memory and apply the *optimum kVp* for every procedure, phototimed or otherwise.

Optimum mA must also be set manually for automatic exposures. For "manual" technique, optimum mA was defined as the maximum mA available for a given focal spot size, which does not overload the x-ray tube heat capacity. Defining the optimum mA is actually a bit more complicated for automatic exposure control than it is for "manual" technique, because there is the additional consideration of *minimum response time.*

MINIMUM RESPONSE TIME

All electronic devices require a mini-mum amount of time and "signal" or input in order to operate. The automatic expo-sure control is no exception. It takes time, albeit thousandths of a second, for the cir-cuit to detect and react to the radiation received.

Minimum response times vary greatly from one radiographic unit to another and between manufacturers. When a new unit is installed, it is a good idea for the quality control technologist to ensure that staff radiographers are made aware of its minimum response time (MRT), especially if this unit will be frequently used for pediatric radiography. Perhaps the best way to ensure this over time is to post it in writing on or near the control panel of the unit. Typical MRTs range from 0.002 seconds for state-of-the-art equipment up to 0.02 seconds for older units.

With extremely high-speed screens, such as 800-speed rare earth screens, the exposure times required for proper radiographic density can be reduced to such an extent that they are too short for the AEC circuit to respond to. The delay caused by the circuit would result in a dark, over-exposed image. In such a circumstance, the best alternative is to decrease the mA station used until sufficient exposure times are produced.

It is common for pediatric radiology departments to maximize the efficiency of the overall imaging system by using 3-phase or high frequency generators and very high speed screen-film combinations, in order to shorten exposure times as much as possible and thus control motion. Such situations are particularly vulnerable to the risk of overexposure due to the minimum response time. The following example will illustrate:

Let us assume an MRT of 0.005 seconds for a modern 3-phase machine, when using the AEC. To keep exposure times short, the radiographers are in the habit of using the 300 mA station. At the 300 mA station, the minimum total *mAs* this machine can produce would be:

$$300 \text{ mA} \ X \ 0.005 \text{ sec.} = 1.5 \text{ mAs}$$

Suppose that the ideal technique for a PA chest on a child was 65 kVp and 1 mAs. If the radiographer "phototimes" the expo-

sure on this child using the 300 mA station, the radiograph will turn out dark: The AEC cannot shut off in less than 0.005 seconds–it cannot produce less than 1.5 mAs at this mA station.

Note that in this situation, *adjusting the density control knob to a "minus" setting will not help.* Regardless of the density that it is set to, the machine still cannot respond in less than 0.005 seconds. The solution is to *lower the mA station.* Reducing the mA to 200, the minimum achievable mAs would be:

$$200 \ X \ 0.005 \text{ sec.} = 1.0 \text{ mAs}$$

This is right at the desired technique, and should work if the machine is calibrated accurately. Note that if 0.8 mAs were needed, a further reduction to the *100 mA* station would be necessary. Minimum response time is of concern whenever the following factors compound: High-speed receptor systems, high-power generators, high mA stations, and small anatomy.

Optimum mA for automatic exposure control, then, would be defined as high enough at a given focal spot size to minimize motion, but not so high that the needed exposure times are shorter than the AEC can handle.

BACK-UP TIME

Whenever the automatic exposure control circuit is activated, the main exposure time control, whether a knob or a set of buttons, becomes a "back-up timer" for the AEC. A back-up timer is crucial to prevent extreme overexposure to the patient if some electrical component of the AEC circuit should fail. In such an event, the exposure might otherwise continue until the radiographer realized that something was amiss and released the exposure button. Consider the implications of such an event for patient exposure: If the required time was one-half second, and it took the radiographer 4 seconds to realize, comprehend and react to the situation, the patient would receive *8 times* the normal exposure. If the required time was $1/40$ second, and the reaction time for the radiographer was an unlikely 2 seconds, the patient would receive *80 times* the necessary exposure. Clearly, a safeguard must be built into the electronic systems.

Fortunately, many recently-manufactured x-ray machines now include circuitry which automatically sets an appropriate back-up time or back-up *mAs* for all AEC exposures. For older equipment, proper back-up times must be determined. The most recommended approach is for the quality control technologist to determine a specific back-up time for each view and have this written on an *AEC technique chart* posted in each room (see the preceding chapter). If it is left to individual staff radiographers in daily practice, they should at least employ some rules of thumb. Both types of information will be presented here.

It is a common practice to simply set the back-up time at 1 or 2 seconds on all procedures. For torso radiography on unusually large patients, the radiographer must be mindful to increase the back-up time to 3 or even 4 seconds. Otherwise, the back-up timer will shut off the exposure before the AEC would have, before an adequate density is produced. The result will be a light radiograph *and a repeated exposure to the patient.*

On the other hand, modern chest techniques, even on adult patients, often require only 2 or 3 mAs for a good image density. Note that using the 200 mA station, 2 mAs can be achieved with an *extremely short* exposure time of only a hundredth of a second (0.01 sec.). In chest radiography, it is not uncommon to find exposure times measured in *thousandths* of a second. Note the implications, then, of the common practice of setting the back-up time at 1 second. Suppose that the average chest radiograph requires $1/100$ second exposure. If the AEC fails to function properly, and the exposure continues to the back-up time of 1 second, the patient will receive 100 times the necessary exposure! *In effect, the patient received an exposure equivalent to 100 chest x-rays in order to obtain a single chest radiograph.* Clearly, when it comes to *chest* radiography, even one second is excessive as a back-up time. The same argument holds for proximal extremities that are "phototimed." A useful rule of thumb for these procedures is to generally set the back-up time at 0.2 ($1/5$) second. (This is 20 times the "average" and thus encompasses even large chests or single-phase equipment.)

Thus, radiographers must be conscious of the two extremes when setting back-up times: chests and extremities on the one hand, which require much less than one second, and torso procedures on very large patients on the other hand, which may require much more than one second. Since most radiographers are not likely to know from memory the specific manual exposure

TABLE XXIV
"Rule of Thumb" AEC Back-Up Times

All Chest and Proximal Extremities:	0.2 second ($1/5$ sec.)
Average Torso and Skull Procedures:	1 second
Very Large Torso Procedures:	2 to 4 seconds

times for various procedures, some broad rules of thumb for setting back-up times are useful. These are presented in Table XXIV and should be committed to memory.

It is better, still, for the quality control technologists to determine *specific* back-up times for *each view*, and write these onto AEC technique charts for each room. To calculate these, a workable rule is to approximately *double the expected manual exposure time* for that particular anatomy, *if the same mA station were used.* For example, if a typical manual technique for an AP abdomen projection were 15 mAs, what would be an appropriate back-up time using AEC at 300 mA? The manual exposure time is:

$$15 \text{ mAs} / 300 \text{ mA} = 0.05 \text{ second}$$

An appropriate back-up time then would be 2 X 0.05 = 0.1 second. For very large or very thin patients, the 4 centimeter rule can be used to adjust: *Change technique by a factor of 2 for every 4 centimeters change in thickness.* For example, for a very large patient measuring 30 cm through the AP abdomen, double the average technique of 15 mAs in 4 cm steps as follows:

$$22 \text{ cm (average)} = 15 \text{ mAs}$$
$$22 \text{ cm to } 26 \text{ cm} = 30 \text{ mAs}$$
$$26 \text{ cm to } 30 \text{ cm} = 60 \text{ mAs}$$

Now find the exposure time required at 300 mA to obtain 60 mAs:

$$60 \text{ mAs} / 300 \text{ mA} = 0.2 \text{ sec}$$

Doubling this figure, an appropriate back-up time for this very large patient would be 0.4 second, or rounding it up, about $1/2$ second. This calculation only needs to be done once for each view, if these specific back-up times are then included on AEC technique charts in each radiographic room. In this way, on a daily basis staff radiographers and students need only follow the charts, rather than determining back-up times case by case.

A common error while using the AEC is to forget to activate the correct *bucky* mechanism, such as when doing a chest at the vertical chest board but leaving the table bucky on. The bucky selection button also activates the AEC detectors for that bucky. In this case, the exposure would continue at the chest board, while the detectors at the table are "waiting" to receive adequate exposure. The result is an overexposed chest radiograph, since the exposure will continue until the back-up timer stops it. Always check all stations at the console before making an AEC exposure, including the bucky selection and the density control to make sure it was not left on a *plus* or *minus* setting from the previous patient.

THE A.E.C. DENSITY CONTROL

A knob or series of buttons labelled *Density* may be found on the console which applies to the AEC circuit. This control increases or decreases the preset sensitivity of the thyratron by specific percentages, so that the exposure time will automatically be extended or shortened by those amounts. There are various formats for this control: Some have only three settings, for small, average, and large patients. In this case the "small" setting will usually cut the exposure time to one-half, and the "large" setting will double it. Others are labelled as $1/2$, $3/4$, N, $11/2$, and 2. The "N" represents "normal" or average, $3/4$ would be a 25 per cent decrease, and $11/2$ would represent a 50 per cent increase as expected. The most common format is to have seven settings which may be labelled 1 through 7, or -3, -2, -1, N, +1, +2 and +3, or in some cases there is no labeling but symbols showing a bar or light that becomes wider to indicate an increase and narrower to indicate a decrease. In this format, each station usually represents a *25 per cent increase or decrease* in technique. For example, the +2 setting would indicate a 50 per cent increase in technique (two 25% sets), *not a doubling of technique.*

When using the density control, it is essential to remember rules of thumb used for manual technique change, especially the rule of thumb for *minimum density change* discussed in Chapter 5: *Technique must be changed at least to $^3/4$ or to $^4/3$ the original in order to see a visible difference image density. Always increase technique by at least one-third, or decrease it by at least $^1/4$.* In this regard, note that if the AEC density control is formatted in steps of 25 per cent, *the +1 station or 25 per cent increase may not darken the film enough to even see a visible change.* This is illustrated in Figure 191: Note that the radiograph exposed using the +1 setting is not visibly darker than the radiograph exposed with the "N" setting on this machine. On the other hand, the -1 setting did result in a visibly lighter exposure.

In Chapter 5, it was recommended that one generally increase mAs by 50 per cent to obtain a darker image. On AEC density controls that are formatted in 25 per cent steps, this corresponds to the +2 setting. As with manual technique, so with AEC: Often additional repeats are caused by being too timid and not changing the technique enough. To obtain a darker film, it is recommended that you skip the +1 (or 1 $^1/4$) station, and go straight to the +2 (or 1$^1/2$) station. To obtain a lighter image, the -1 or $^3/4$ station will usually result in a visibly lighter radiograph. As with manual technique, when a radiograph is *substantial-*

ly too light or too dark, it is advisable to adjust technique by a *factor of 2*, doubling it or cutting it to one-half.

As long as the AEC circuit is functioning properly, the density control should only need to be used infrequently. Constant adjustments are indicative that the AEC is being misused by the technologist or that there is a calibration problem with the equipment. For example, always setting it to +1 for oblique positions and +2 for lateral positions most likely indicates poor positioning: The AEC should normally compensate for the differences in thickness between these views. However, if sloppy positioning on oblique L-Spines causes them to frequently be off-centered by just one inch, this error alone is enough to cause the radiograph to turn out too light. (Almost one-half of the center detector would lie under soft tissue rather than bone, and the density produced will be a compromise between these two tissues, Figure 199.) The solution is not to get into the habit of using the +1 density setting, but rather to improve one's centering skills for the oblique position. The density control should generally not be used for changes in part thickness, nor to compensate for adjustments in kVp.

It *is* appropriate to adjust the density control up or down when the position and configuration of the detector cells cannot be adapted to placement of the anatomy of interest. For example, on a unilateral "frog-leg" position of a hip, a problem is created by the fact that the acetabulum and head of the femur, which must be demonstrated dark enough on the film, are not near the center of the film. When the center detector cell is activated, it will produce a good density in the femoral neck area that lies over it, but frequently the acetabulum and femoral head area will turn out too light because this anatomy lies in a corner of the

Figure 191. Demonstration that the minimum density change rule also applies to AEC exposures: Compare each set of radiographs by observing the middle of the upper tibia. Note that in radiograph **A**, using a density control setting of **-1** (a 25% decrease in exposure), is just visibly lighter than radiograph **N**, but in the following set the **+1** setting (a 25% increase in exposure) *did not produce a visibly darker image in* **B**. In the third set, radiograph **C** was produced at the +2 setting (a 50% increase in technique), and produced a visibly darker film. An increase of at least 1/3 or 30% is required to ensure a visibly darker image.

film rather than over the detector. When using manual technique, we generally settle for the neck area being a bit dark in order to have the acetabulum area dark enough. Selection of the +2 density setting (a 50% increase) will often darken up the acetabulum area enough without overexposing the neck area to an unacceptable degree.

Another example would be "phototiming" a smaller pediatric chest, perhaps on a six-year-old: If the two side detectors are used on this small a chest, there is often a risk that the upper portions of the cells might extend above the shoulders of the child, thus being exposed to the "raw" x-ray beam, and shutting the exposure off too

early, resulting in an underexposed film. This problem is precluded by activating the center cell only, but since this cell lies over the heart and spine, the resulting image would likely be too dark in the lung fields. A minus-2 setting would correct this.

When equipment is out of calibration, the density control can provide a *temporary* coping tool while waiting for service. The density control *itself* can be out of calibration, and there is a simple way for a radiographer to check this: Most AEC units include a digital mAs indicator on the console which reads out the actual total mAs used *after* the exposure is completed. No film is required, but a knee, skull, or torso phantom, or some other absorber to simulate a body part, is needed. For a knee phantom, select the "knee" button or setting on a preprogrammed machine. Take an automatic exposure of the phantom part without any film in the bucky, with the density control set to "N." Immediately after the exposure, write down the digital mAs readout. Do the same for all density control settings, without changing any other variables. Now for each *plus* or *minus* setting, perform the following calculation:

$$\frac{N - A}{N} \times 100$$

where *N* is the mAs readout for the "N" setting, and *A* is the mAs readout for the plus or minus station. This calculation will yield the percentage by which the technique was changed up or down from "N."

Observe the following results for one modern machine tested by the author:

+1 = +17%	-1 = -14%
+2 = +42%	-2 = -51%
+3 = +75%	-3 = -67%

It seems clear that this machine was designed for each setting to be an increment of 25 per cent; The -2 and the +3 settings fit almost exactly. The +2 setting falls 8 per cent short of a 50 per cent increase, and the -3 setting falls 8 per cent short of a 75 per cent decrease. Most interesting, though, are the +1 and -1 settings: The +1 setting is only increasing technique by 17 per cent, only $2/3$ of the expected 25 per cent. It has already been said that a 25 per cent increase may not be visible—a 17 per cent increase would certainly not be. The -1 setting is the most inaccurate; it is 44 per cent off! This 14 per cent reduction in technique may well not be visible either. Radiographers using this machine would do well to go right to the +2 or -2 settings when needed.

On another machine tested by the author, it was discovered that the -2 and -3 settings actually *increased* the mAs readouts to almost double! Radiographers using these stations would be guaranteed to have to take yet another repeat. This should serve as a wake-up call to radiographers and quality control technologists alike: Density controls can be and often are out of calibration. The procedure to check them is easy to do and well worth the short time it takes. Stations that are far out of calibration could be marked to avoid use until a service technician corrects the problem.

The AEC circuit is automatically engaged when the machine is set for spot-filming. Overhead radiographs may also be phototimed at the option of the radiographer. In many procedures, the use of the automatic exposure control will reduce repeat rates and improve radiographic quality and consistency. Nonetheless, there are many limitations to automatic exposure controls, and unknowledgeable use of them can actually cause higher repeat rates on some procedures.

LIMITATIONS OF AEC

Automatic Exposure Controls are used by some radiographers as an escape from the mental work needed to set manual techniques. Patient dose has indeed been reduced in many procedures. But AECs were not intended to be used on *all* procedures, and radiographers who use them inappropriately actually increase their repeat rate and overexpose patients. The major technique constraints on using AECs are:

1. AECs should never be used on anato-

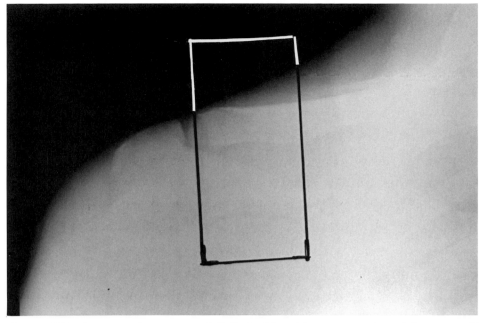

Figure 192. Automated exposure of (*left*) clavicle with upper portion of detector cell exposed to the raw x-ray beam, and (*right*) lateral sinus with portion of detector cell exposed to raw x-ray beam near bridge of nose, both resulting in underexposure.

my that is too small or narrow to completely cover the detector cell. This includes most distal extremities and extremities on small children. Detectors measure the average amount of radiation striking the area they cover. Portions of the detector cell not covered will receive too much radiation and the AEC will shut off too soon, resulting in a light, underexposed radiograph.

2. AECs should not be used on anatomy that is *peripheral* in relation to the x-ray beam, such as the clavicle, mandible or lateral projections of the scapula, sternum, or sinuses. In each of these situations the central ray is centered close to an edge surface of the body part, so that portions of the detector cell may extend beyond the part into the raw x-ray beam. As it averages the measured exposure, the detector cell will terminate the exposure early, resulting in a light radiograph Figure 192).

3. Even when automated exposure is

Figure 193. Automated exposure attempted for a lateral-oblique mandible. Detector cell is over thicker skull anatomy, so that mandible is grossly overexposed (arrow).

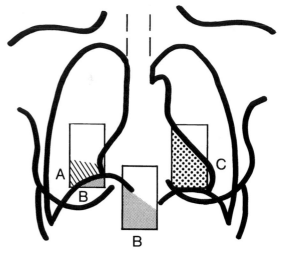

Figure 194. Diagram of the critical importance of superior-inferior centering during AEC chest radiography: Centering even an inch low may place the detector cells over (A) thicker breast tissue and (B) abdominal tissue below the diaphragm, and (C) more heart tissue, all of which darkens the radiograph. Simply by centering higher the radiograph will be significantly lightened, as shown in Figure 195.

used for proper applications, positioning and centering must be perfected within the limits of human ability. For the correct density level to be produced, *the detector(s) used must be covered with the anatomy of interest,* not just covered with any anatomy (Figures 193 and 199). The *tissue of interest* must cover most of the collective detector area. For example, using the two side photocells for the PA chest radiograph, centering must not be so low that the cells overlap abdominal tissue below the diaphragm (Figure 194), or a dark density will result.

Perhaps the single most common cause of repeated AEC exposures is *centering the bucky and film too low for PA chest projections.* This is especially common on short patients, and is probably due to the fact that so many radiographers center chests in terms of where the *top of the film and the top edge of the field light* fall in relation to the patient's shoulder shadows, rather than in terms of the cross-hair indicator for the central ray. Suppose you form the habit of allowing one inch of field light above the shoulders: On a short or a small patient, the lung field will not be as long, and leaving the same amount of light above the shoulders will result in both the central ray and the detector cells effectively being centered lower in relation to the *diaphragms* (Figure 194). If even the bottom one inch of the detector cells extends below the diaphragm, the cells will be recording abdominal tissue and will average the density between the abdominal tissue and the lung fields. This results in a longer exposure and an overexposed image. Figure 195 demonstrates how much lighter the

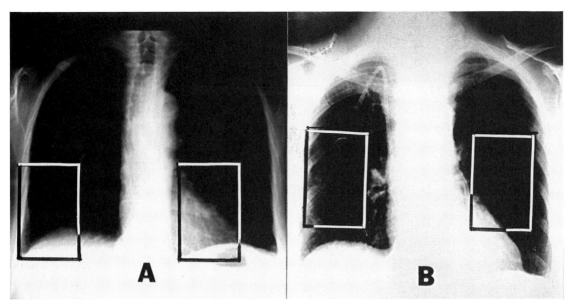

Figure 195. Automated PA chest exposures illustrating the sign)ficance of the density change caused by simply centering higher, as diagrammed in Figure 194. In (A) overexposure resulted from the detector cells lying partially over abdominal tissue below the diaphragm and over too much heart tissue. Note how much lighter the repeat (B) resulted, when the only correction made was to center about 1 1/2 inches higher (technique was not changed).

exposure will result solely by allowing more film above the shoulders so that the detector cells are completely over the lung/heart field. There was no adjustment in technique between these two radiographs, only the change in centering.

Centering *even one inch* low on a PA chest projection can make enough difference to cause a repeat. This is because there are *three* different tissue factors which all compound with low centering: First, the position of the diaphragm is critical. Centering low may place a portion of the detector cells over abdominal tissues below the diaphragm. There is such a great difference between abdominal tissue and lung tissue that even a small amount of abdominal tissue over the cells will significantly darken the exposure. Note also that if the patient takes poor inspiration, the diaphragms will be higher and worsen the situation. A good inspiration is essential.

Second, the amount of heart tissue over the left detector cell is a very significant factor. There is almost always some heart "shadow" over the left cell, but centering one inch low can result in one-half of this entire cell being covered with cardiac soft tissue. Note here that many patients have a condition of cardiomegaly which can place the upper border of the ventricles an inch higher than normal. If the patient has an enlarged heart, *and* the chest board is centered one inch low, the bulk of the left detector cell might fall under heart tissue. Third, on female patients, centering low places the detector cells under thicker portions of the breasts. For patients with pendulous breasts, centering even one inch low can make a significant difference in tissue thickness affecting *both* side cells. When using the AEC for chest radiography, technologists must constantly bear all three of these factors in mind: Breast tissue, the effect of the heart, and the location of the diaphragm, in respect to the detector cells.

4. As shown in Figure 199, demands of positioning for some phototimed procedures are *not* within the reasonable limits of human ability. Off-centering adjustments attempted for such procedures might result in an unacceptable projection of the anatomy (e.g., "closed joints," superimpositions or distortion), or in unacceptable collimation adjustments. *Proper positioning should never be compromised* for automated exposures. In such cases, manual technique must be employed.

5. The x-ray field must be collimated to the anatomy of interest, because excessive scatter radiation from the table or body will also cause the AEC to shut off prematurely.

6. The AEC should never be used when there is any type of radiopaque surgical apparatus, orthopedic corrective devices, orthodontic dental work, or other artifacts which cannot be readily removed from the area of interest. Figures 196 and 197 show two classic examples of this problem, both of which resulted in gross overexposures. In Figure 196, not only is there bridge work but also a metal tooth over the detector cell. As the AEC averages the exposure from the surrounding tissues with these areas where virtually no radiation is reaching the cell, it stays on too long and the odontoid anatomy is overexposed. In Figure 197, the AEC stays on for an extended time as it attempts to achieve some shade of gray under a radiopaque hip pin, resulting in an excessive exposure to the bones of the femur and pelvis. Radiographers must be conscientious enough to screen patient's charts and x-ray requisitions, and to verbally communicate with the patient regarding the presence of any surgical, orthopedic or orthodontic hardware prior to radiographing the patient.

Given these various technical constraints on the employment of automatic exposure controls, it is recommended that they be used primarily for procedures in the trunk of the body, the femurs, neck and cranium. They should never be used for mastoids, mandibles, distal extremities or other complex, peripheral or small anatomy.

7. Automated exposure should never continue to be used when repeating a radiograph unless the radiographer fully understands the cause of the improper density on the first attempt and is confident in the adjustment needed. If there is any uncertainty in analyzing the initial radiograph, manual technique should be used

Figure 196. Automatic exposure of odontoid projection with dental hardware absorbing beam. The detector cell increased exposure time in an attempt to average the densities between the dental work and the anatomy, resulting in overexposure to the spine.

Figure 197. Automatic exposure of hip with surgical pin present. As the AEC attempts to produce a density under the pin, the surrounding anatomy is overexposed. Manual technique should be used on all patients with previous hip surgery.

for the repeated exposure. If further repeats are necessitated, the manual approach will assure predictability which automatic exposure control cannot provide.

DETECTOR CELL CONFIGURATION

Figure 198. Typical configuration of detector cells in Bucky mechanism, with center cell lower than two side cells. (*Left*) center cell activated for procedures such as skull or abdomen, (*right*) two side cells activated for typical PA chest, such that cells are covered with *tissue* of interest.

The location of the detector cells is often demarcated by a triad of rectangles drawn on the radiographic tabletop or on a wall-mounted Bucky mechanism (Figure 198). Sometimes it is demarcated by dark lines in the field light, projected from a plastic insert in the collimator. For this type, the indicated size of the cells will be accurate *only* at a specified distance (usually 72 inches for chest units).

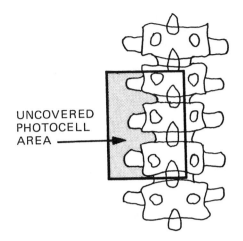

UNCOVERED
PHOTOCELL
AREA ——

Figure 199. Diagram showing how off-centering of oblique spine by only 3/4 inch places one-fourth of detector cell outside of tissue of interest (bone). Underexposure will result.

The actual detectors are located behind the tabletop. For older machines, photo-multiplier tubes were placed behind the bucky tray, so as to not cause any artifact on radiographs. To maximize efficiency, this placement required a large hole in the bucky tray and special phototiming cassettes that allowed more of the remnant beam to reach the detectors. The modern development of ionization chambers that are made of extremely thin aluminum allowed such detectors to be placed direct-ly behind the tabletop, in front of the bucky tray and cassette. At extremely low kVp techniques, these chambers can show up as artifacts on the finished radiograph, but are not normally visible with most techniques.

Positioning of the patient for an auto-mated exposure must be done in relation to the detector as well as to the film cassette, in order to assure a proper density out-come. This means that the selection of the detector cell configuration to be used (e.g., middle cell only, side cells only, or all three), effectively becomes part of position-ing.

It should be further pointed out that it is not adequate to position for automated exposures with an eye to simply covering the detector cell with *any* anatomy. *For proper density results, the detector cell must be fully covered with the tissue of interest.* It is fre-quently said that AEC technique requires good positioning, and this is generally true. But, in some cases the implied positioning skills are unrealistic, and automated expo-sure should not be attempted at all.

Let us assume, for example, that the lumbar spine is approximately 2 inches in width, and that the detector cells used are also 2 inches wide. Activating the middle cell only, it is easy to secure an AP projec-tion with proper density, assuming that the field light center markings are accurate. For oblique views of the lumbar spine, however, estimating the exact alignment of the spine with the detector is much more difficult. If the spine were off-centered by *only $1/2$ inch*, fully one-quarter of the detec-tor would be under soft tissue rather than bone (Figure 199).

In this soft tissue area, the detector will pick up additional radiation, "assume" that the bone image is darker than it really is, and shut off sooner than normal. A light image would result.

There is no question, then, that radiog-raphers must be much more conscientious about centering of the anatomy of interest exactly over the detector cells used. This requires not only good positioning skills, but a better appreciation of all related anatomy and the relative densities of these tissues. With such an appreciation of the anatomy, there are several parts of the human body where an astute radiographer can become creative with the configuration of the detector cells used, and to great advantage. A classic example is the unilat-eral "frog" position or Lauenstein method for the hip. This position was discussed in the previous section on the density control.

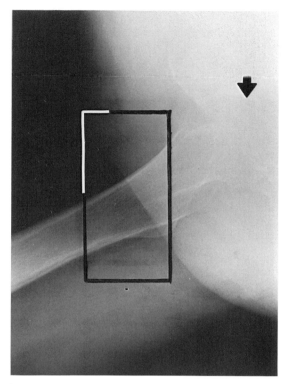

Figure 200. Automated exposure attempt for "frog" lateral hip. Anatomy over center detector cell is properly exposed, but anatomy of interest includes femoral head and acetabulum (arrow) which are underexposed.

The problem encountered is that, as shown in Figure 200, the *anatomy of interest includes the head of the femur and acetabulum of the pelvis,* and that these structures are not normally positioned over the center of the film. Thus, when only the center detector cell is activated, a very nice density will result for the femoral neck area over that cell, but this will often be too light in the acetabulum area.

Observe Figure 200 and ask yourself if a *different* detector cell might have been used to achieve a darker image. There are two distinct possibilities: The "side" detector cell which lies more *medially* into the thicker portion of the pelvis could be activated alone, which should darken the image substantially. Or, this medial cell could be activated *in combination* with the center cell to obtain a slightly darker film, where the exposure is averaged between the femoral neck area and the pelvis area (Figure 201). The author's experience is that such a combination does not adequately darken the image, and it is recommended that the medial cell be used alone. In fact, even though using the medial cell darkens the image significantly, it is often *still* not quite enough, and so it is recommended that this cell be used *along with a density control setting of +2.*

The lateral rectum view for a barium enema is another example where one of the side detector cells, the cell lying under the posterior half of the pelvis, might be used to advantage on some patients rather than the center cell. The radiographer must be observant of the position of the cell in relation to the patient's pelvis and be sure that no portion of the cell would extend behind the patient's body. Certainly for most projections the center cell alone should be used. Some confusion may result when considering anatomy such as the stomach which lies predominantly to one side of the body. With proper centering even on a small film, the center cell will be over the barium filled stomach, and the left detector should *not* be used. The same logic applies to a coned-down view of the left ribs. On a lateral L-spine, it is *not* appropriate to use the posterior cell—If the position is centered correctly, the spine should lie directly over the center cell.

Screening chest radiography, which we do so much of, is in fact one area where radiographers can and should be much more creative about cell selection. Probably the most common practice on the PA chest is to activate both "side" cells without the middle cell. Use of *all three* cells results in an exposure averaged between the lungs and the heart tissue, with

Figure 201. Options for resolving the problem demonstrated in Figure 200: The detector cell lying *medially* into the thicker anatomy should be activated either in combination with the center cell (*left*) or by itself (*right*). In addition, the density control should be set to +2.

the lungs getting "two-thirds of the vote." This provides a chest view that is slightly darker than if the two side cells are used. Do not be intimidated about trying this combination–it is not likely to overexpose the film, and is in fact the preferred configuration in some departments. To obtain views that are slightly lighter, the *right* cell (that is, the cell over the patient's right lung) may be selected by itself. This works well, because typically the left cell is partially covered with heart tissue, and by eliminating that input, the right cell will provide a density base solely upon lung tissue which is somewhat lighter. Again, do not hesitate to employ this method to obtain lighter films–it is not likely to overcompensate. For chest radiography, cell selection provides just the kind of flexibility to meet the individual preferences of radiologists. Without changing the mAs or kVp used, simply use all three cells for radiologists who like their films a little darker, and the right cell only for those who like their films a bit on the light side. For the lateral chest

projection, the center cell should always be used, squarely centered within the heart shadow, to ensure that the image will be dark enough when penetrating laterally through two lungs and mediastinal structures.

Table XXV is a sample automatic exposure technique chart which includes suggested cell configurations for each anatomical part. Anatomical parts not listed on this chart are not recommended for AEC use–manual techniques should be used on these. For example, the humerus is not listed because the bone is too thin to cover the center cell with the *tissue* of interest. Upright abdomens are excluded as well– they should not be "phototimed." The centering of the upright abdomen is such that the diaphragm is close to the center of the film. Almost no matter which cells are selected, it becomes a guessing game as to which portions of these cells will lie over lung and which over abdomen, and so the resulting density will be unpredictable.

Manual technique skills are still very

TABLE XXV
A E C   TECHNIQUE CHART

PROCEDURE	VIEW	kVp	mA	BACKUP TIME (s)	DETECTOR SELECTION	DENSITY SETTING	NOTES
CHEST	PA/AP	106	200	0.1	■□■	N	72"
	LAT	116	200	0.2	□■□	N	72"
6-YR CHEST	PA	90	200	0.05	□■□	- 2	72"
RIBS ↑DIAPH	AP/OBL	60	400	0.2	□■□	-1	72"
RIBS ↓DIAPH	AP	76	400	1.0	□■□	N	**72"**
ABDOMEN	AP	80	400	0.2	■■□	N	
IVP	AP/OBL	80	400	0.2	■□■	N	
G.B. / Coned	AP/OBL	80	400	0.2	□■□	N	
PELVIS	AP	80	400	0.2	□■□	N	
HIP Unilateral	AP/LAT	80	400	0.2	*■□□	+2	*medial cell
LUMBAR SPINE	AP	80	400	0.2	□■□	N	
	OBL	80	400	0.4	□■□	N	
	LAT	80	400	1.0	□■□	N	
	L5/ S1	90	400	1.0	■□□	N	
THORACIC SPINE	AP	74	400	0.2	□■□	N	
	LAT	60	10	5	□□■	N	breathing
TWINING C/T	LAT	76	400	0.4	□□■	N	
CERVICAL SPINE	AP	76	200	0.2	□■□	N	40"
	Odontd	76	200	0.2	□■□	N	40"
	Lat/Obl	76	200	0.5	■□□	N	72"
SKULL (SINUS) (FACIAL)	PA/Cald	80	400	0.2	□□■	N	
	Waters	80	400	0.2	□□■	N	
	Townes	80	400	0.3	□□■	N	
	LAT	76	400	0.1	■□□	N	
Mastoid/Coned	LAT	76	400	0.1	□■□	N	
SHOULDER	AP	76	200	0.2	□■□	N	
FEMUR	AP/LAT	76	200	0.2	□■□	N	
KNEE / LEG	All	70	200	0.1	□■□	N	
U.G.I.-A.C.	All	90	400	0.2	□■□	N	air con
B.E.-A.C.	AP/OBL	90	400	0.2	□■□	N	air con
	Sigm/Lat	90	400	0.2	□■□	N	air con

much needed and will continue to be, for tabletop "extremity" procedures, for decubitus views, mobile radiography, and for those anatomical areas that have been discussed in this chapter which are not amenable to the centering required for automatic exposure. Radiographers must use excellent judgment in deciding when to use the AEC and when to opt for manual technique.

AEC TECHNIQUE CHARTS

In the foregoing discussion, we have seen that the use of AEC does not obviate the need for the radiographer to set technique factors–the only the AEC sets automatically is the exposure time and the resulting total mAs. Optimum kVp must still be set "manually" to ensure adequate penetration and gray scale. An optimum mA station must be selected by considering the minimum response time for the machine, the associated focal spot size, the probability of motion and x-ray tube heat load. The small focal spot should be selected for extremity procedures. An intelligent choice from various options of detector cell configurations and density control settings must be made. An appropriate back-up must be selected for machines that do not do this automatically, such that the patient is protected from excessive exposure in the event of AEC circuit failure. For all these reasons, it makes good sense to construct and use *AEC Technique Charts* for all AEC units. An example of an AEC chart is presented in Table XXV, showing columns for all of this information. Additional guidance such as the recommended SID or film/screen combination may also be included on charts like this. They are strongly recommended. Appendix II provides a blank AEC chart in identical format, which you may wish to copy for personal use.

TROUBLE-SHOOTING

Whenever an AEC exposure turns out too light or too dark, the radiographer should have a "mental checklist" of possible causes to run down. Table XXVI presents a checklist of possible causes for overexposure, and Table XXVII is a checklist for underexposure. When an unacceptable AEC exposure is produced, the radiographer should mentally go through the checklist, identify the probably cause, correct it, and repeat the exposure. If the second exposure is still too dark or too light, further repeats using the AEC *should not be attempted unless the radiographer has confidently identified the cause and corrected it.* If there is any uncertainty about the cause after two exposures have been attempted, the appropriate action is to *revert to manual technique at that time.* Even if a repeat is necessitated after changing to manual technique, only one such repeat should be required. This is better than continuing to "phototime" when there is no clear understanding of the exposure problem, which can lead to a multiplication of unnecessary exposures.

The use of automatic exposure control does not require any less knowledge on the part of the radiographer than does manual technique. Different types of information are needed, but the radiographer must be just as astute. Thus, the modern radiographer must learn *both AEC and manual technique skills* thoroughly, and maintain clinical proficiency in both. Because of the advent of AEC, there is *more* to learn about radiographic technique and exposure, not less, in our school curriculum and continuing education.

TABLE XXVI
Causes of Dark AEC Exposures

-Wrong bucky activated

-Needed exposure time *less* than minimum response time (small anatomy, high mA, high screen speeds)

-Density control left on *plus* setting from previous patient

-Electronic malfunction of AEC, (back-up buzzer sounds)

-Incorrect detector cell configuration, such that activated cell(s) lie under tissue *denser* or *thicker* than tissue of interest

-Presence of radiopaque artifacts or appliances within the anatomy (hip or knee prostheses, orthopedic rods, pins, plates, or screws, dental appliances, pacemakers, bullets, etc.)

-Presence of external radiopaque artifacts such as lead sheets or sand bags over sensor

TABLE XXVII
Causes of Light AEC Exposures

-Backup time shorter than needed exposure time, (esp. on large patient)

-Density control left on minus setting from previous patient

-Inadequate collimation, (excessive scatter radiation reaching cells)

-Incorrect detector cell configuration, such that activated cell(s) lie under tissue less dense or thinner than tissue of interest

-Detector cells not fully covered by tissue of interest:
    -Anatomical part too small
    -Anatomy too peripheral
    -Specific tissue area too small
    -Specific tissue area not centered over selected detector cell(s)

PROGRAMMED EXPOSURE CONTROLS

Some modern equipment has been designed to simplify technique manipulation for the radiographer by programming preselected technical factors into a computer-type memory for each anatomical procedure. The control buttons on the console are marked with anatomical drawings rather than numbers. The radiographer first selects the procedure button and then may make a programmed technique adjustment upward or downward by selecting a patient-size button. The patient-size selection available is usually limited to average, small and large. The anatomical programmer may also be overridden so that manual techniques may be selected if desired.

The benefit of programmed exposure controls is their simplicity. The inevitable disadvantage is their lack of flexibility. Just as technique charts cannot be universally applied to all patients without the radiographer's professional assessment of patient status and condition, preprogrammed techniques cannot take into account all of the many variations of habitus and condition that occur.

No amount of computerization or automation can ever totally replace the necessity for the professional judgment of a well trained radiographer.

SUMMARY

1. *Automatic exposure controls* can reduce repeat rates and *patient exposure* on many procedures, particularly in the trunk of the body. They cannot be used properly on all procedures, however, and should not become a *crutch* for radiographers trying to avoid mental work. Such a practice may actually increase repeat rates.

2. Automatic exposure controls should not be used on *complex*, peripheral or very *small anatomy*, as improper density levels will result.

3. When phototimers are used, *positioning* must be perfected, the x-ray field must be properly *collimated* to the anatomy of interest, and the correct combination of *photocells* must be used.

4. Activated photocell detectors must always be completely covered with the *tissue of interest*, not just any anatomy.

5. In unique situations, such as where hardware or prosthetic devices might interfere with the photocell measurements, it is more reliable to use *manual technique* rather than automatic exposure. Whenever there is any doubt regarding the cause of a poor quality automated exposure, manual technique should be used.

6. *Optimum kVp, optimum mA*, and *appropriate back-up time* must be manually set for automated exposures, along with the correct photocell configuration.

7. *Technique charts* are required for the proper use of automatic exposure controls, and should include the information in #6 above as a minimum, along with photocell configuration, density setting, etc.

8. If excessive mA or receptor system speeds are used, the required exposure time may be less than the *response time* required by the AEC for accurate control.

9. *Density controls* on AECs should be checked periodically for accuracy by noting the readout mAs values at each setting. Most density controls are formatted in increments of 25 per cent up or down from average.

10. The *density control* may be used whenever the detector cells cannot be configured so that the specific anatomy of interest is completely positioned over them for proper density, or temporarily when the AEC is out of calibration until it can be fixed.

11. When using high power generators, high mA stations and high speed image

receptors, radiographers must be aware of the *minimum response time* for the machine, especially on pediatric patients or small body parts. Optimum mA will be *low* enough to ensure that the needed exposure time is *longer* than the MRT.

12. When adjusting the *density control,* remember that a $1/3$ increase or $1/4$ decrease is the minimum change required to see a difference in density. The +1 station may not provide enough increase to be visible.

13. *Back-up time* should generally be set at about double the expected manual exposure time. Quality control technologists should include back-up times on AEC technique charts. As a rule of thumb, use 0.2 seconds for all chests and proximal extremities, 1 second for abdominal and skull projections, and 2 to 4 seconds for very large torso projections.

14. The most common cause of repeats on *PA chest* projections is *low centering* of the film. To avoid this, allow more film above the shoulders on smaller patients. Beware of placing any portion of the cells *below the diaphragm, or over excessive heart or breast tissue.*

15. *Programmed exposure controls* are simpler but less flexible than a standard technique console. They do not replace the need for the radiographer to evaluate each patient for habitue and condition.

REVIEW QUESTIONS

1. Programmed exposure controls were designed to simplify technique. What is their disadvantage?

2. Why does it take the AEC longer to shut off the exposure on a larger patient?

3. A radiographer uses AEC a 6-year old pediatric chest using the two *side* photocells. Explain why the radiograph might come out light.

4. A radiographer uses AEC an AP thoracic spine using the middle photocell. *Why* might inaccurate positioning result in a light radiograph?

5. A radiographer uses AEC an AP cervical spine on a wall-mounted bucky, and uses a 72-inch SID instead of the normal 40 inches. Why will the radiograph NOT come out light?

6. When changing to a new film/screen system, why must the AEC be completely recalibrated?

7. A radiographer uses AEC on a pediatric chest. The detector cells are covered completely but the field size is left uncollimated much larger than the patient size. Describe how the density of the radiograph will come out *and* why:

8. If any radiopaque prosthesis or hardware cannot be removed from the detector cell area during an automated exposure, how will the image density turn out?

9. How can extremely high speed image receptor systems lead to inaccurate automatic exposures?

10. As a rule, the back-up time should be set at _____ the expected exposure time required.

11. A radiographer repeats an automated exposure that came out too light, increasing the density control setting. The second image turns out light again. What should he/she do next?

12. List four items that an AEC technique

chart should include information about:

13. Are there any procedures which should never be "phototimed," even though the positioning skills of the radiographers are high?

14. The needed total mAs for a particular procedure is 0.8 mAs. The minimum response time for the machine is 0.006 seconds. Using AEC at the 200 mA station, will the radiograph turn out light, dark or correct density?

15. Why might it be a good idea *not* to use the +1 setting (+25%) in order to obtain a darker exposure?

16. How can the radiographer quickly check the accuracy of the density control settings without exposing any films?

17. What is the most common cause of overexposed PA chest radiographs using AEC?

Chapter 29

MINIMIZING PATIENT EXPOSURE

The *entire focus of radiographic technique is to produce the best diagnostic image quality at minimum risk to the patient.* The second part of this task is as important in professional practice as the first, and is in fact the greatest justification for the first, since high quality precludes repeated exposures to the patient. The properly educated radiographer has both the concern for the patient and the knowledge to practice good radiation protection.

The implications of technique factors for patient exposure have been discussed in detail in each of the foregoing chapters, so this chapter will only broadly review each of these variables as it relates directly to patient exposure.

MILLIAMPERE-SECONDS (mAs)

The *total* mAs used to produce a radiograph is *directly proportional* to patient exposure. Twice the mAs will deliver twice the skin entrance exposure to the patient. Other factors, such as kVp, distance and screen speeds must be optimized with an eye to keeping mAs levels as low as image quality will allow (for example, without quantum mottle).

It is appropriate to change mAs as needed, however, to obtain proper image quality for different views within a given procedure and for patient thicknesses that vary from average. The alteration of kVp for these two functions can cause inconsistencies in penetration, fog levels and image contrast that may necessitate repeated

exposures. Generally, image quality should not be sacrificed as a means of lowering patient exposure, as it can defeat its own purpose. One example of an exception to this rule is in doing encephalo-pelvimetry or fetography, where the primary goal is to obtain a measurement rather than produce a pathological diagnosis: by using high kVp instead of increased mAs, the image will be overpenetrated and fogged, but the measurements can be made, and important fetal dose is saved in this manner. The radiographer should consult with the radiologist in making this decision.

KILOVOLTAGE-PEAK

All other factors equal, an increase in kilovoltage results in a net increase in patient exposure. The higher energy of the electrons striking the anode in the x-ray tube results in more x-rays being produced (see Chapter 6). Since these x-rays are collectively more penetrating, a lower percentage of the x-ray beam is absorbed within the patient, but this effect is not enough to cancel out the added numbers of x-rays produced in the tube. The net result is more exposure.

However, when higher kVp levels are compensated by reducing other factors in order to maintain image density, the net result is a *decrease* in patient exposure. For example, if the kVp is increased by 15 per cent, approximately 25 per cent more x-rays would normally be produced, having more penetrating power. If the mAs is then reduced by one-half to compensate, the net intensity of the x-ray beam would be about one-half of 125 per cent, or 63 per cent of the original. In addition to this net loss of x-rays, the increased penetration ability of the rays will further reduce internal dose to the patient. From the standpoint of maintaining image density, *high kVp techniques result in less net patient exposure than low kVp techniques.*

PHASE AND RECTIFICATION

A common misconception is that 3-phase, high-frequency or CPG equipment produces much lower patient exposure because lower mAs values can be used. These designs are more *electrically* efficient in producing x-rays, but compensatory techniques used in practice cancel out any difference in skin exposure. For example, 3-phase equipment produces almost twice the exposure rate of 1-phase for a given selected mAs, and thus requires only one-half the mAs. Exposure times are shorter for 3Φ because there are more x-rays *per second* at the same mAs value. A *slight* savings in patient dose is achieved because of higher average energy levels in the 3Φ beam.

A battery-powered mobile unit also achieves higher average kV levels, but it is common practice to use a set kVp on these machines that is much lower than one would use with a fixed unit, such as 70 kVp instead of 80 kVp for chest radiographs. In practice, the electrical efficiency of equipment has little effect on net patient exposure.

FILTRATION

Protective filtration is designed for the express purpose of reducing unnecessary patient exposure. It does so by eliminating low-energy x-rays that would not make it through the patient to the film, and are therefore diagnostically useless. When filtration levels increase enough to affect radiographic density in the image, such as with compensating filtration, technique must be adjusted upward to restore density, and the net change in patient exposure is nullified.

A minimum of 2.5 mm Aluminum filtration is required on all x-ray equipment operating above 70 kVp.

FIELD SIZE LIMITATION

Although limitation of the field size contributes to image quality, it should be regarded by the radiographer as an essential component of good radiation protection practice. Even if mAs is increased by 30-50 per cent to compensate for collimation, this is outweighed by the reduction of the amount of tissue irradiated. This is further supported by the fact that highly radiosensitive organs may be spared exposure by collimation. This reduction is on the order of *100 times* less when the exposure just outside the edge of the primary beam is compared to the exposure within the beam. Such a change eclipses any compensatory increase in technique.

Radiographers should therefore be ever-mindful of proper collimation. However, students will learn from experience that *overcollimation* is worse than insufficient collimation. If anatomy of interest is "clipped off" by collimating too tightly, the exposure must be repeated, doubling the exposure to the patient. Because, field lights are not always accurate, a very good rule of thumb is to *always allow at least 1/2-inch of light beyond each border of the anatomy of interest.*

Proper collimation is the most effective means for the individual radiographer to control patient exposure.

PATIENT STATUS

For thicker patients, higher mAs values are required to maintain image density, with a correspondingly higher exposure. Additive diseases, casts, and splints also require higher techniques and higher patient exposure. In most cases, these circumstances are outside of the radiographer's influence. *Compression* using a suitable device is one example of an exception where intervention by the radiologist or radiographer can reduce the required technique.

GRIDS AND CASSETTES

It has been traditionally taught that the use of grids results in higher patient exposure. This is generally true, since mAs may be increased to compensate density when a grid is introduced into the remnant beam. But, it should be remembered that the relationship of the grid is an *indirect* one—it is the change in mAs, not the grid itself, that increases patient exposure. The same can be stated for cassette materials which may be more or less radiolucent to the x-ray beam.

IMAGE RECEPTOR COMBINATIONS

Intensifying screens were developed for the purpose of reducing patient exposure. Like grids, screens *indirectly* affect patient dose by allowing a reduction in mAs which is very substantial at high speeds. The usable speeds are limited by mottling effects and loss of sharpness in recorded detail. Within these limitations, *the higher the screen speed, the lower the patient exposure required to produce radiographs.*

Radiographic films are also available in various speeds, and the highest speed should be generally be used *within* the limitations of the gray scale and detail levels required by the radiologist.

Screens must be properly matched with the films they are designed for, as discussed in Chapter Fifteen. Any type of mismatching results in a loss of image density, and unnecessary increases in technique may ensue.

Conversion of a radiology department to "rare earth technology" does not guarantee any reduction in patient exposure levels. Many departments, in order to avoid the rewriting of technique charts, have adopted rare earth screen systems with the same speed index as their older screens. ("Medium" rare earth screens are about equal in speed to "high-speed" calcium tungstate screens.) These departments have no basis for advertising state-of-the-art practice. Any reduction in patient exposure hinges upon the actual mAs values used. If these are not reduced, there would seem to be little justification for making a change in screen technology.

Aside from establishing a quality control program, the selection of appropriate screen-film combinations is the most effective means for the technical manager to control patient exposure.

DISTANCES

In practice, distances have no direct bearing upon patient exposure. Any change in SID must be compensated with mAs in order to maintain image density. The compensated technique will always precisely cancel out the inverse square law effects of modified distance, and result in the same net patient exposure.

POSITIONING AND INSTRUCTIONS

Positioning considerations necessary to proper diagnosis do not frequently lend themselves to modification for protective purposes. There are some exceptions: radiographing the skull with PA rather than

AP projections reduces dose to the eye lenses by placing them behind the major volume of tissue, which acts as a natural filter. Male gonadal dose may be similarly reduced for some procedures.

Proper and clear instructions to the patient regarding breathing, swallowing, and holding the position are essential to avoiding repeated exposures. Timing of the exposure, particularly for chest radiographs on small children, is a crucial ability that comes only with supervised practice.

TECHNIQUE SELECTION

In selecting an appropriate technique, the guidelines for optimum kVp and mA and the concepts in Chapter 24 should be followed. Technique selection should be *systematic* and *scientific*. Radiographic technique is *not* an art in the sense of being a creative act of imagination, or a guessing game—it is an art only in the sense of a skill requiring specialized knowledge, and it is a science of estimation.

TECHNIQUE CHARTS

Studies have demonstrated that the proper use of technique charts reduces repeat rates by as much as 30 per cent *even when no other quality control methods are used.* The implications for patient exposure reduction should be motivation enough for every radiographer to use charts. Technique charts are fully discussed in Chapter 26.

For the student, it is worth noting that many radiographers who *appear* to set techniques without the benefit of charts are indeed using a chart—they have simply memorized it by repeated use, so that they no longer have to look it up. You can be assured that the techniques they use did not originate in their imagination, but ultimately came from a chart. A chart is simply a written record of what works—why deprive others of this knowledge by refusing to write it down?

AUTOMATIC EXPOSURE CONTROLS

As described in the last chapter, the mere use of phototimers or automatic exposure controls does not guarantee any reduction in patient exposure, and the *abuse* of them can increase patient exposure. Optimum kVp, optimum mA, and an appropriate back-up time must be combined with proper collimation of the x-ray beam and knowledgeable positioning to minimize repeated exposures.

The AEC must be used only for those procedures which fall within its limitations to produce correct radiographic densities—those procedures involving relatively simple tissues, and thick enough, axially located anatomical parts that will properly cover the correctly chosen detector cell configuration. Technique charts should be provided for AEC units.

It cannot be overemphasized that, *when the radiographer is unsure of the cause of poor quality on phototimed radiographs, he should immediately revert to "manual" techniques, rather than continuing to attempt automated exposures.* Even if a manual technique results in an additional repeat, the needed adjustment can be predicted with confidence. This is not true of repeats using the AEC. Electrical malfunctions of the AEC are outside the expertise of the radiographer, and attempts to compensate for unfamiliar problems can lead to a string of repeated exposures. This is yet another reason why *every radiographer should be comfortable with manual technique.*

FLUOROSCOPY AND
MOBILE PROCEDURES

Protection of the patient during fluoroscopy is discussed in Chapter 33, and only key points will be emphasized here. It must be remembered that true fluoroscopy and spotfilming are two distinct operations. Traditional cassette spotfilming is essentially identical to phototimed "overhead" radiography. Optimum kVp and mA should be used so that exposure time is minimized, and the back-up timer must be set as described in Chapter 27 for phototiming. The control marked "fluoro mA", listed in multiples of 100, is actually the spotfilming mA applied to the x-ray tube under the table. The overhead kVp control becomes the spotfilming kVp and must be set for adequate penetration of the anatomy and contrast agents employed.

For dynamic fluoroscopy, the "fluoro kVp" control should be set to correspond to the spot-filming kVp level. The true fluoro mA is not normally changed and not always accessible, *but the radiographer is responsible for being aware of the actual mA readout when Fluoroscopy is underway. This readout is obtained from the same mA meter that one watches during routine exposures to ensure that the exposure took place.* If this actual value ever exceeds 8 mA, the first reaction should be to increase fluoro kVp if possible. Fluoroscopic kilovoltage should always equal or exceed the optimum kVp for the procedure as listed in Table IV. For example, at least 110 kVp should be used for solid column barium studies, and at least 90 kVp for air contrast barium studies. The actual kVp can be much more than this, but should never be allowed to drop below the optimum amount.

Fluoroscopic exposure rates to the patient must never exceed 10 Roentgens per minute measured at the tabletop. This rate can be checked with an ion chamber as described in Chapter 30.

Fixed fluoroscopy units must have a 5-minute timer which sounds an audible signal when this amount of fluoroscopy exposure to the patient has been reached. While the time of fluoroscopy is under the control of the radiologist, *the radiographer is responsible for monitoring fluoro time and for communicating with the radiologist when the recommended limit of 5 minutes is exceeded.* It is strongly recommended for legal and professional reasons that the total accumulated fluoro time for each patient be noted on requisitions or patient records for future reference.

An understanding of this responsibility should discourage the practice of constantly resetting the timer without noting the reading in order to avoid annoyance of the physician. There are at least two reasonable options open to the radiographer: (1) Be sure to be in the control booth when the timer approaches zero, allow the audible signal to begin to sound, but immediately reset it, or (2) reset the timer each time it reaches, say, one minute remaining, *but note the accumulated time, and tell the physician when 5 minutes has been exceeded.* This second approach may be illegal in some states, so consult with administrative radiographers prior to engaging in such a practice.

When the radiographer fluoroscopes a patient, he must use good collimation and remember to bring the fluoro tower down in near-contact with the patient in order to minimize patient dose.

Mobile C-arm fluoroscopes often do not have fluoro timers. The distance from the C-arm x-ray tube and the surface of the patient must never be less than 12 inches.

QUALITY CONTROL

Quality control methods for equipment are discussed in Chapter 30 and those for processing conditions in Chapter 41.

Quality control is the use of diagnostic tools to detect trends that will eventually cause repeated exposures to the patient, and correct them *before* such unnecessary exposures come about. By definition, then, *QC* plays a vital role in minimizing patient exposure.

Studies show that radiology departments employing comprehensive quality control programs, with technique charts, processor monitoring and repeat analysis can reduce the number of repeated exposures by 35-50 per cent. The budgetary savings of such an achievement, combined with the reduction in patient exposure and increase in professionalism, would seem more than adequate incentive for any administrative radiographer to take heed.

SUMMARY

1. Screen speeds, grids, distances and many other variables only indirectly affect patient exposure, in that they alter the amount of total *mAs required* for proper density results. The mAs is *directly proportional* to patient exposure.
2. *High-kVp, low mAs* exposure techniques reduce patient exposure.
3. Higher *phase* or more electrically efficient equipment does NOT necessarily reduce patient exposure. While lower mAs values are used, the *exposure rate* is proportionately higher for the mAs.
4. At least 2.5 mm of total aluminum equivalency is required as *filtration* in all machines operating above 70 kVp.
5. The most effective way for the individual radiographer to minimize patient exposure is through proper *collimation. Overcollimation* can result in clipping the anatomy of interest and cause unnecessary repeats and patient exposure.
6. The two most effective ways for the technical manager of a radiology department to help reduce patient exposure for routine procedures is to select appropriate receptor systems and to establish a quality control program with technique charts, equipment checks and processor sensitometry.
7. Used improperly, automatic exposure controls can result in increased repeat rates and patient exposure.
8. To reduce patient exposure, fluoroscopy requires the use of optimum kVp just as overhead radiography does.
9. Fluoro timers should be allowed to run out and sound the audible signal when 5 minutes is accumulated.
10. Fluoroscopic exposure rates to the patient must never exceed 10 R/min. as measured at the tabletop.

REVIEW QUESTIONS

1. What effect do high-kVp, low mAs exposure techniques have upon patient exposure ?
2. How much total aluminum equivalency is required as filtration in all machines operating above 70 kVp?
3. The most effective way for the individual radiographer to minimize patient exposure is:
4. The two most effective ways for the technical manager of a radiology department to help reduce patient exposure for routine procedures is to select appropriate _____ and to

establish a _____ program.

5. When available, does the use of automatic exposure controls always result in saving patient exposure?

6. To reduce patient exposure, fluoroscopy requires the use of optimum _____.

7. Generally, fluoro timers should be allowed to run out and sound the audible signal when 5 minutes is accumulated, but if the radiographer resets the timer prior to the sound, he/she should at least _____ when 5 minutes has lapsed.

8. The use of technique charts can generally reduce patient exposure by _____ per cent.

9. Fluoroscopic exposure rates to the patient must never exceed _____ as measured at the tabletop.

Chapter 30

QUALITY CONTROL

THE REDUCTION of repeat rates in a radiology department has professional, ethical, biological and economical benefits. The objective of all quality control programs is to minimize the repeat rate through ensuring consistency in the quality of radiographs produced.

A complete quality control program has no less than six different components. They include radiation exposure monitoring, radiographic unit monitoring, sensitometry and darkroom monitoring, the use of technique charts, the analysis of repeat rates and continuing education.

RADIATION EXPOSURE MONITORING

All radiology departments should employ a system for monitoring the cumulative occupational exposure to employees who work with ionizing radiation. Thermoluminescent dosimeters or film badges should be provided to all such employees and the monthly dosages posted on a bulletin board.

In addition, many departments also monitor patient exposure to radiation through simple mechanisms as both a patient advisement tool and as a legal precaution. For example, the total fluoroscopy exposure time accumulated during a fluoroscopic procedure can be taken from the fluoro timer and *noted* on patient records. The number of overhead exposures taken for each procedure can also be noted on patient records. Radiation procedure record forms are available from the government which can be given to patients to maintain themselves.

RADIOGRAPHIC UNIT MONITORING

Most of the quality control and fundamental calibration checks for radiographic equipment can be performed by the radiographer. The importance of this kind of monitoring is illustrated in the fact that the radiation output per milliampere has been found to vary as much as 50 per cent from one unit to the next within a radiology department and as much as 100 per cent between units in different radiology departments.

Tests that are able to be carried out by radiographers such as mA linearity, kVp accuracy, timer accuracy, focal spot damage, alignment, collimation and distance checks should be done monthly or bimonthly. This does not preclude the need for professional backup and additional checks on fluoroscopes and other more complex equipment by certified radiation physicists. It is recommended that all equipment in a department be thoroughly checked by a radiation physicist at least once each six months.

SENSITOMETRY AND DARKROOM MONITORING

This aspect is described in Chapter 40. Most of these functions can be and should be performed by staff radiographers, with occasional backup from processor specialists. When no quality control program is in place, processing errors and conditions account for well over 35 per cent of all repeats. All quality control programs should begin with the processor.

USE OF TECHNIQUE CHARTS

Radiology departments using a systematic approach to the development of techniques and enforcing their proper use often reduce repeat rates by as much as 25 per cent. Seventy-three per cent of all repeats are caused by radiographs coming out either too light or too dark. Part of this is from darkroom and processing variables; the rest is from improper selection of technique. When technique charts are used in combination with processing sensitometry, repeats can be literally cut in half. The construction of technique charts is discussed in Chapter 27.

These tests will be explained in this chapter.

ANALYSIS OF REPEAT RATES

There would be little sense in implementing any other aspect of a quality control program without the benefit of repeat analysis. Table XXVIII graphically illustrates the effect that quality control programs can have on the accountability of both the medical imaging department and the individual radiographer.

The greatest value of repeat analysis lies in the identification of continuing education needs for the imaging staff. By addressing those needs through inservice education, repeat rates can be reduced and patient exposure spared. Education is an integral part of any quality control effort, but the *specific* educational needs of the staff must be identified if it is to be effective.

TABLE XXVIII
Nationwide Radiograph Repeat Analysis*

Reason for Repeat Exposure	Per Cent of All Repeats for Department Without Quality Control Program	Per Cent of All Repeats for Department With Quality Control Program
Positioning Errors	13	41
Density Too Light	41	18
Density Too Dark	32	15
Blank Film	12	11
Motion	1	5
Other	1	10

*Taken from *Nationwide Evaluation of X-Ray Trends, United States Bureau of Radiological Health.*

CONTINUING EDUCATION

There would be no sense at all to monitoring radiographic quality if no intention of acting upon the results existed. When the technological variables are all monitored and controlled, the greatest factor determining radiographic consistency and quality is the skill of the radiographer. The field of radiography is advancing so rapidly, with new image receptor systems, computerization, and whole new subspecialties in imaging techniques, that continued learning should be a matter of survival as well as professionalism.

Every radiology department should explore both traditional and nontraditional methods of encouraging and providing opportunities for the staff to update their knowledge and skills and to better appreciate the plight of the modern patient. Every radiographer must realize that there is no *arrival* at total competency or total knowledge, that certification is not the end but the beginning of growth and improvement, and that there is always somebody else who knows something we could use. Developing an attitude of continued learning leads not only to professionalism, it leads to greater enjoyment and fulfillment in a career.

REPEAT ANALYSIS

The national average repeat rate for all operators of x-ray equipment (registered and unregistered) is about 13 per cent. More than one out of every ten radiographs must be retaken. Many radiology departments have succeeded in bringing their overall repeat rates down to 5-7 per cent by employing complete quality control programs. Such departments represent the epitome of professionalism in radiography.

The analysis of repeat rates amounts to nothing less than accountability—accountability to employers, to the public, and to ourselves. Repeat rates can be analyzed in a fashion which is not threatening to each individual radiographer. At the end of each month, all of the repeats for the staff as a whole may be sorted according to cause: too light, too dark, positioning error, blank, motion, darkroom error, etc. The staff can then identify the need for in-service education or quality control programs dealing with *specific* areas for improvement. As another alternative, each individual radiographer may be asked to sort and analyze his own repeats for the month, after which the radiographs are discarded. There are several variations possible for a repeat analysis program. Whatever method is used, it provides accountability and a mechanism for continuing professional improvement.

Such analysis has been done on a nation-wide level by the government. The results for departments with quality control programs intact and for those without quality control programs are presented in Table XXVIII. Note that where no QC program exists, most repeats are caused by poor technical quality of the radiograph, but where a QC program is used, 41 per cent of all repeats (the greatest percentage) are from positioning errors. This places the burden of radiographic quality directly upon the shoulders of the staff radiographer, where it belongs. In a positive way, the staff of a radiology department may then turn their attention to continuing education and the further development of positioning skills by identifying those areas of need. No longer can poor radiographs be vaguely attributed to electrical line surges, unpredictable processors and the darkroom technician. The radiographer is clearly accountable for manipulating the equipment and working with the patient in producing radiographs of high quality.

DETERMINING REPEAT RATES

There are many methods of obtaining repeat rate figures, some more accurate, others easier to implement. There are also several ways of categorizing these figures according to the needs and interests of the department and its staff: The two most useful methods of categorizing repeat rates are (1) by *type of cause*, such as positioning errors versus technique errors, or (2) by *type of procedure*, such as head procedures versus spine procedures. This second method has been largely neglected by texts on quality control, perhaps because it can be threatening to staff radiographers if used by management to "point fingers." Yet, it can be extremely helpful to the *individual* radiographer as a self-analysis which does not have to be divulged to any one else, and thus is included in this discussion.

It should be pointed out as well that *repeat rate studies can and should be modified as needed to target specific problems.* For example, suppose a department doing a monthly repeat analysis by *cause* finds that repeats due to positioning errors are much higher than desired. An analysis *by procedure* is now in order to determine if there is a particular type of procedure with which the staff radiographers are having difficulty positioning. A higher rate in pediatric procedures would be expected, but an unusually high rate in head procedures might indicate a need for some inservice education or sharing of case studies in that area. Having identified a specific category of procedures, such as head positioning, still another modification might be to acquire data for one evaluation period categorizing all repeats due to head positioning errors into categories of improper rotation of the part, improper flexion/extension, improper tilt or abduction/adduction, improper centering or angling of the x-ray beam, improper collimation or artifacts such as markers superimposing the anatomy. Note that the categories used in Tables XXIX and XXX can be exchanged between the two forms.

Departmental Repeat Analysis

To determine the overall repeat rate for a department, there must be a way of ascertaining (1) the total number of views taken during the evaluation period, and 2) the number of films used for repeated exposures during the period.

If an actual film count is not available, the total number of each type of radiographic procedure performed during the evaluation period (a statistic which most departments track) may be multiplied by the average number of overhead views taken for each procedure, as in Table XXIX. For the individual radiographer, or if a log of procedures is not already kept in the department, Table XXX may be used. The period of the study must be relatively long, at least one month, in order to provide reliable statistics.

Old rejects must be discarded and a new "throw-away" box or "reject bin" must be started at the beginning of the study period. Some departments keep individual boxes for each radiographer. At the end of the period, count the total number of films in the throw-away box. Subtract those which are green, blank or cannot be attributed to radiographer error, such as sensitometry films or dark room errors as in Table XXXI. Sort and count the remainder according to the desired categories. For example, if categorizing by *cause*, sort those which were *primarily* rejected because they were too light, those that were poorly positioned, and so forth. Many will present more than one problem, and the *primary* cause for the repeat, the most significant error, must be determined.

A "total waste" figure may be of economic interest to management and can be calculated by adding the number of all films in the throw-away box (including green and blank films) to the total number of "good" films used, and then dividing the number of throw-aways by this total of all films used, as shown in Table XXXI. Multiply the result by 100 to obtain a percentage.

For radiographic quality control, the total repeats (after subtracting the number of green and blank films) should be divided by the sum of repeats and good films used

TABLE XXIX

Repeat Analysis: Log of Total Views

At the end of each working day, fill in the number of each *type of procedure* performed that day. At the end of the study period, fill in the routine number of views taken for each type of procedure. Multiply the number of views by the number of each procedure done to obtain a total.

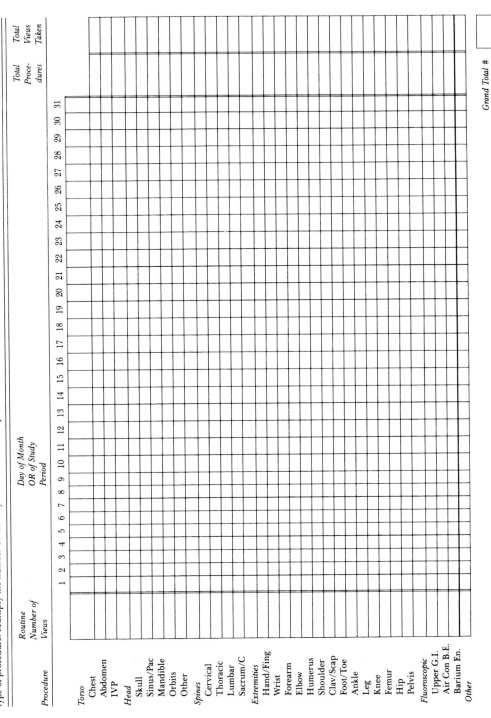

Grand Total #
Views for Period

TABLE XXX

Repeat Analysis: Log of Repeated Exposures
(by type of procedure)

After *each procedure performed,* fill in the number of *repeated* exposures taken according to the categories of procedures below. Use more than one log sheet as needed for the evaluation period. At the end of the period, total the repeats in each category, then divide *each* category total by the grand total of all repeats to obtain percentages.

NOTE: "Torso" includes chest, abdomen, and IVP. "Extremity" includes pelvic and shoulder girdles. "Fluoroscopic" includes UGI, BE and air contrast BE.

Type of Procedure:	*Torso*	*Head*	*Spine*	*Extremity*	*Fluoroscopic*	*Other*	
Fill In Number Of Repeats Taken							
							B
							Grand Total # Repeats For Period (Add All Columns from **A**):
A Totals for Period:							
Percentage of All Repeats: (A/B × 100)							

TABLE XXXI
Repeat Analysis By Cause

Name/Department: _____ Period — From: _____
To: _____

CAUSE	NUMBER OF FILMS	PERCENTAGE OF ALL REPEATS
1. Positioning Error		
2. Patient Motion		
3. Too Light		
4. Too Dark		
5. Artifacts (including fog, markers, static)		
6. Acceptable Films*		
7. Other		

A. Total Number of Views Taken for Period.............................: _____
(from Log in Table XXIX, or film count)

B. Total Number of Repeats for Period ....: _____
(Sum 1–7 above, OR from Log in Table XXX, OR total films in throw-away box minus clear, green, and unrelated films)

C. **OVERALL REPEAT RATE:** ....**B/A** × 100 = _____

D. For each category, divide the number of repeats taken in that category by the total number of repeats for the period (B) to obtain the percentage of all repeats in the last column.

E. Total Waste (total films in throw away box divided by total films used OR
B + green and clear films divided by A + B + green and clear films) .....: _____

*Refers to films of good quality in the opinion of the quality control technologist, which may have been rejected by radiologists or technologists for reasons other than image quality, or where there is disagreement regarding the acceptability of the radiograph.

for the period. Again, multiply this number by 100 to obtain the repeat percentage for each category of the analysis as in Table XXXI.

Individual Repeat Analysis

Potentially one of the most beneficial uses of repeat analysis is for each individual radiographer to perform their own. A department may encourage staff radiographers to do so, and provide the forms, yet allow each radiographer to keep his/her own results private. Every radiography student should have the experience of analyzing his/her own repeat rates for a period of time as a part of their radiography education.

The Repeat Analysis Logs in Tables XXIX and XXX are particularly suited for individual analysis. The log in Table XXIX is filled in once each day to track the total number of views taken during the evaluation period. Table XXX should be filled in on a procedure-by-procedure basis to keep an accurate count of repeated views taken.

By using Table XXX, the individual is then allowed to discard the rejected films in a collective throw-away box, and does not have to maintain an individual throw-away box, reducing obtrusiveness (threat) and embarrassment.

IMPLEMENTING A REPEAT ANALYSIS PROGRAM

Obtrusiveness refers to the effects of the radiography staff knowing that they are being evaluated upon their performance. When a repeat analysis program is started, obtrusive effects must be expected in the initial stages–repeat rates may increase due to a sense of higher standards, or suddenly decrease from various attempts to manipulate the rate downward. The results are therefore unreliable until the staff has accustomed itself to the program. Some authors recommend not informing staff that an analysis is underway, but suspicions of such activity will cause more severe obtrusive effects than knowledge of the study. To assure reliability:

1. The analysis program should be planned as an ongoing, regular study, not a one or two-time event, and the staff should be told this.
2. Staff must be assured that results of repeat analysis will be used to help meet departmental needs, and not in employment or advancement decisions.
3. The results of the first month should not be used to make any conclusions or decisions–rather, the first period of evaluation should be used as a "practice run". It may be wise to extend this "practice period" to two months. Staff should *not* be told that there is such a practice period, much less when results will begin to be used, or a new obtrusiveness effect will result.
4. After the practice period, baseline data should be accumulated over the next couple periods to which future trends can be compared. Minor fluctuations must be expected, and only gross deviations from national norms or baseline data should be regarded as "problem areas."

GOALS AND RESULTS

Each department must determine its own goals, but realistically, an overall repeat rate of 5 per cent or less should be considered as ideal. Repeat rates above 10 per cent in *most* categories (excepting pediatrics, for example) should be considered as problem areas needing some kind of remedial action. Recall that *uncertified* radiographic technicians can achieve repeat rates as low as 13 per cent. Certainly, properly trained equipment operators might be expected to achieve rates well below (e.g., one-half of) this amount.

The proper use of the information obtained by repeat analysis is to identify gross trends within the department which substantially deviate from either national norms or from the baseline data obtained for the department, and determine corrective action needed for equipment and continuing education needs for staff.

The final column in Table XXXI calculates the percentage of all repeated exposures attributed to each cause. It must be remembered that as some of these percentages are reduced due to corrective actions taken, other percentages in this column will increase, even though the actual number of repeated exposures for those causes has *not increased.* Such changes must not be misinterpreted as problem areas. The general goal would be for this column to appear roughly in line with column two in Table XXVIII. Implementation of a quality control program primarily reduces repeats for technical causes, and is *expected* to increase percentages under the positioning category.

The emphasis should be upon reducing the overall repeat rate, and this last column should be interpreted only in relation to norms, and as a way of identifying trends.

RADIOGRAPHIC EQUIPMENT

TIMER QUALITY CONTROL

The precision of exposure timers has developed a great deal in the last several decades, from spring-wound timers to electronic impulse timers which can measure one pulse of electricity as short as $1/120$ second in duration. Nonetheless, modern exposure timers are found to be inaccurate and requiring adjustment quite often. In the worst situation, for example, the time knob may loosen and slip one notch, so that the actual time set is a whole step away from that actually achieved. Inaccurate exposure times lead to unpredictable technique and a loss of control over image density.

Guidelines for Accuracy

It is suggested that a workable range of accuracy for regular timers would be plus or minus 5 per cent.

Test Procedures

SINGLE-PHASE TIMER. Single-phase timers may be checked with a simple manual spinning top (Figure 202). The moving hole in the top records each separate pulse of x-rays from the tube in a different location on the film. Since electrical current flows at 120 pulses per second, simply divide 120 into the number of dots you count on the film to get the exposure time. For example, $1/4$ second should produce 30 dots $(30/120 = 1/4)$ (Figure 203). If the dots are not fully separated, you spun the top too slowly; if the dots complete a circle

Figure 202. Photograph of electric and manual spinning tops used for quality control checks of the exposure timer.

and begin to overlap each other, you spun the top too fast. (Note: If you should get exactly one-half of the dots you expected, this indicates the failure of a rectifier, not the timer.)

THREE-PHASE TIMER. For a three-phase machine, you cannot use a manual spinning top because the electrical pulses overlap. You must use an electrical spinning top (Figure 202) (which can also be used for a single-phase machine). Most electrical spinning tops revolve consistently at 360 degrees (one revolution) per second. A slit in the top records a black arc on the x-ray film. To find the true time, carefully measure the degrees of the arc with a protractor centered to the center of the image of the top. Divide 360 degrees into your

Figure 203. Radiograph of manual spinning top test for single-phase machine showing an accurate 1/4-second time. Thirty dots equals 1/4 of the 120 x-ray impulses per second emitted by the tube.

Figure 204. Radiograph of electrical spinning top test for three-phase machine showing an accurate 1/4-second time. At a speed of one revolution per second, a 90-degree arc equals 1/4 of the 360 degree cycle.

measured degrees to obtain the time. For example, 1/4 second should produce a 90-degree arc $(90/360 = 1/4)$ (Figure 204).

MILLIAMPERAGE QUALITY CONTROL

Milliamperage is an electrical function. There are normal statistical variations in the generation of electrical current, which may be added to fluctuating demands on electricity throughout the hospital, and to wear, aging, and abuse of the x-ray equipment itself, which may cause inconsistencies in the actual mA obtained at a given setting over time. Such fluctuations in milliamperage output can cause significant changes in the density recorded on radiographs.

The direct relationship between milliamperage and image density remains true, but control over density is totally lost when the actual milliamperage obtained is different than the milliamperage set at the machine console. The technologist must be able to trust the accuracy of the mA controls. When they are out of calibration, radiographic technique becomes unpredictable.

Guidelines for Accuracy

Linearity refers to the proportionate accuracy of the output of one mA station in relation to another station. In other words, the 200-mA station should put out twice as great an intensity of x-rays as the 100-mA station, the 400-mA station should emit four times more, etc.

Federal standards require that each mA station be linear to within plus or minus 10 per cent of each *adjacent* mA station. On step wedge images, this translates to an acceptable *density* deviation of plus or minus 0.1 as measured on a densitometer.

Reproducibility is the consistency with which a given mA station emits the set output from one exposure to the next. The set output should not vary up and down significantly between uses. Such fluctuation would result in unpredictable techniques and a loss of control, just as poor linearity would. Federal standards require that a given exposure setting be reproducible to within plus or minus 5 per cent, or a density deviation of 0.05, when repeated 10 or more times. Although this repeatability generally applies to a total technique setting, including the set kVp and exposure time, these two factors do not tend to fluctuate significantly from one exposure to the next in comparison with milliamperage. Milliamperage, in fact, is somewhat notorious for fluctuating. Further, separate tests allow the kVp and timer to be calibrated, so that reproducibility tests may be considered to be primarily applicable to the mA stations.

Output between different rooms of the same phase within a radiology department may also be measured in mR/mAs and should fall within 10 per cent of each other, or 0.1 density, at the same mA and kVp settings.

Test Procedures for Linearity

The most accurate way to check the calibration of the mA stations is to use a good ionization chamber with digital readout. The intensity rate of the radiation in

Figure 205. Photograph of a step wedge penetrometer and a densitometer (*right*) used to produce and measure densities on test films.

mR/second, or the total intensity in mR for a given exposure time, should double when the mA station is doubled and vice versa.

A less accurate but very practical and useful method which may be employed by radiographers is to expose a *penetrometer* step-wedge and measure the recorded densities with a *densitometer*, two devices likely to be found in most radiography departments (Figure 205).

METHOD A. If there are only three or four mA stations to check and you begin with a radiograph with a relatively light, (0.3-0.4) density level, you can simply increase the mA station from one exposure to the next and take densitometer measurements off of one of the middle steps of the penetrometer. You must be sure to use the same step for each measurement. All other variables (screens used, processing, distances, field size, etc.) must be maintained equal throughout the experiment. To ensure equal processing factors, make all of the exposures on one 14- x -17-inch film, so that they are all developed at the same time. Within the accuracy ranges described, each change in mA station should produce a proportionate change in film density. Density measurements above 2.5 are unreliable using this method, and should not be used.

METHOD B. If several mA stations are to be checked for calibration, you must use an equal mAs approach, reducing the exposure time by an inverse proportion to each increase in milliamperage. For example, 100 mA at $1/10$ second, 200 mA at $1/20$ second, and 300 mA at $1/30$ second might be used. The measured density from each exposure should then be equal to the others within plus or minus 0.1 (Figure 206). Although this approach allows several stations to be checked, it is dependent upon the assumption that the exposure timer is accurate. Therefore, this method should always be performed in conjunction with a timer accuracy test. If a particular time is found to be inaccurate, the percentage of inaccuracy may be calculated and subtracted from subsequent inaccuracies measured during the mA test to find the actual mA accuracy. Again, the same middle step should be used on the penetrometer image for each measurement and all other variables must be carefully stabilized.

Test Procedure for Reproducibility

To check for reproducibility of exposure, simply repeat the same exposure eight or ten times, using a penetrometer on one 14- x -17-inch film, for all exposures so that processing will be equal and measure a middle step with the densitometer to determine if it varies significantly from an average. To find the average, divide the sum total of all of the density measurements by the number of measurements taken; then compare each individual measurement to this average. *No single measurement* should deviate by more than 5 per cent, or 0.05 density, from this average.

Test Procedure for mR/mAs Output

The unit mR/mAs is useful in comparing different machines *of the same phase and type of generation* to see if they are linear from one room to another. This is important to know because if these machines are within the recommended limits, then the same technique chart should be able to be used in all of the different rooms. Single-phase machines must *only* be compared to other single-phase machines, $3\Phi^{12}$ machines to other $3\Phi^{12}$, and $3\Phi^6$ to other $3\Phi^6$.

The actual output from the x-ray tube can be measured using an ion chamber. All compared measurements must be done at the same kVp, since kVp can affect the output of the tube. It is recommended that at least three series for comparison be done, one at 60 kVp, one at 80 kVp and another at 100 kVp. Comparisons can also be done for each mA station. At a given mA, a relatively long exposure time (at least 0.5 seconds) should be used for the ion chamber to obtain an accurate measurement in mR (set for the "integrated dose" mode). This total mR is then divided by the mAs used (mA station multiplied by the exposure time) to find the mR/mAs. For most accurate results, three or more exposures should be repeated at each setting and an average taken, by adding the amounts and dividing by the number of exposures. The result should not vary by more than 10 per cent from one room or machine to another of the same phase.

A practical quick check can be made by radiographers using a penetrometer and

Figure 206.   Radiograph of milliamperage linearity test using a.penetrometer. Factors left to right: 100 mA at 1 second, 200 mA at $1/20$ second, and 300 mA at $1/30$ second. Observing medium- density step 4 or 5, it is apparent that the 100 mA station is slightly darker than the other two, but within acceptable limits as measured on a densitometer.

densitometer.   Simply expose the step wedge penetrometer using identical techniques in the different rooms. It is best to use the same film for all exposures so that processing consistency will be assured. Collimation, distances, and all other variables must be kept constant. On the resulting radiograph, the measured density on a selected medium-density step should not vary by more than plus or minus 0.1 from one machine to another of the same phase.

KILOVOLTAGE QUALITY CONTROL

Penetration is the single most important quality of an x-ray beam. It is directly dependent upon the energy spectrum of the beam, which is controlled by the electrical kilovoltage applied across the x-ray tube. Since the energies of the x-rays in the beam vary across a heterogeneous spectrum, beam energy cannot be directly measured as a discrete quantity. However, the penetration ability of the beam may be directly measured and, because of its direct relationship with beam energy, the energy may then be extrapolated from the penetration data. It is essential to the radiographer that such monitoring of the obtained energy take place, so that the selected kVp setting on the equipment may be trusted to produce the desired kVp.

The *Wisconsin kVp Test Cassette* (Figure 207) was developed to derive the actual peak energy of the x-ray beam from its penetration characteristics. Inside the cassette, each exposure passes through two devices: on one side is a copper step-wedge; on the other is an intensifying screen with an *optical attenuator*—a simple light filter designed to always attenuate or stop exactly one-half of the light which the screen emits (Figure 208). Both sides are covered by a lead mask with round holes in it so that two columns of round spots are recorded on the film.

After exposure and development, each kVp area on the radiograph will show two columns of density spots (Figure 209). In the column which was under the optical attenuator, all of the spots will be of the same density. This density represents an exposure to exactly one-half the light emitted from the intensifying screen. The opposite column will consist of spots with a graduation of different densities, representing the exposure under each of the steps on the copper step-wedge, the lighter spots being under the thicker steps. By comparing these spots with the optical attenuator column and finding a *match*, it may be determined what thickness of copper was required to attenuate one-half of the x-rays. The thicknesses of copper required to absorb one-half of the beam are known for the various kVp levels, with greater thick-

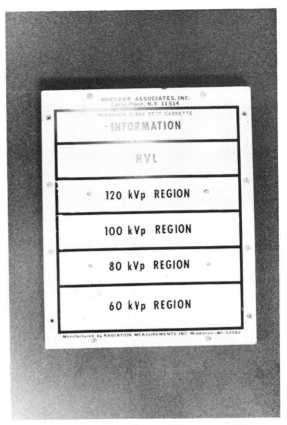

Figure 207. Photograph of a Wisconsin kVp test cassette showing demarcated exposure areas.

Figure 208. Photograph of opened Wisconsin kVp test cassette showing optical attenuator light filters (dark areas).

Figure 209. Radiograph produced with Wisconsin kVp test cassette showing matching density spots (circled) used to find the actual kVp output of the x-ray machine.

nesses being required for higher kVp levels. So, once the half-value thickness is measured, a chart may be consulted to find the corresponding actual kVp of the beam.

Guidelines for Accuracy

It is suggested that actual kVp values should fall within plus or minus 2 kVp of the indicated kVp setting. If they are not within this range, a serviceman should be called to make electrical adjustments.

Test Procedure

The Wisconsin kVp Test Cassette must be used to determine actual kVp accuracy. Four exposures are made on one film, collimating to a marked area for each, in steps of 20 kVp from 60 to 120 kVp, using the following techniques, respectively, for a single-phase machine: 150 mAs at 20 inches SID, 20 mAs, 5 mAs and 3 mAs at 40 inches SID. For a three-phase machine, the mAs values must be cut in half.

To determine the kVp, first you must identify the two dots which most closely match in density. You may do this either visually or using a densitometer for accuracy. The column under the optical attenuator will have spots of all the same density, representing one-half the original exposure. The other column under the step-wedge will have spots of increasing density. The spot in this column which matches the other column represents the *half-value layer* (Chapter 8) in copper for the beam. Half-value layer is a measurement of the penetration or energy of the beam, and kVp can be directly extrapolated from it. Graphs of the kVp/HVL relationship are provided with the cassette. To find the kVp, you simply locate the matching step number on the graph (which may fall between two spots on the film) and read across to the graph line and then down to the kVp axis.

Table XXXII lists the typical matching step numbers for each kVp setting tested with the Wisconsin kVp Test Cassette when the kVp is accurate. If the actual matching step number you measure is above this number, the actual kVp is greater than the kVp station indicates. If the measured step number is lower, the actual kVp obtained is less than indicated.

TABLE XXXII
Wisconsin kVp Test Casette; Matching Step
Numbers for Accurate kVp Settings

kVp	Single-Phase Step Number	Three-Phase Step Number
60	5.0	5.6
80	5.2	6.0
100	5.1	6.1
120	5.0	5.75

HALF-VALUE LAYER AND FILTRATION

The most important quality of the x-ray beam is its ability to penetrate through a substance. Protective filtration is used to remove low-energy x-rays from the beam because they cannot penetrate through the patient. Optimum kVp levels are necessary to assure adequate penetration through the anatomy. Beam penetration may be raised in two distinct ways: (1) by increasing the *minimum* energies present in the beam through the use of filtration and (2) by increasing the *maximum* energies present in the beam through the use of higher peak kilovoltages. Either of these methods results in an increase in the *average* energy of the beam and in higher penetration.

Since kilovoltage does not tend to vary much from that value set at the control panel and can often be checked and adjusted by the service representative, any measured inadequacies in beam penetration usually reflect upon the amount of protective filtration placed in the collimator. If the kVp is found to be accurate but the penetration of the beam is too low, more protective filtration should be added to the collimator. Radiographers must be aware of any such need as a matter of profession-

alism and patient safety.

The only true measure of beam penetration is the *half-value layer*, abbreviated *HVL*. Half-value layer is defined as that thickness of absorber (usually aluminum) needed to reduce the intensity of the beam mR) to one-half of the original intensity. The higher the HVL, the more penetrating the beam.

Guidelines for Accuracy

Although NCRP regulations require a minimum of 2.5 mm aluminum equivalency in total filtration (inherent plus added) for most diagnostic x-ray machines, more filtration is required when the half-value layer does not exceed HVL recommendations at each kVp level. HVL is the direct measurement of actual beam penetration and indicates whether filtration levels are adequate.

At 80 kVp, the HVL must be at least 2.34 mm of aluminum equivalency. Required HVL values at other kVp levels may be found in governmental regulations, but one simple test at 80 kVp will often suffice.

Test Procedures

The Wisconsin kVp Test Cassette has an area on it for finding the beam HVL directly, using the same process of matching the resulting columns of spots as discussed in the last section. A technique of 4 mAs for single-phase or 2 mAs for three-phase must be used in this area at 60 kVp.

HVL can also be found by using pocket ion chambers with sleeve filters or large ion chambers and several thin sheets of aluminum filtration. First, for a given technique of average kVp level, a reading is taken of the beam intensity (mR) without using the sleeve filters or aluminum sheets.

Then, readings are taken with increasing thicknesses of the filters added until less than one-half of the original reading is obtained. The readings may be plotted against the thicknesses of absorber on graph paper to form an absorption curve. To find the HVL in aluminum, simply find the dose which is one-half or 50 per cent of the original dose, read across to the curve and down to the absorber thickness—this is the HVL.

COLLIMATOR QUALITY CONTROL

When the actual size of the x-ray field is greater than that indicated on the collimator control knobs, unnecessary patient exposure and additional scatter fogging of the radiograph occur. When the actual field size is less than that indicated, anatomy of interest may be cut off from the field of view, necessitating repeat exposures. It is essential to the radiographer, therefore, that both the field size control knobs on the collimator and the projected visual light field accurately indicate the size and location of the actual x-ray beam.

It is important to understand that the projected light field may not accurately represent the actual x-ray field location. Further, recall that the tabletop is at a different distance from the x-ray tube than the Bucky tray. For these two reasons, the practice of simply measuring the light field on the table to determine field size can lead to several errors. X-ray field size should be determined by directly measuring the exposed area on a radiographic film.

Inaccuracies in the field size indicator on the collimator may be caused by slippage of the collimator shutters. These shutters are usually turned by gears and can occasionally slip, especially on older collimators.

Guidelines for Accuracy

It is recommended that each dimension (length and width) of the actual field size measure within plus or minus 2 per cent of the SID being used (2 centimeters at 40 inches SID) from the size indicated on the collimator control knobs for that distance. It is suggested that each half of the field be symmetrical to within 1 centimeter of the opposite half.

It should be noted that light field edges are frequently as much as one-half inch off of alignment from the actual edges of the x-ray beam (Figure 210). Where the actual beam edge is inside the light field edge, anatomy of interest may be cut off when tight collimation is used.

Test Procedures

Collimate to any size smaller than the film you are using and make a very low

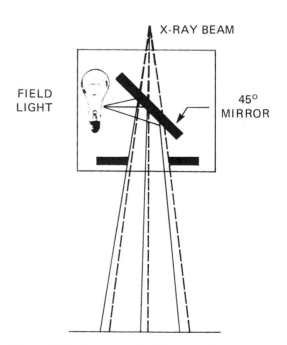

Figure 210. Diagram of collimator mirror responsible for alignment of the light field with the actual x-ray beam.

mAs exposure without anything in the beam. Process the film and simply measure the exposed rectangle in both axes with a ruler to compare it with the collimator indicator. If there is a measured discrepancy, a collimator shutter has slipped and the collimator needs service. Proper alignment of the collimator shutters may be determined by measuring with a ruler the light field on the table from the midline to each edge and checking for symmetry. If one edge measures farther from the midline than the opposite edge, the shutter has slipped.

This test for field size accuracy is usually done in conjunction with the light field alignment test and vertical beam alignment test which follow. All three tests can be made with one exposure, as shown in Figure 211.

LIGHT FIELD ALIGNMENT QUALITY CONTROL

Inside modern collimators there is a light bulb and a mirror aligned in such a manner as to project a field of light in the same path as the x-ray beam. The light bulb cannot be placed in the path of the x-ray beam or it will appear as an artifact on radiographs, so it is set to the side at right angles to the x-ray beam central ray. Its light is then reflected by the mirror into the path of the x-ray beam. The mirror, although it acts as added filtration in the x-ray beam, does not create any artifacts on the film because of

Figure 211. Radiographs of light field alignment checks using paper clips to demarcate light beam edges (*left*) and using the Wisconsin beam alignment device (*right*). Both examples demonstrate the light field misaligned to the *north* and *west* of the actual x-ray beam, so that the corresponding markers are not within the darkened area. The tool to the right also shows a true central ray angle out of vertical toward the *east* since the screw in the center is projected outside the outer edge of the washer, indicating an angle greater than 2 degrees.

its even thickness and homogeneous composition. Normally, the mirror should be placed at exactly 45 degrees from the central ray, so that the light field will be projected precisely where the x-ray field is. When the mirror or the light bulb is misaligned, the center and edges of the light field will not accurately represent where the actual x-ray beam is directed (Figure 210).

It should be noted by every radiography student that it is not uncommon for the light field to be misaligned by as much as one centimeter or one-half inch at the usual 40-inch SID. To avoid cutoff of anatomy, which could lead to repeat exposures, therefore, it is advisable to use the following rule of thumb: *Always allow yourself one-half inch of light beyond each border of the anatomy of interest.* Although collimating the beam down as closely as possible to the size of the anatomy of interest is a commendable professional practice, it must be remembered that to risk cutting off any portion of that anatomy is to risk a repeat exposure and therefore additional patient exposure. This rule of thumb will prevent many of the cutoff problems arising from the use of different x-ray machines with different degrees of alignment accuracy.

The accuracy of the light field alignment is an essential component of patient protection. Some machines are as far as one full inch off of alignment and cause frequent repeat exposures. Once the misalignment is detected, it can often be remedied by a simple adjustment of a screw in the collimator which controls the mirror angle (Figure 81 in Chapter 9). If not, a service specialist should be called in.

Guidelines for Accuracy

Each edge of the actual x-ray beam must be within plus or minus 1 per cent of the SID from the edge of the light field. The central ray of the x-ray beam must also be within 1 per cent of the SID from the center of the light field. At the typical 40-inch SID, then, each of these should be within 1-cm accuracy.

Test Procedures

The edges of the light beam must be demarcated with radiopaque markers. Unfolded paper clips or wire serve well enough for a homemade check. Test plates may be purchased which indicate the exact percentage or amount by which the beam is off of align. Also, be sure that there is a marker in one corner of the light field so that you can orient the exposed film in the proper direction to match the collimator.

Make an exposure with one of the devices explained above marking the edges of a light field which is well less than the film size being used. Process the film. The exposed black rectangle on the film is the actual x-ray field, whereas the markers outline the light field (Figure 211). Be sure to orient the film to North-South and East-West so that it matches the collimator you are checking. If the black area is one

Figure 212. Photograph of Wisconsin beam alignment test tool.

inch to the West of the markers, then the *light field* must be adjusted toward the West one inch. The center of the beam may be checked against the center of the light field by drawing diagonal lines from the corners of the film and from the corners of the exposed area. Where the diagonals cross in each case marks the central ray, light versus x-ray beam.

If the light field central ray is found to be one-quarter inch off from the x-ray field central ray, while the edges of the light field are found to be one-half inch off, or perhaps off in a different direction, then the indication is for *two* distinct problems: light field misalignment and possible shutter slippage. The central ray location should be used as the criterion for adjusting the light field alignment first. Vertical beam alignment should also be checked (see next section). Finally, collimator shutters should be checked for conformity of edges.

VERTICAL BEAM ALIGNMENT QUALITY CONTROL

Occasionally, a light field which appears to be off-centered to the x-ray table transversely is not, in fact, off-centered but misangled. This can occur when the transverse tube angle lock has been used for some procedure by a radiographer who did not take special care to restore it to an exact vertical position afterwards. Normally, this transverse angle lock should not be used for any procedure. It is possible to achieve the same results by first swivelling the tube on its axis and then utilizing the usual longitudinal angle lock.

It is critical to radiographic procedures that the central ray of the actual x-ray beam be exactly perpendicular to the planes of the tabletop and Bucky mechanism. This should be checked in combination with field light alignment and field size tests, so

that one problem will not be misconstrued with another.

Guidelines of Accuracy

The x-ray beam must be within two degrees of perfect vertical alignment.

Test Procedures

To check vertical alignment of the beam, you need two radiopaque objects fixed in perfect vertical alignment. Six-inch Plexiglass™ test cylinders may be purchased (many come with the light field test plates mentioned previously) which have a small screw embedded in perfect center on the top and a washer embedded similarly on the bottom (Figure 212). An exposure is made centering the light field to the screw, and the film is processed. On observing the radiograph, if the edge of the screw lies outside of the *outer* edge of the washer (Figure 211, *right*), then the beam is off of vertical more than two degrees and must be adjusted by using the locks on the tube head or, if the tube is fixed in position, by a service specialist.

DISTANCE INDICATORS

Newly installed distance indicators rarely present inaccuracies, but older equipment or reinstalled equipment should be checked for slippage.

Guidelines for Accuracy

It is recommended that SID indicators be accurate to within plus or minus one-half inch or two centimeters.

Test Procedures

Distance indicators on the x-ray machine

may be checked for accuracy by simply
using a tape ruler. The measurement must
be taken from the exact location of the
focal spot within the cylindrical tube housing (*not* from the collimator). Most anodes
are 3-4 inches in diameter, placing the focal
spot about $1^1/2$ inches toward the collimator from the middle of the cylindrical tube
housing.

FOCAL SPOT QUALITY CONTROL

It is important to understand that the
nominal focal spot size quoted by tube manufacturers is a measurement obtained
under the most ideal conditions with a low
mA setting. The actual size may be as
much as 50 per cent larger than the nominal size for several reasons. To estimate
how small a thrombus or embolism may be
resolved during an angiogram, you must
know the true size of the focal spot at the

Figure 213. Photograph of star pattern focal spot
test template used to obtain accurate measurements of focal spot size.

mA stations normally used for the procedure. The most significant reason for this
problem is *blooming* of the focal spot. At
high mA settings, many electrons are
boiled off of the cathode to form the *space*

Figure 214. Radiograph of star template to measure focal spot
size. Diameter measurements taken between the marked *first*
blur points are multiplied by a constant to obtain the actual
size.

charge or electron cloud. Being of the same electrical charge, they repel each other so that the size of the cloud *blooms* or expands beyond the normal diameter. When they are propelled across the tube, they strike a larger area on the anode, creating a larger actual focal spot. Although manufacturers of x-ray tubes generally consider a 30 per cent margin of error as allowable, and government regulations allow for 50 per cent deviation, special procedures technologists will want to know more accurately the real focal spot sizes they are using.

Still more important is the simple monitoring of the x-ray tube over time for possible damage to the focal spot on the anode. Small cracks in the surface of the anode focal track, called *etching*, occur over time with the thermal shock produced from bombardment of high-speed electrons. Abusive use of the x-ray tube can cause acute problems such as fractures or melted pits on the anode surface. Since any of these conditions cause an uneven surface to the focal spot, changing its apparent projected size or configuration, they can be detected by sudden changes in the resolution or sharpness of detail in an image.

Test Procedures

STAR PATTERN TEMPLATE METHOD. The most accurate and practical method of obtaining an actual measurement of the focal spot size is to use a *star*-type test template (Figure 213). The template should be placed at an object-film distance equal to one-half of the SID. Recommended distances are 12 inches from the film to the template and 24 inches SID. It is important that the middle axes passing through the line pairs of the pattern be aligned with the length and width of the x-ray tube (hence, the focal spot) and that they not be placed diagonally. A light exposure is made and the radiograph processed.

A blur pattern will result on the finished radiograph. The radiographer should scan from the periphery of the pattern *inward* until the *first* point where the line pairs are not distinguishable is located. A mark should be made at this point of blur (Figure 214). It may be seen that further inward the line pairs seem to resolve again and then blur again. This phenomenon is *false resolution* and occurs from the overlapping of blurred line images. Thus, it is essential to measure only the outermost points of blur. A mark should be made at these points for each of the four arms of the star.

Using a millimeter ruler, record the measurements between the two *pairs* of marks across the pattern–length and width. If the template has the typical two degrees of arc per line, then these two measurements may simply be multiplied by the factor 0.035 to obtain the actual size, length and width, of the focal spot.

PINHOLE CAMERA METHOD. A second method for measuring focal spot size is with a pinhole camera. The pin-sized hole in a metal plate is placed one-half way between the tube target and the film, resulting in a magnification factor of one, so that the size of the density spot projected on the film represents the actual size of the focal spot itself (Figure 215). (The geometry of the pinhole camera method is completely different from the geometry of normal image magnification discussed in Chapter 20. The two must not be confused.)

The pinhole camera method is less accurate than the star pattern template method because the shadow being measured has penumbral edges. It is also much less practical because excessively high exposures are required to record a density through the pinhole, which may lead to tube anode damage.

WISCONSIN FOCAL SPOT TEST TOOL.

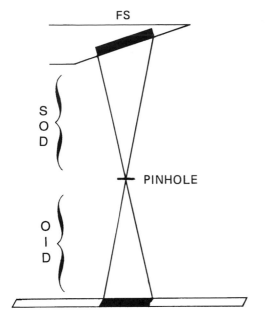

FS

S O D

PINHOLE

O I D

Figure 215. Geometry of pinhole camera focal spot test, showing the SOD and OID as similar triangles. With the pinhole at the mid-point, the projected image will measure precisely the same as the actual focal spot size.

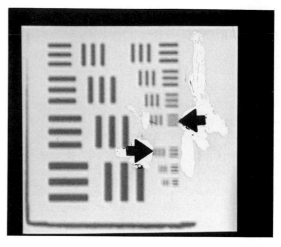

Figure 217. Radiograph of focal spot check using Wisconsin tool. Note that blur points (arrows) indicating focal spot size are different for width and for length.

The Wisconsin Test Tool consists of a metal template with groups of vertical and horizontal line pairs cut into it (Figure 216). This template is placed six inches off of the film and a light exposure is made with a SID of 24 inches. In similar fashion to the star pattern template method, the radiographer should scan the finished radiograph from the thickest line-pair groups down to locate the *first* group which is blurred enough to make the individual lines indistinguishable. The last group resolved *before* this blur point indicates the maximum res-

FOCAL SPOT TEST TOOL

RADIATION MEAS. INC.
P.O. BOX 44
MIDDLETON, WI

Figure 216. Photograph of Wisconsin focal spot test tool using line-pair groupings for both length and width measurements.

olution (Figure 217). There should not be more than three lines resolved in this group–four lines would be caused by false resolution when blurred lines overlap. Since the resolution of sharpness is a direct function of focal spot size at given distances, a chart may be consulted to find the effective focal spot size from the smallest line-pair group resolved. With the listed distances, the chart should be one adjusted for ⁴/₃ magnification.

Like the star pattern template, a measurement is taken for each dimension of the focal spot–length and width. The template must be positioned so that the line pairs run with the length and width of the x-ray tube (hence, the focal spot). Each line-pair group is indicative of the focal spot measurement lying *perpendicular* to the lines in that group. That is, lines running cross wise are used to find the length of the focal spot, while lines running lengthwise indicate the width of the focal spot (Figure 217).

The Wisconsin method is particularly useful in an ongoing program of checking for focal spot damage within a radiology department: An initial check is made in which the line-group number resolved is recorded. Without the necessity of consulting a chart to translate the line-group number into an actual measurement, a monthly check may be made to simply detect any sudden change in the line-group number resolved. Such a sudden change would be indicative of damage to the focal spot.

This method is not as accurate in taking actual measurements as is the star pattern template method. Since the line pairs are in *discrete* groupings, the actual point of blur lies somewhere between the last group resolved and the first group blurred. This means that the measurement taken is an estimate which may be more than 10 per cent inaccurate. The star pattern template, on the other hand, has *gradient* line pairs,

gradually thinning toward the center of the pattern, so that an exact point of blur may be found and an exact measurement obtained.

IMAGE RECEPTOR SYSTEM QUALITY CONTROL

For the purposes of quality control, or of selecting appropriate recording media for a particular radiology department, radiographic film, intensifying screens and cassettes should always be considered in combination as a system. Some film/screen combinations are incompatible, and their characteristics must be carefully matched to obtain the optimum image quality. In determining resolution (the capacity to record sharp detail), speed, contrast or the proclivity to produce quantum mottle, one complete film/screen/cassette system should always be compared to another complete system.

By far, the intensifying screens are the most important component of the receptor system in controlling resolution, speed and contrast. That is, changing from one speed or type of screen to another has a much more dramatic effect upon these image qualities than a change in film type does. Therefore, when these qualities are measured, they primarily reflect the characteristics of the intensifying screens used, even though the film also has some bearing on them.

Regardless of the system used, it is critical to radiographic quality that the intensifying screens be in direct contact with the film across its entire surface. Poor screen contact results in a severe blurring of recorded detail in that area of the radiograph, along with a slight loss of density. The felt and metal backings provided by the cassette are responsible for proper screen/film contact, so that poor contact is always indicative of cassette damage. Hence, the condition of the cassette itself is essential as a component of the receptor system.

Guidelines for Accuracy

No specific standards are set for evaluating receptor performance or screen contact. Screen contact should be perfect across the entire surface. Measurements of resolution, speed and contrast in the system are valuable only from the standpoint of comparing them to other systems. Naturally, the most desirable system is that combination of film, screens and cassette which produces the highest resolution, greatest speed, optimal contrast and least mottling. In reality, some of these must be traded off for each other (for example, higher speeds often lead to excessive mottling) and some may only be evaluated arbitrarily by the individual radiologist, such as *optimal* contrast. Therefore, the selection of a specific system and the assessment of its performance depends upon the values and needs of a particular radiology department.

Test Procedure

To check for proper *screen contact,* place a fine wire mesh on top of the cassette and expose it to a light technique. Laminated wire meshes avoid the problem of the wire itself being bent in spots. When observing the processed radiograph, it is often difficult to distinguish areas where the edges of the wire are slightly blurred. It is much easier to step back away from the illuminator and observe the film from a five- or six-foot distance, from which the blurred areas will stand out clearly as areas of *darker density* on the film (Figure 218). If there is a blurred area, it indicates that the screen

is warped in that area, usually from physical damage to the cassette. The cassette must be repaired or discarded.

To compare different kinds of screens for resolution of detail, place a straightline resolution test pattern directly on the cassettes and expose lightly. On the exposed films, scan with the eye from the thicker lines toward the thinner ones until you find the first point where the line pairs are blurred into each other. You can simply compare this point on each film visually or you may find the actual line pairs per millimeter resolved (LP/mm) by looking up the blur point line-pair numbers on a table. It may be desirable, in addition, to expose anatomical phantoms and evaluate the sharpness of detail visually.

To compare different kinds of screen/film combinations for speed and contrast, simple exposures of a penetrometer step-wedge are made and measure-

Figure 218. Radiograph of wire mesh test for screen-film contact showing areas of poor contact. From a distance, the blurring of the white lines of the mesh causes an appearance of increased density in these areas.

ments taken off of a densitometer. For speed, simply compare the same step between both films. For contrast, a lighter density step should be divided into a darker one, using the same two steps on both films.

VIEWING CONDITIONS

A radiograph is only as good as its illumination. The manner in which radiographs are viewed is as important to the radiographer as it is to the radiologist. Radiographs are made with translucent densities of varying tone value and details only become visible when they are transilluminated by light of conventional color and intensity.

THE ILLUMINATOR

The modern illuminator is designed for viewing radiographs up to 14-x-17-inches in size and consists of two fluorescent tubes suitably mounted in a reflecting box and behind opal diffusing glass. The quality and quantity of light transmitted through the radiograph by the illuminator determines the diagnostic worth of the image. The radiographer should provide a standard level of density that is translucent when the radiograph is viewed on the illuminator. The radiologist should view the radiographs on an illuminator that provides comparable color and intensity. To maintain the same quality and intensity of light, the illuminator should be cleaned regularly and old fluorescent tubes should be replaced with new, 15-watt bulbs.

To obtain the best transmission of illuminator light through a radiograph, all light that might pass *around* the radiograph should be blocked out. For example, when small CT or MRI films are viewed on a 14-x-17-inch illuminator, a mask may be used with an aperture cut to suit the size of the film being viewed. If this is not done, the density of the radiograph appears greater than it actually is.

AMBIENT LIGHTING

When radiographs are being read, the level of general illumination in the viewing room should be sufficiently low so that extraneous light is not reflected from the surfaces of the radiographs, thus lessening the brightness of image details.

AUTOMATIC EXPOSURE CONTROLS

Several electronic and radiographic checks can be made for automatic exposure controls, most of which should properly be done by a qualified physicist. Tests for reproducibility, kVp and other parameters common to regular radiographic units are essentially identical to those described in preceding sections of this chapter. AEC exposures must be repeatable within an accuracy range of plus or minus 10 per cent. To check repeatability, five exposures should be taken using a step-wedge penetrometer, and a densitometer should be used to measure and compare the densities obtained. AECs should also be linear to within 20 per cent between different rooms. Three basic tests can be done by the radiographer to determine proper functioning of the unit:

Density Control

As described fully in Chapter 28, the density control settings can be checked for accuracy without using any film, by exposing a phantom knee, skull or abdomen to a series of exposures and simply reading off the digital mAs readouts. Make the first exposure with the density control set to "N" or "O." Immediately after the exposure, write down the readout on the mAs indicator. Do the same for each *plus* or *minus* station on the density control. For each readout, perform the following calculation:

$$\frac{N\text{-}A}{N} \text{ X } 100$$

where *N* is the mAs readout for the "N" station and *A* is the readout for the *plus* or *minus* density setting being checked. This will yield the percentage of increase or decrease in technique from the normal or average setting. These percentages can then simply be compared with what the buttons or knob on the density control indicate. These stations should not be more than 10 per cent off from the indicated increase or decrease in technique.

Linearity

Place thick sheets of plexiglass or a plastic pail of water so that the detector cells activated are completely covered. Each detector chamber can be checked individually if all three cannot be covered at once. Make two exposures at the same kVp and with all other factors constant. For the first exposure, fill the pail with at least 3 inches (8 cm) of water or use a 3-4 inch thickness of plexiglass sheets. For the second exposure, fill the pail with 6 inches (16 cm) of water or double the amount of plexiglass thickness. Resulting densities should fall within 10 per cent of each other as measured on a densitometer. For a more complete check, repeat the experiment at different kVp settings.

Back-Up Timer

Cover the activated photocell(s) with three sheets of leaded rubber. Set the back-up timer at 1 or 2 seconds, and expose. The exposure should automatically terminate at the set back-up time, or before the accumulated mAs readout exceeds 600 mAs.

TOMOGRAPHIC UNITS

Tomographic units must comply with the same linearity, reproducibility, kVp, and other radiographic parameters as other equipment. Special checks on exposure angle, section thickness, and resolution can be performed by a qualified physicist. A simple test can be done by the radiographer to determine the level of the section as indicated on the unit.

The test tool is a simple radiolucent wedge with wires and a set of numbers to indicate the height of each wire with respect to the maximum height of the wedge (25cm). Or, an aluminum step wedge with lead numbers placed on each step will do for a less complete check.

When linear movement is to be evaluated, the wedge must be positioned so that it is 45 degrees to the tube and film motion. Having placed the central ray to the center of the inclined part of the wedge, a section level on the unit (say 9cm) is set to correspond to that on the wedge (9cm). The wedge is subsequently exposed using appropriate technique factors.

When the film is processed, it should show a sharp image of the wire located at the 9cm mark if the indicator on the machine is correct. The section level should be within plus or minus 5mm of the setting on the machine indicator.

FLUOROSCOPY

Testing and maintaining the fluorography unit for quality control is the job of a physicist, checking to assure that the following are present and/or operational and meet NCRP recommendations: Source-to-table distance (15" for the stationary unit and 12" for the mobile unit), primary barrier of 2mm of lead in the intensifier housing, filtration of no less than 2.5mm of aluminum equivalence, proper collimation to allow for an unexposed border on the monitor, bucky slot cover and protective curtain present, cumulative timer checked, and the x-ray output intensity should be checked yearly or more often as required by state regulations.

It should also be noted that in some states the technologist is required to record the amount of fluoro-on-time the patient was exposed to and compute the estimated total exposure by multiplying the intensity output rate by the number of minutes. As an example, if the physicist has determined the output intensity to be 2.1 R/min and the fluoro on time was 3.5 minutes, then the total estimated exposure would be computed as follows:

$$2.1 \times 3.5 = 7.35 \text{ R}$$

Furthermore in some cases the number of overhead and spot radiographs taken, including repeats, must also be recorded.

SUMMARY

1. A complete *quality control* program includes radiation exposure monitoring, radiographic unit monitoring, sensitometry, the use of technique charts, analysis of repeat rates and continuing education.
2. The proper construction and use of *technique charts* can reduce repeat rates by as much as 25 per cent.
3. The *analysis of repeat rates*, especially in a department which employs a quality control program, can be used to identify the *continuing education* needs within a radiology department.
4. Exposure *timers* should be accurate to within 5 per cent of the indicated time and may be checked with manual or electrical spinning tops.
5. *Adjacent milliamperage stations* should be linear to each other within 10 per cent. The same mA stations between two machines of identical phase and rectification should be within 10 per cent of each other in output. A given exposure should be reproducible to within 5 per cent. All of these may be checked by exposing step wedge penetrometers or by using ion chambers for higher accuracy.
6. Kilovoltage settings should be within 2

kV of the actual peak beam kilovoltage. This can be *checked* by using the Wisconsin kVp Test Cassette.

7. Half-value layer *tests*, using the Wisconsin kVp Test Cassette or ion chambers and filters, can be used to determine the actual penetration quality of the x-ray beam. When the HVL is inadequate, it is more likely to be from insufficient protective filtration in the collimator than from inaccurate kVp stations. Although 2.5 mm of aluminum is the required minimum protective filtration for machines, more filtration may be needed if the HVL falls below 2.34 mm Al.

8. Field size indicators should be accurate to within $1/2$-inch (2% of the SID) and can be *checked* with a simple ruler measurement of the exposed black field on the film. The edges of the light field should be within $1/2$-inch of the edges of the actual x-ray field, and both should be within 2 degrees of vertical. These can be *checked* with field edge markers and an alignment test cylinder.

9. SID should be within $1/2$-inch of that indicated and can be *checked* with a tape ruler.

10. The actual focal spot size must be within 50 per cent of the size listed by the tube manufacturer. It is important to know the actual size, because objects smaller than it may not be reliably recorded on radiographs. Damage to the focal spot may be detected by the use of the Wisconsin line-pair focal spot test tool. Accurate measurements may be made by using a *star* focal spot test template. The pinhole camera may also be used but is not recommended because of the high exposure required and possible tube damage.

11. A laminated wire mesh may be used to *check* proper screen/film contact. Resolution patterns may be used to compare the sharpness of detail obtained between different types of screens.

12. *Illuminators* must be kept clean and functional, and peripheral and ambient lighting must be reduced to optimize the viewing of radiographs.

13. Phototimed exposures should be *repeatable* within a 10 per cent accuracy, using a densitometer. Density control stations should also be within 10 per cent accuracy of the indicated increases and decreases in technique. These can be easily checked by the radiographer simply using the mAs readouts at the different stations.

REVIEW QUESTIONS

1. What is the acceptable range of deviation for the linearity of adjacent mA stations?

2. What is the acceptable range of deviation for exposure timers?

3. An electric spinning top revolves at a rate of 1 rps. For a three-phase timer test, what should the arc produced by an exposure time of one-half second measure in degrees:

4. Define "reproducibility" as it relates to mAs:

5. Why is it important for reliability on mA quality checks, to take all exposures on one film?

6. What is the acceptable range of inaccuracy for kVp settings?

7. What is the purpose of the optical attenuator in the Wisconsin kVp test cassette?

8. What is Half Value Layer and what does it measure:

9. At 80 kVp, the HVL for a particular x-ray machine is found to be 1.9 mm. A1. If the kVp control is accurate, what does this HVL indicate needs to be changed?

10. The borders of the light field must be within plus-or-minus _____-inch (or _____-cm) of the actual borders of the x-ray field.

11. What device in the collimator is responsible for alignment of the light field with the x-ray beam?

12. The intersection of two diagonal lines drawn from the opposite corners of the black area on a light field alignment test radiograph will locate the center of the:

13. In a light field/x-ray field alignment test radiograph, the borders of the black area overlap the paper clips used on the east and south sides by 1 inch, and cut off those on the North and West sides by 1 inch. In which directions is the light field misaligned from the x-ray beam? Is this an acceptable amount of misalignment?

14. The x-ray beam must be vertical within plus-or-minus _____ degrees.

15. What is the purpose of putting black masks around radiographs?

16. Old plastic covers on illuminators can cause _____ on the apparent image:

17. It is determined that a given time setting lasts about 10 per cent too long. During a film density test to check the mA stations, this time was used with the mA station in question, but was not used for the original reference technique. The exposure on the mA station in question produced 23 per cent more density than the reference exposure. What is the actual accuracy of the mA station in question?

18. In repeat analysis, what is "obtrusiveness":

19. A radiographer used 120 films and made 110 exposures to obtain 80 diagnostic quality radiographs of the skull during a one-month period. What is her repeat rate for skull work?

20. Automatic Exposures must be reproducible within what per cent?

21. An AEC density control check is done by exposing a knee phantom and yields the following mAs readouts:

$$N = 10.5 \text{ mAs}$$
$$+1 = 12.1 \text{ mAs}$$
$$+2 = 17.3 \text{ mAs}$$
$$-1 = 7.9 \text{mAs}$$
$$-2 = 5.3 \text{ mAs}$$

Which station is much too *low* for the indicated change? Which station is much too *high*?

Chapter 31

SOLVING MULTIPLE TECHNIQUE PROBLEMS

Multiple technique problems like those about to follow are valuable, not only in preparation for similar problems on certifying examinations, but also as a concise review of the most basic and important relationships in radiographic technique. The problems presented here will seem overwhelming at a glance, but the whole point of this exercise is to demonstrate that, *taken one step at a time*, even the most complex problems can be solved. See Table XXXIII.

Although you may wish to attempt solving them "on your own" first, this is not necessary. The discussion following the table of problems takes you step-by-step through their solution. At each point where you are unsure, refer to the discussion for guidance.

There are several approaches to solving the kind of multiple technique problems that are presented on certification examinations. The author has used and taught four different types, including the *function* system, and the method presented below is recommended highly because of its simplicity. All of the various methods are workable and accurate enough, but many are unnecessarily complex. It is asserted that the easiest approach will also be least likely to result in errors.

Regardless of the method used, the student must begin with a thorough understanding of the principles in each section of this book. Screen and grid factors for density must be thoroughly memorized. Also, an appreciation for which factors have a greater or a lesser effect upon image qualities such as contrast or sharpness of detail must be developed.

Remember that for each type of problem, you must first select only those columns of variables which directly affect the image quality. For example, if you are solving for image contrast, cross out any columns for mAs, phase, SID, tube angles, or focal spot size—these variables either are not related to contrast at all, or they make too little difference to consider. After eliminating unrelated variables, take the remaining columns one step at a time, following the directions.

1. SOLVING FOR DENSITY

Most multiple technique problems encountered on certifying examinations are for solving the net resulting density of the radiograph. In solving for density, use the following rules:

For mA, time or mAs:	*Direct proportion*
For machine phase:	*3Φ or CPG = 2 x 1Φ*
For kVp:	*The 15 per cent rule*
For SID:	*The inverse square law*
For OID:	*Estimate + or -*
For Screen Speed:	*See Tables XV and XVI*
For Grid Ratio:	*See Table XI*
For Filtration:	*Estimate slight + or−*

Always determine the total mAs first by multiplying the mA and time. Then, for each column, simply multiply the mAs value by the appropriate factor to obtain a *density value* number. For example, if A has 15 per cent more kVp than the other choices, double the density value for A and then cross off that column and do not go back to it; if A has a 400-speed rare-earth screen, multiply the density value by four times; if *A* has a 15:1 ratio grid, divide the density value by 5, and so on. The *density value* becomes, as you adjust it, a number representing the relative density that will result from the technique and must not be confused with actual mAs. The density value simply tells you relatively how dark the film will be. When you finish, the greatest density value is the darkest film.

2. SOLVING FOR PATIENT SKIN DOSE

These may be solved in exactly the same method as the density problems as discussed above. However, different factors will be considered—filtration becomes a significant column to evaluate, while screen speeds and grid ratios should be completely ignored (since they are behind the patient and after the fact) if the mA and time are already given. *Exposure values* will replace density values.

For machine phase, recall that 3Φ equipment is about 70 per cent more efficient in actual mA output than single-phase. For the purpose of these problems, this amount can be rounded upward to roughly a doubling. Consider 3Φ equipment to produce roughly twice the patient skin dose as 1Φ equipment for the same mAs setting. For kVp: Skin dose increases about *25 per cent* for each increase of 15 per cent in kVp, and decreases 25 per cent for a 15 per cent reduction in kVp.

Thicker patients absorb more radiation in accordance with the 4-centimeter rule used for technique. However, when estimating *skin dose*, the only significance in patient thickness is that the larger patient's surface will be slightly closer to the x-ray tube, reducing the effective SOD. This is usually a small percentage of the overall distance and may be ignored for these problems.

3. SOLVING FOR CONTRAST

The effect of the variables upon image contrast cannot be accurately quantified. Hence, you are reduced to using a system of *pluses* and *minuses* to solve for which film is the most contrasty or the least contrasty. It is essential that you develop a sense of the relative magnitude with which each variable affects contrast from the units in this book. For variables that have a great effect, use larger, bolder, or more pluses and minuses. A review of which variables affect contrast to a greater or lesser degree follows:

1. Grids have a dramatic effect.
2. Patient thickness has a considerable effect.
3. OID has a considerable effect.
4. Changing from direct exposure film holders to intensifying screens or vice versa has a dramatic effect; however, the difference in contrast from one speed of screen to the next is very minimal.
5. Changes of 6 or 10 kVp are not significant in their effect upon contrast when compared to the effects of grids or OID; but, kVp changes of 30 kVp or more have a considerable effect.
6. No other factors have a noticeable effect on image contrast.

4. SOLVING FOR SHARPNESS OF RECORDED DETAIL

The effects of SOD/OID ratio and focal spot size upon image sharpness of detail can be *quantified* as follows:

Distances: To find the SOD, subtract the OID from the SID. Divide the OID into the SOD. The

TABLE XXXIII
Sample Multiple Technique Problems

#1. Which of the following produces the greatest density? _____

	mAs	Machine Phase	kVp	SID	OID	Patient Thickness	Screen	Grid	Filter
A.	400	1Φ	72	40"	2"	22cm	Rare Earth Reg.	16:1	2.5mm
B.	200	1Φ	82	40"	2"	14cm	Extremity	12:1	2.5mm
C.	100	3Φ	94	80"	2"	30cm	High	6:1	1.5mm
D.	200	3Φ	72	80"	4"	24cm	Dir. Exp.	None	2.5mm

#2. Which of the following produces the greatest density? _____

#3. Which of the following produces the greatest contrast? _____

#4. Which of the following produces the greatest sharpness of detail? _____

#5. Which of the following produces the greatest patient skin dose? _____

	mA	Time	kVp	Screen	Grid	SID	OID	Focal Spot	Filter
A.	400	3/5	82	High	12:1	40"	2"	0.6mm	2.5mm
B.	300	4/5	94	Par	6:1	60"	6"	1.2mm	2.5mm
C.	600	0.4	72	Rare Earth Reg.	None	80"	2"	1.2mm	1.5mm
D.	200	1.2	80	High-Plus	16:1	30"	2"	1.2mm	2.5mm
E.	300	0.4	82	Slow	None	80"	2"	0.6mm	2.5mm
F.	800	0.6	94	Dir. Exp.	None	20"	2"	1.2mm	2.5mm

resulting number gives you a relative measure of sharpness–the greater the number, the sharper the detail.

Focal Spot: If the smaller focal spot listed is one-half the size of the large one listed, the detail will be twice as sharp and you can double the number you derived from the distance ratio above.

However, the effects of screen speed and film speed upon image sharpness cannot be easily quantified. Here, you must use a *plus-and-minus* system combined with the number obtained from the distance ratio and focal spot. Bear in mind that the effects of screen and film speeds are very minimal compared to the geometrical factors of distance and focal spots.

Using the two lists of variables that follow, five sample multiple technique problems are presented in Table XXXIII. The solutions follow.

SOLUTIONS TO PROBLEMS IN TABLE XXXIII

Solution to # 1: A is the Densest Radiograph.

Method:

1. In phase column, double mAs value for C & D. Write this to the side.
2. In kVp column, double B, double C twice (two sets of 15 per cent increase).
3. In SID column, cut C & D to 1/4 density value.
4. In OID column, you may place a minus by D or ignore it entirely if the final density values are not close to

each other.

5. In patient thickness column, double the density value for B twice (two sets of 4 cm thinner), cut C in half twice, and ignore D because it is too close to 22.

6. In screen column, multiply the density value of A by 4 times, that of B by $1/2$ (divide it by 2), that of C by 2 times, and leave D as it is.

7. In grid column, divide the density value for A by 5, that of B by 4, that of C by 2, and leave D as it is.

8. In filter column, you may place a plus by C or ignore it if the final density values are not close to each other. The final density values you should arrive at are:

A = 320   C = 50+
B = 200   D = about 3-

Solution to #2: D is the Densest Radiograph.

Method

1. Multiply all of the mA's and times to get the total mAs for each.

2. In the kVp column, use the two 82's and the 80 (essentially the same) as standards, thus leaving A, D & E as they are, double the mAs value for B & F, and cut the mAs value for C to $1/2$.

3. In the screen column, par will be the standard so leave B as it is, double the density value for A, multiply the density value for C by 4 times, that of D by 3 times, that of E by $1/2$ (divide it by 2), and that of F by $1/30$ (divide it by 30).

4. In the grid column, use non-grid as the standard so leave C, E & F as they are, divide the density value for A by 4, that of B by 2, and that of D by 5.

5. In the SID column, use 40 inches as the standard because all the rest are rounded out fractions of it ($1^1/2$X, $3/4$, $1/2$, etc.) so leave A as it is, divide the density value of B by 2 and that of C & E by 4, multiply the density value of D by

2 times and that of F by 4 times.

6. In the OID column, place a minus by B or ignore it if the final density values are not close to each other.

7. In the focal spot column, do nothing– this factor does not directly relate to film density.

8. In the filter column, place a small plus by C or ignore it if the final density values are not close. The final density values you should arrive at are:

A = 120   C = 120+   E =16
B = 120-   D = 288   F = 128

NOTE: If you choose different *standards* in some of the columns which you compare the others to, your actual density value numbers may come out different than these, but they will be proportionately related in the same way and you will still get the right answer as long as you do not err in making comparisons in each column. When two answers come out very close numerically, then you must go back and carefully consider the pluses and minuses, the less significant factors.

Solution to #3: D has the highest contrast.

Method:

1. The mA, time, SID, focal spot and filter columns should be ignored, as they are not directly related to contrast. (If two answers come out very close to tying, you may go back to the time column and consider it as a *potential* effect on motion and contrast.)

2. In the kVp column, the two 82's and the 80 should be used as the standard to save time, a small minus should be placed next to the two 94 kVp's listed, and a small plus placed by the 72.

3. In the screen column, simply use an additional plus or minus for each screen speed increase, except that three or four minuses should be used for the direct-exposure technique because it is

dramatically grayer than even the slow-est speed of screen. Thus, you should put a small plus next to the high, noth-ing next to the par, three pluses next to the rare earth, two by the high-plus, one minus by the slow, and four minus-es by the direct exposure. All of these should be relatively small.

4. In the grid column you should use large pluses and minuses. The three, non-grid techniques should have noth-ing by them, as they are standard. Using a similar approach to the screens above, there should be three large plus-es by the 12:1, one large plus by the 6:1, and four large pluses by the 16:1.

5. In the OID column, a large plus should be placed by the 6-inch OID (this is *air gap technique*). Tallying everything up, you should arrive at something similar to this:

A = 1 small plus & 3 large pluses
B = 1 small minus & 2 large pluses
C = 1 small plus & 3 large pluses
D = 6 large pluses
E = 1 small minus
F = 5 or 6 minuses

Solution to #4: E has the sharpest recorded detail.

Method:

1. Eliminate the mA, time, kVp, grid, and filter columns, as these are not directly related to sharpness of recorded detail. (If you get two results that are close, you may go back to the time column and consider it as a *potential* for reduc-ing sharpness.)

2. Divide each OID into its accompany-ing SOD to obtain a sharpness ratio. You should get 19, 9, 39, 14, 39, and 9, respectively.

3. On the focal spot column, double the sharpness ratio for the two 0.6 focal spots; thus, A will now be 38 and E will

be 78.

4. In the screen column, place a small minus by the high speed, nothing by the par, two small minuses by the rare-earth and the high-plus speeds, one small plus by the slow, and four pluses by the direct exposure. Your final result should be:

A = 38+   C = 39- -   E = 78+ +
B = 9   D = 14- -   F = 9+ + + +

Solution to #5: F produces the highest dose to the patient's skin.

Method

1. Since the technique used is stated, screens and grids which are behind the patient have no bearing on surface skin dose, and may be ignored. Focal spots may also be ignored.

2. Calculate the total mAs value from the mA and time columns for each tech-nique just as you would for a density problem. These numbers will then be considered as *exposure values.*

3. For the kVp column, recall that the 15 per cent rule must not be used for skin dose, but only for radiograph density. For skin dose, we must know the actual change in radiation output from the x-ray tube when kVp is changed. This output is proportional to the square of the change in kVp, but as a rule of thumb, *it changes by about 25 per cent for every 15 per cent increase or decrease in kVp.* For example, if kVp is increased from 80 to 92, the skin dose would increase by approximately 25 per cent or one quarter, and vice versa.
Since there are three techniques close to 80 in the kVp column, select A, D and F as standards and leave their exposure values (mAs) unchanged. The new *exposure values* should be:
A. 240
B. 240 mAs x 25% (0.25) = 60; 240 +

60 = 300

C. 240 mAs x 0.25 = 60; 240 - 60 = 180

D. 240

E. 120

F. 480 mAs x 0.25 = 120; 480 + 120 = 600

4. On the SID and OID columns, although it would be more accurate to subtract the OID from the SID to obtain the SOD (from the tube to the patient's surface), it is easier to ignore the 2-inch OIDs, in effect, *rounding out* the SOD's to equal the SID's, and only consider the 6-inch OID. Leaving the 40-inch exposure value at 240 as the standard, the 60-inch exposure value is roughly cut in half to 150, the 80-inch one in one quarter to 45, the 30-inch doubles to 480, the 80-inch one on E cuts to one quarter at 30, and the 20-inch one quadruples to 2400.

Regarding the OID on B, you may estimate that moving the patient 6 inches closer to the tube would increase patient skin dose by roughly one-fourth or 25 per cent, making the exposure value about 190, or you may plug the numbers into the inverse square law to get an exact value of 185 (set up as $X(54)^2 = 150(60)^2$).

5. On the filtration column, the 1-mm less filter that C has will cause a significant increase in skin dose, probably between 50 and 100 per cent. To take the extreme case, you may double the exposure value for C to roughly 90. The final results are:

A = 240   C = about 90 E = 30

B = about 190 D = 480   F = 2400

Try the following review questions for practice. (An answer key is available in the Appendix.)

REVIEW QUESTIONS

1. Which of the following produces the greatest density:

a. b. c. d.

	mA	Sec	Phase	Patient Thickness	kVp	SID	OID	Ratio Grid	Screen	Focal Spot Size	m.m. Filter
a.	150	$1/2$	3Φ	25 cm	48	60"	2"	12:1	400	1.0	2.5
b.	200	$1/5$	1Φ	25 cm	48	40"	2"	8:1	300	1.0	3.5
c.	400	$1/10$	3Φ	29 cm	56	30"	4"	none	Direct Exposure	1.0	2.5
d.	300	$1/4$	1Φ	20 cm	40	40"	4"	16:1	200	0.5	2.5

3. Which of the following produces the highest contrast:

a. b. c. d.

2. Which of the following produces the highest patient skin dose:

a. b. c. d.

4. Which of the following produces the sharpest detail:

a. b. c. d.

	mA	Sec	Phase	Patient Thickness	kVp	SID	OID	Ratio Grid	Screen	Focal Spot Size	m.m. Filter
a.	150	$1/2$	3Φ	25 cm	48	60"	2"	12:1	400	1.0	2.5
b.	200	$1/5$	1Φ	25 cm	48	40"	2"	8:1	300	1.0	3.5
c.	400	$1/10$	3Φ	29 cm	56	30"	4"	none	Direct Exposure	1.0	2.5
d.	300	$1/4$	1Φ	20 cm	40	40"	4"	16:1	200	0.5	2.5

Part V

SPECIAL IMAGING METHODS

Chapter 32

MOBILE RADIOGRAPHY

Because of the many additional variables involved in mobile radiography, such as other equipment and furniture being in the way, limited space, and immobility of the patient, mobile or "portable" radiography frequently presents the greatest challenges faced by radiographers in securing quality images. The adaptability and creativity required to maintain all radiographic variables at the optimum level possible for mobile and trauma procedures is what sets the most skillful radiographers apart. Following are special technique considerations that will help enhance image quality.

MOBILE GENERATORS

Generators for mobile units are of two common types: battery-powered units and capacitor-discharge units. The battery-powered units are the state of the art, producing a very efficient current similar to a 3-phase, 12-pulse machine. Comparing techniques with the most common type of stationary unit, *a modern battery-powered mobile unit typically requires approximately 6 kVp less than the 3-phase, 6-pulse machine* to produce the same density for any given procedure.

Modern capacitor-discharge mobile units use precharged batteries to charge a capacitor to a preset voltage level selected at the console. Older CD units must be plugged into an electrical outlet during each use in order to charge the capacitor. In either case, the stored electrical charge is released and discharges across the x-ray tube when the exposure button is depressed. As the exposure progresses, the electrical charge drains off of the capacitor, and the remaining voltage drops. Therefore, the average voltage is much less than the starting kV peak. For this reason, capacitor-discharge units require roughly twice the total technique than battery-powered units to produce the same density on a radiograph.

Exposure on the battery-powered unit is initiated identically to stationary machines—rotor and expose. The capacitor-discharge unit, however, requires a special protocol: the total mAs value and kVp must be selected prior to charging the capacitor. A charge button is then depressed and held down until the preset technique is indicated on a meter (Figure 219). At this point, the charge button is released and rotoring may begin with exposure shortly following. If exposure is delayed for more than a few seconds, the charging button must be pressed again to recharge the capacitor. This is due to the fact that capacitors quickly lose their stored charge through electron "leakage." (Since electrons repel each other, it is difficult to

419

keep them concentrated on a single small device.)

Both types of mobile units must be plugged into an electrical outlet between uses in order to recharge their batteries. Some older portable units are half-rectified, and require twice the mAs of a single-phase unit, or four times the mAs of a three-phase unit. Such equipment requires twice the mAs values as the capacitor discharge unit, or four times the mAs of a modern battery-powered unit. Generators are more fully discussed in Chapter Seven.

mAs SELECTION

Most mobile units have a single "mAs" control, rather than mA and exposure time being selected separately (Figure 219). The units are usually designed to operate at a high, fixed mA value, so that exposure

Figure 219. Console of a capacitor discharge mobile unit, showing line voltage meter at upper left (arrow) with line voltage compensator knob directly below. Charging button is on exposure switch (*left*, arrow). Controls to preset kVp and mAs, and kVp meter are alsow visible.

time becomes the main variable. For capacitor-discharge units, the mAs selected should not exceed about one-third of the kVp selected, or the actual mAs produced becomes unreliable. Any mAs value available may be selected for battery-powered units.

KVP AND LINE VOLTAGE COMPENSATION

Modern battery-powered units require about 6-8 kVp *less* than typical three-phase equipment. Capacitor discharge units are comparable to single-phase equipment, which produces an *average* keV at about one-third of the kV peak.

Optimum kilovoltage is essential for proper penetration of the anatomy and for sufficient gray scale in the radiograph, and the radiographer must be able to rely on the equipment to produce the kVp selected. Capacitor discharge units which must be plugged in during each use have a *line voltage meter* and a *line voltage compensator* control (Figure 219). This meter indicates whether the incoming voltage from the wall receptacle is sufficient. Variations in the supply voltage can easily occur in a hospital environment, where renal dialysis, radiology, and other departments make high demands on electricity. If the meter indicates that the line voltage is not adequate, the line voltage compensator must be turned up until the meter reads sufficient voltage. This adjustment actuates a capacitor circuit that stores additional charge to "boost" the electrical supply to the x-ray tube.

GEOMETRICAL FACTORS

Radiographers must often perform "cross-table" projections during mobile procedures, and in working around other equipment and the patient with all attached devices it seems that every conceivable angle of tube and cassette can be encountered. In this process, all proper distances and alignment must be preserved to the extent possible to maximize image sharpness, and to minimize magnification and distortion.

DISTANCE CONSIDERATIONS

The SID must often be estimated during mobile procedures. If a measuring tape is attached to the tube or collimator, it should be used, or the radiographer may wish to carry a compact tape measure in a pocket. *To estimate 40 inches,* the *average* person may extend one arm, and *measure from the contrary side of the body to the fingertip. To estimate 72 inches, measure from fingertip to fingertip with both arms extended.*

For angled projections, the *one inch for* *every 5 degrees* rule should be used to maintain SID. These rules of thumb are more fully discussed in Chapter 18.

The radiographer must remember to make every effort to place the film in contact with the part during mobile procedures. If this is not possible, the minimum OID possible should be achieved, and an increased SID should be considered as compensation. Changes in SID can be compensated with mAs to maintain density, according to the following rules of thumb:

Changing From 40 inches To:	Increase mAs by:
50 Inches	50 per cent
60 Inches	2 x
72 Inches	3 x

These factors can be inverted to compensate for distance reductions. For example, use one-third the 72-inch technique for

Figure 220. Diagram illustrating typical alignment problems encountered in mobile AP chest radiography, when the axis of the body (dashed line) is not parallel with the film or bed. The proper x-ray beam angle is **A**, perpendicular to the patient, rather than the film **B** or the bed **C**. For demonstration of fluid levels, patient should be raised up as much as possible.

a 40-inch chest radiograph. For a 60-inch chest radiograph, use $2/3$ the 72-inch technique. *Any distance change of more than 20 per cent will require technique compensation to maintain density.* All of the concepts in Chapters 18 through 20 should be fully appreciated and applied in mobile radiography.

ALIGNMENT AND POSITIONING CONSIDERATIONS

The radiographer must become adept at visually estimating the alignment of the x-ray beam with the patient and film cassette. This skill is necessary to minimize shape distortion and avoid superimposition of unwanted anatomy over the anatomy of interest. While the light field provides an easy approach to centering, it does *not* give an obvious indication of off-angling unless it is very severe. The radiographer must always carefully observe the angle of the x-ray tube in relation to the patient, from *two perspectives.* (1) side-to-side angle as observed from behind the x-ray tube, and (2) cephalic/caudal angulation as observed from the side of the patient and the x-ray beam.

A rule that is very helpful to accurately determine the angulation of the x-ray beam in relation to the film and patient is to *stand back as far as you can* away from the machine and patient. *Alignment is always easier to see from a distance.*

The caudal angulation of the x-ray tube for sitting mobile chest radiographs provides a classic example of the awareness needed for proper alignment. As illustrated in Figure 220, in spite of all positioning efforts the lower back of the sitting patient is frequently not in contact with the film cassette. This means that the long axis of the patient's body and the cassette are at different angles. Should the x-ray beam be

angled perpendicular to the cassette or perpendicular to the patient's body? Without thinking, a radiographers may angle perpendicular to the cassette (and the bed), resulting in the common "lordotic chest" radiograph, with straightened ribs and diaphragm (Figure 221). In this case the central ray should be angled caudally until it is truly perpendicular to the axis of the *body.*

Figure 221. Lordotic mobile AP chest radiograph taken at angle **C** in Figure 220. Note straightened, linear appearance of ribs.

When long bones or extremities cannot be positioned parallel to the film, *Ceiszynski's law of isometry* should be used as explained in Chapter 21, splitting the difference between the angles. However, many projections are designed to "open" joint spaces or demonstrate anatomical relationships. For these, as with the mobile chest in Figure 220, *it is always more important for the central ray to be perpendicular to the* anatomy than it is to be perpendicular to the film, if one must choose.

If the purpose of the procedure is to rule out possible fluid levels, the central ray must be horizontal, regardless of part or film angulation.

OTHER CONSIDERATIONS

Some radiology departments prefer to use wide exposure latitude receptor systems for mobile radiography in order to reduce the probability of repeated exposures. These would include slightly slower screen speeds, wide-latitude films, and low ratio grids. Low ratio grids (5:1 or 6:1 ratios) can be especially helpful because their low selectivity allows a much wider margin for error in angulation, centering and especially distance variations. As described in Chapter 13, any grid must be carefully aligned with the x-ray beam to avoid grid cut-off. The mobile radiographer must watch for off-centering or off-angling of the beam, tilt of the grid/cassette, SID within the grid radius, and even upright placement for focused grids: It is not uncommon in surgery, for example, for the radiographer to place a grid-cassette into a sterile cover held by a nurse, and for the nurse to then place the covered cassette upside-down, or for a "wafer" grid to be taped onto a cassette upside-down.

Many portable units have added filters that can easily be removed from the collimator (see Figure 74 in Chapter 8). The radiographer should ensure that proper filtration is in place at all times to protect the patient from unnecessary exposure to useless, low-energy radiation.

MANUAL VERSUS AUTOMATED TECHNIQUE

Automatic exposure controls have been available for use with mobile units in the form of phototiming "paddles" which are placed behind the cassette during portable exposures. These have been recalled by manufacturers because the placement of the photocell detectors in relation to the anatomy of interest has proven too unreliable for consistent results. They may lead to more repeated exposures than manual technique, and are not recommended for use. Most technologists continue to prefer manual technique for mobile procedures.

When manual technique is used for mobile radiography, a *systematic approach* is as important as ever. Using the concepts from Chapters 25-27, *concise technique charts*

Figure 222. Modern mobile unit showing attached manual technique chart on back of tube stand (arrow).

should be developed for mobile units. There are many workable approaches to this need, but these charts must be compact and *permanently attached* to the mobile machine. They can be laminated or covered with clear x- ray film for protection, and chained or taped to the unit (Figure 222).

Although mobile radiography can test one's skills and knowledge, the same high standards of image quality that apply to general radiography should be sought after for mobile procedures.

SUMMARY

1. Battery-powered mobile units require slightly less *technique* (6 kVp less) than 3Φ equipment. Capacitor discharge units require about twice the technique of battery-powered units.
2. With *capacitor discharge* mobile units, one must always check the kVp meter immediately prior to exposure to ensure adequate charge. Recharging may be necessary if more than a few minutes have passed. Insufficient incoming line voltage is indicated and may be compensated on these machines.
3. Skill in estimating various *distances* and knowledge of the technique adjust-

ments required for changes in distance are essential in mobile radiography.
4. Skill in visually aligning the x-ray beam to the anatomy of interest is also essential for mobile radiography. *Alignment* can always be better seen by positioning oneself at a distance from the equipment.
5. If the anatomy and the film cannot be placed parallel, it is essential to *align the x-ray beam properly to the anatomy* rather than to the film.
6. Manual technique is recommended for mobile radiography. *Technique charts* should be provided for all mobile units.

REVIEW QUESTIONS

1. How do techniques for battery-powered mobile units compare to those for 3Φ equipment?
2. For a capacitor discharge unit, what must the radiographer do if more than a few minutes have passed between charging and exposure?
3. Inbetween uses, what should be done with most mobile machines?
4. Before making an exposure with a capacitor-discharge unit, what two meters must both be checked?
5. If a 72-inch technique is used with a 60-inch actual SID, will density be

altered enough to require a repeated exposure ?
6. How can the radiographer best position himself to assess proper alignment of the x-ray beam during mobile procedures?
7. For a projection of a joint space, if you have to choose between placing the x-ray beam perpendicular to the anatomy or perpendicular to the film, which would be best?
8. Is it practical to require technique charts for mobile units?

Chapter 33

FLUOROSCOPIC IMAGING

WILLIAM HEATHMAN

In 1896, the year following Roentgen's discovery of x-rays, Thomas Edison introduced what would be the first dynamic imaging device in radiology. Edison's device allowed the physician to image a body part in real time. This first fluoroscopic (fluoro) unit was a simple system comprised of an under-the-table x-ray tube and an over-the-table intensifying screen, both of which were attached to a movable carriage. The user would lean over the screen while the tube was energized in order to view the image. This fluoro system had two major drawbacks. First, the image on the screen was extremely dim and required a near blackened room in order to be able to see the displayed image. Second, it required a very high radiation exposure to the patient and the radiologist. This system remained relatively unchanged for the next 50 years, except for the addition of a mirror system which allowed the user to stand to the side and out of the primary beam.

In the late 1940s the first electronic image intensifier tube was introduced. The image intensifier brought with it improved image visibility, lower patient and user dose, and the ability to add multiple devices for recording permanent images during the fluoro procedure. It is important for the technologist to have a basic understanding of how an image intensifier functions, and how to operate the fluoroscopic system and its many ancillary recording systems in order to assist the radiologist in the performance of fluoroscopic procedures.

Fluoroscopic procedures normally include three distinct components: the actual *fluoroscopy*, several *spot film* exposures and some *overhead* exposures. Fluoroscopy provides dynamic real-time imaging in which the physiological functioning of organs may be observed. For example, the functioning of the muscles of the esophagus in deglutition (swallowing) may be observed as a bolus of barium passes downward to the stomach in a peristaltic wave. Fluoroscopy also allows the radiologist to move and reposition the patient during observation of the image in order to better demonstrate anatomy and pathology of interest. Fluoroscopy does not provide a permanent record of the image, however, unless special options such as cine-filming or videotaping are used.

Spotfilming is devised to provide the radiologist with permanently recorded images of selected anatomy or pathology of interest during the fluoroscopic procedure. Each time the radiologist notes something important on the fluoroscope screen, he may activate the spotfilmer to quickly place a film cassette into the beam and make an exposure onto a small area of the film for later reference. Spotfilm exposures are similar to overhead exposures in every way, except that the fluoroscopic x-ray tube under the table is used and the film is placed above the patient in the fluoro tower rather than under the patient. The fluoroscopic x-ray tube is usually placed only 15 inches from the tabletop. This small source-to-object distance, combined with a large object-to-image distance often caused by placing the film in the fluoro tower, degenerates the image. Magnification is substantial and the sharpness of image detail is dramatically reduced. Because of the poor geometric quality of spotfilm imaging, nearly all fluoroscopic procedures also include some regular overhead exposures in order to provide some radiographs with high resolution of detail.

IMAGE INTENSIFIERS

Modern image intensifiers, though they are complicated devices, can be explained in a simple general manner. An x-ray tube under the table exposes the patient, and as the beam passes through the patient it is received by the image intensifier (the round portion of the fluoro tower just above the patient). X-ray photons received by the image intensifier are converted into light photons at the input phosphor, and this light then causes electrons to be emitted at the photocathode (Figure 223). The electrons are both accelerated and focused as they travel upward in the intensifier tube. Their energy is then converted back into light at the output phosphor. Details of this process are provided in most radiographic physics textbooks, and will not be covered here.

The result of this conversion and amplification is an image which can be 1000 to 20,000 times brighter than that image at the input phosphor. This dramatic increase in the brightness of the image, termed *brightness gain*, is the prime factor in reducing the patient exposure, and improving the visibility of the image. Once the image is intensified it can then be reflected through a series of mirrors to be viewed by the radiologist, or it can be received by a TV camera tube positioned above the output phosphor and then transmitted to a TV monitor (Figure 223). Additional ancillary recording devices such as conventional cassette spot films, rolled and cut spot film cameras, cine cameras, or even a VCR or video disc recorder, can be attached to the unit to provide a means to permanently record fluoroscopic images (Figure 223).

BEAM SPLITTER

In order to record the fluoro image with spot film cameras and cine film, the fluoro unit must be able to divide the light coming from the image intensifier and direct it in two separate paths. This system of reflecting light in two directions is called *beam splitting*. A semitransparent mirror is placed between the image intensifier and the TV camera tube or mirror optics system. Part of the light (up to 90%) is reflected to the recording system while the remaining light passes through the mirror and is received by the TV camera tube (Figure 223). Enough light is transmitted through the beam splitting mirror to the TV camera to allow the radiologist to view an image on the monitor during the exposure.

FLUOROSCOPY TECHNIQUE

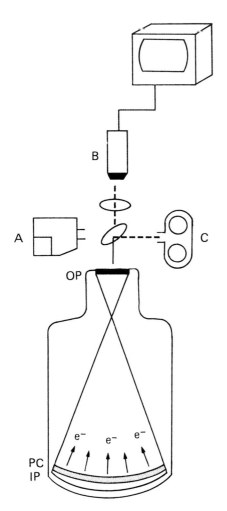

Figure 223. Image intensifier and fluoroscopic imaging options. In the intensifier tube, the input phosphor (IP) and photocathode (PC) convert the signal into a beam of electrons which can be accelerated and focused (minified) onto the output phosphor (OP). Options for processing the image include the photospot camera (A), the television camera (B), and the cine camera (C). The beam splitter lens/mirror above the ouptut phosphor allows two of these options to be used simultaneously. As pictured here, the TV and the cine cameras receive the light image. If the beam splitter mirror is rotated 90 degrees, the photospot camera and TV camera would both receive the light beam.

In setting technique for fluoroscopy, a *mode* knob or button should be set at *image intensifier*, the *Bucky* grid must be turned off and the Bucky tray moved out of the way to one end of the table.

AUTOMATIC BRIGHTNESS CONTROL VERSUS AUTOMATIC GAIN CONTROL

In fluoroscopy, the brightness of the fluoroscopic screen or TV monitor must be maintained at an acceptable level throughout the entire procedure. Two separate systems are available to compensate for part thickness changes as the radiologist rolls the patient onto his or her side, or as the physical density of the part changes during the procedure.

The first system is termed *automatic brightness control* (ABC) and it varies the *radiographic* exposure factors according to the changes in the part being examined. With this system a detector is placed in the beam in the fluoro tower. When a significant change in the intensity of the x-rays is detected, a special circuit automatically increases or decreases the exposure factors. This can be done by adjusting the kVp, mA, or a combination of both. This system will increase patient dose at times, but is efficient in maintaining good image quality.

The second type of system is termed *automatic gain control* (AGC). With this system the amplification of the *electronic* signal is increased or decreased as needed. The *radiographic* exposure factors remain unchanged. This system does not increase patient exposure, but may also not provide the best possible image: If an insufficient number of x-ray photons are reaching the image intensifier, no amount of increased *electronic* amplification can overcome the mottle or increased noise produced. A brightness control knob is sometimes found on the fluoro tower, which can be adjusted by the radiologist as needed.

FLUORO TOWER RELEASE

Prior to the start of a fluoro procedure the entire fluoro unit must be brought across the table. The fluoro *park release* button is depressed and the fluoro unit is then pulled across the table until it locks in a centered position over the x-ray tube (Figure 224). If the tower is not locked into center, the tube will not energize when the footswitch is depressed. When the fluoro unit is not in use it should be moved across the table back into the parked position. In some cases the image intensifier can be detached and moved to a corner of the room out of the way of the overhead radiographic tube. To move the tower into the parked position, raise the fluoro unit to its highest level above the table, depress the park release button and push the unit back into the stored position.

MILLIAMPERAGE

An actual fluoroscopic mA control is normally found on the console and is generally not changed from a preselected position. In most cases this mA control is set to allow the fluoro unit to use the highest mA when needed, generally 4 to 6 mA. Using higher mA values will result in excessive patient dose. The mA may be checked by reading the mA meter on the console while the radiologist is depressing the footswitch. A relatively long exposure, more than a few seconds, is needed to allow the meter to stabilize at an average reading. Most modern fluoro units will adjust the mA during fluoroscopy so as to use the lowest possible setting while maintaining an adequate image on the monitor.

KILOVOLTAGE

A fluoroscopic kilovoltage control should be set at the same kVp as the spot-filmer. Most barium procedures require 100-120 kVp for both. This setting acts as a *minimum* limit on most equipment, because the automatic brightness control unit automatically increases the kVp on larger patients or when a patient is rolled onto his side in order to maintain an adequate signal for the TV camera or other imaging devices. Thus, kilovoltage actually varies automatically during fluoroscopy as the patient changes position. Some machines may also automatically adjust the mA up or down slightly, but, as previously discussed, the mA must not exceed regulations, so kVp is usually changed by the automatic brightness control.

EXPOSURE TIME

There is no predetermined setting for fluoroscopic exposure time, since it varies as the length of time the radiologist is depressing the exposure footswitch.

There is, however, a mechanism for *monitoring* the total amount of exposure time acquired during the procedure. Referred to as the *fluoroscopy timer*, this knob should be set at 5 minutes at the beginning of every fluoroscopic procedure. As the radiologist fluoroscopes the patient, it runs down to zero and then sounds a buzzer and disengages the fluoroscopy unit as a reminder to the radiologist that 5 minutes of fluoro time have been used and patient dose is becoming substantial. If further fluoroscopy is needed, the radiographer should immediately reset this timer to 5 minutes.

For both professional and legal reasons, fluoro timers should not be reset continually so that they never reach zero and sound the buzzer. Many radiography departments maintain records of the total fluoro time acquired by each patient as a legal precaution and for patient advisement.

SPOTFILMING TECHNIQUE

The spotfilming mechanism is located at the bottom of the fluoro tower under the image intensifier tube. It is a sophisticated film-placement device which uses mechanical arms to place the film in the x-ray beam, in front of the image intensifier tube, each time the radiologist desires a permanent record of something he sees during fluoroscopy. Several tightly collimated exposures may be made on one film, because the spotfilmer follows a programmed cycle of changing the film centering in the beam. By centering exposures to the corners and edges of the film as well as its center, traditional machines are capable of fitting up to nine different exposures on one film. These nine traditional placements are diagrammed and named in Figure 225.

Newer machines are capable of even more spots on one film and also capable of using several different sizes of cassettes rather than being limited to the conventional 9-inch cassette.

Figure 224. Traditional spot film changer with image intensifier removed so that spot film can be seen in position for exposure to one corner. White arrowheads at bottom left to right mark (1) load/unload button for bringing cassette to removal position, (2) latch for releasing cassette to remove it, (3) park/release button for fluoro tower transverse movement. Black arrow points out spotfilm format selector, with settings for quarters (upper left), vertical halves (upper right), horizontal halves (lower right), and full spot (lower left).

Q1	HH1	Q3
VH1	F	VH2
Q2	HH2	Q4

Figure 225. Diagram of traditional spotfilm settings to obtain nine views on one film. Abbreviations: Q - quarters, HH - horizontal halves, VH -vertical halves, F - full spot. Sequence for nine views: Q1, VH1, Q2, HH1, F, HH2, Q3, VH2, Q4.

Loading the initial spot film and selecting the filming format, along with changing the spot films during the fluoro procedure, is the responsibility of the technologist. The format selection knob or buttons are located on the fluoro tower (Figure 224).

It is important that technologists familiarize themselves with all the different fluoro units in their department. Each unit may have different spot film loading and unloading procedures. There are two basic types of spot film mechanisms, one that loads from the front, where the radiologist stands, and one that loads from the rear or behind the fluoro tower. The rear loading type will provide access to the film when in the *parked* position. The spot film is kept in the parked position at all times until the radiologist depresses the spotfilm exposure switch. This type of unit requires that the technologist reach down into the film holding area and manually remove the film from the carriage. There is a risk of injury to the technologist with this type of unit so care should be taken while changing spotfilms.

With the front loading type of fluoro unit, if the film does not automatically come to the unload position after the spotfilm has been exposed the selected number of times, an unload button must be activated (Figure 224). Once the film has moved into the unload position generally there will be release button that must be used to release the spotfilm from the carriage (Figure 224).

Spot films are phototimed radiographs. Prior to the start of the procedure the phototimer must be changed to the spotfilm selection, and the center cell or chamber must also be activated.

MILLIAMPERAGE

The regular mA control on the console has a section for *fluoroscopic mA* stations, which are usually limited to 200, 300 and 400 mA. The term *fluoro mA* is something of a misnomer as it is used on x-ray machine consoles, because this control actually sets the milliamperage to be used on the *spotfilms*. The real fluoroscopy mA is preset as previously described. Spotfilms are similar to overhead exposures and use the same types of mA stations, but a separate grouping of control settings is required because they refer to the mA to be used in the x-ray tube *under* the table rather than the overhead tube. A fluoro (spotfilm) mA station must be engaged before either the spotfilmer or the fluoro tower will operate.

KILOVOLTAGE

In the fluoroscopy mode, the regular overhead kVp control becomes the spotfilm control. It should be set well above 100 kVp for all barium procedures except esophagrams, which may use 90 kVp.

AEC AND BACKUP TIMER

When the machine is put in the fluoroscopic mode and the spotfilmer is activated, an *AEC* circuit is automatically engaged to control spotfilm exposure times. AEC's employ radiation detectors such as ion chambers or photomultiplier tubes placed in the peripheral beam or behind the film cassette to measure the amount of remnant radiation reaching the film. The energy of the impinging radiation is converted into an electrical charge which may be stored in a capacitor. When a preset level of electrical charge is reached, this capacitor is allowed to discharge its electrons. The ensuing surge of electrical current is used in an electromagnet to pull the exposure switch back open and terminate the exposure.

With larger patients or when the patient is rolled onto his side, more radiation is absorbed in the patient and less remnant radiation reaches the film (and the detector) per second. It takes a longer time for the electrical capacitor to reach its preset discharge level, so that the exposure time is increased. In this way, the x-ray machine automatically adjusts the exposure time to always ensure adequate density on the resulting radiograph.

A *backup* timer, however, must be set by the radiographer as a precaution in patient safety in case the AEC should fail to function properly. In the fluoroscopy mode, the regular overhead timer control becomes this backup timer. It should be set around one second for most patients and around two seconds for very large patients. If the AEC circuit should fail to terminate the exposure at the proper time, which should be considerably less than the backup time, the backup timer will terminate it. This prevents the exposure from continuing for five or six seconds before the radiologist or radiographer realize that anything is amiss.

A *density* control on the console refers to the AEC. If the circuit is not functioning properly so that films are coming out too light or too dark, this density control may be adjusted upward or downward as a *temporary* solution to the problem until a service specialist can be notified of the malfunction. Automatic exposure controls and their limitations are more thoroughly discussed in Chapter 28.

IMAGE QUALITIES

The quality of a fluoroscopic or TV image can be defined in its brightness (tonal value), contrast, noise, sharpness of detail and magnification. It is important to keep in mind that when a TV monitor is used to display the fluoro image, there are *two* separate systems which will affect the displayed image qualities: the radiological system and the electronic TV system.

BRIGHTNESS

The brightness of the displayed image may be easier to understand in terms of the tonal value of the image. Tonal value is the light being transmitted through the monitor system and reaching the human eye. You have probably adjusted the brightness of your TV set at home simply because each person has a different comfort level for the amount of light reaching the eye while viewing television. Radiologists also have a preference for the lighting level at which they view the fluoro image. The brightness control knob on a TV monitor adjusts only the amount of light transmitted within the monitor and does not change the fluoroscopic technique factors. The change in brightness is equal in all areas on the screen, so image contrast is unchanged. Brightness is usually adjusted so that the darkest area on the monitor is black.

CONTRAST

The contrast seen on a spot film, overhead radiograph, and any of the other film type of image recording devices, is affected by the technique used, scatter radiation produced, and the physical density of the anatomical part being radiographed. In fluorography contrast is not only affected by these factors but also by the electrical components of the image intensifier and TV monitor. Light is given off isotropically (equally in all directions) from the input phosphor. Some of the off-angle light photons form a type of scatter and cause the photocathode to produce a scatter electron. This scatter electron will be converted back into a scattered light photon at the output phosphor and cause a loss of contrast in the displayed image. Even the electrons which carry usable information will produce scattered light photons at the output phosphor. All of these scattered light photons will reduce the displayed contrast on the monitor.

The displayed contrast is mostly out of our control, but can be adjusted somewhat on the TV monitor. When the contrast is increased electronically at the TV monitor, the amount of visible background noise on the monitor increases with it. *The contrast knob should be turned up until the background noise is visible, then turned down slightly to reduce the noise effect. The brightness should then be adjusted* to the preference of the radiologist or until the darkest areas of the image are black. Both the contrast and brightness should be adjusted together to produce the best possible displayed image.

NOISE

After the x-ray beam passes through the patient, the more systems it must be processed through until it is viewed or recorded, the more image noise is produced. Noise is inherent in every type of electrical device, and appears as a grainy or salt and pepper appearance on a TV monitor. Noise can be thought of as the "quantum mottle" of image intensification. Both noise and mottle are increased when there is an insufficient number of photons reaching the recording system. Image intensifiers are designed to operate at the lowest possible exposures. So the amount of noise displayed is a combination of the inherent electrical interference and the use of low exposure factors. There is very little that can be done to reduce the amount of noise produced in the system since it is a result of the electrical amplification of the image. The displayed noise can be limited by properly adjusting the TV monitor as mentioned above.

The amount of inherent noise produced in a system is rated as its signal-to-noise ratio. The higher the ratio, the better the displayed image will be. For example, a 500 to 1 ratio means that the actual information output signal will be 500 times greater than the inherent signal noise. A system with a 500 to 1 ratio will produce a clearer image on the monitor than a system with a 200 to 1 signal-to-noise ratio.

LAG

Lag is another electrical property which limits the dynamic ability of the fluoro system. It is that time it takes for an image to build up on a TV screen and then decay. Lag time is also affected by the automatic brightness control going through a series of technique changes while attempting to maintain the brightness on the monitor. Lag is not noticeable when the fluoro unit is stationary, but becomes very obvious as a "ghost image" when the unit is moved. Since this ghost image superimposes the newly desired image, it should be considered as a type of image noise.

RESOLUTION

The ability of the system to display the actual image is rated in the number of line pairs per millimeter (LP/mm) that it can visualize. The image intensifier at the input phosphor has the ability to display 3 to 6 LP/mm, depending on the amount of magnification that is used. As the amount of magnification increases, the number of line pairs displayed also increases for Fluoroscopy.

The older optical mirror system for viewing the image is the best method as far as resolution is concerned, but presents a low level of brightness and small image size. The TV monitor is limited to about 2 LP/mm, but is now the preferred system of viewing due to its ability to enhance contrast and brightness and to provide a large displayed image. When all viewing and recording components of the fluoroscopic chain are compared for resolution, the *TV monitor* is the weakest link.

VIGNETTING

Vignetting is the loss of sharpness and brightness at the peripheral borders of a TV monitor caused by the physical and electrical components of the fluoro system. The problem starts with the divergence of the x-ray and is increased with the flaring of the outer electrons in the intensifier tube and divergence of the light photons from the output phosphor. It is more noticeable with larger fields of view.

MAGNIFICATION

Magnification in radiography is generally associated with degradation of the sharp-

ness of detail on radiographs, but in image intensification it can be advantageous. Most modern image intensifiers have the ability to select a magnification factor on the control panel and on the fluoro tower.

When a magnification factor is selected the area of input phosphor being used is changed. The smaller area used on the input phosphor, the larger the image will be on the display monitor. A fluoro system may have a 25cm, 15cm, and 10cm selection of input phosphors. The normal size selected is 25 cm, while a selection of 10 cm would provide an image which is 2.5 times larger $(25/10 = 2.5)$. The advantage to the use of this system of magnification is that with the increased magnification comes an increase in resolution. The resolution can be increased from 3 to 6 LP/mm. The radiologist may use several different magnification selections throughout a procedure. The least amount of magnification (the largest input phosphor) is used for surveying during the procedure, while a magnification selection may be used during spot filming. The use of a magnification selection throughout the entire procedure would only serve to increase the patient exposure: Due to a smaller field of view on the screen it would take longer to view the entire anatomical structure. More importantly, at increased magnification the fluoro unit has to increase the exposure factors to maintain brightness on the monitor. Image intensifiers with two different field sizes are referred to as *dual-focused*, while units with 3 field sizes are called *tri-focused*.

Electronic magnification, as a control factor built into the fluoro system, is a benefit to the radiologist. But when magnification occurs due to *distance* changes, the displayed and recorded image will be degraded. The prime factors to consider when controlling unwanted magnification are the SID, SOD, and the OID, as described in

Chapters 18, 19, and 20.

In fluorography, to minimize the amount of magnification on the displayed or recorded image, keep the OID to a minimum by lowering the fluoro tower as close to the object being radiographed as possible.

IMAGE RECORDING DEVICES

Static or "still" images can be recorded, during fluoroscopic procedures either by the traditional spot film cassette changer or by photospot (105 mm) camera. Recordings of dynamic (moving) images during actual fluoroscopy can be made using cinefluorography (*cine* for short, pronounced "sin-ay"), or using video recording. Video recording can now be done with either videotape or with videodisc. It should be remembered that generally, the more devices an image is processed through, the poorer will be the resolution and the greater the noise. The advantages and disadvantages that each of these options presents for fluoroscopic image quality will now be discussed.

time. The response time is slowed by the need for the x- ray tube to change to the higher mA setting, (200 to 600 mA, versus the 4 to 6 mA for fluoro), and the time for the spot film carriage to position the cassette below the image intensifier and align it with the tube. A one- to two-second delay from the time the radiologist depresses the exposure switch to the time the film is actually exposed is not unusual. Some of the other advantages to cassette spot films include their ease in viewing along with overheads on a standard view box, no special storage needs such as containers for cine, and the larger film size, 9 x 9 inches versus 105 mm rolled film or 16 and 35 mm cine film.

SPOT FILM CASSETTE CHANGER

Even the most basic fluoro machine will have a *cassette spot film* device. This system allows the radiologist to position the image intensifier over an anatomical part and record what they see in the form of a standard radiograph. The traditional spot film cassette is 9 x 9 inches but all other sizes of cassettes up to 14 x 14 can be used in many newer units. When compared to the spot film camera, video disc and tape, and cine film recorders, the cassette spot film provides the highest resolution, but also the highest patient dose (both because the image is not processed through the intensifier tube). The system is easy to use and maintain, but may not be the best choice for dynamic studies due to its slow response

SPOT FILM CAMERAS

An increasingly popular recording device is the *spot film camera* or *photospot camera*, so named because it takes "spot films" of the *light* image from the intensifier tube. This system is generally of the rolled film type though there are clipped film cameras also. The size of film ranges from 70 to 90 to 105 mm in width. The camera is mounted to the side of the beam splitter (Figure 223), and can be activated by the radiologist on the fluoro control panel. A rolled reel of film is loaded into the camera carriage system and wound through a system of tension rollers and positioned in front of an aperture (Figure 226). The film is advanced through another set of tension rollers and fed into the opened receiver

Figure 226. Photograph of photospot camera with cover removed. The aperture or shutter where the film is exposed is at the top of the camera (white arrowhead), and various rollers for film threading are shown (compare to Figure 227.)

where it is guided onto the take up spool by a small guide wire. Figure 227 shows a typical threading path for loading the film. Once the camera housing is closed the load/unload knob is turned to the load position and the film is advanced a several more frames by pushing the advance button on the outside of the housing (Figure 228). During the exposure a window opens in front of the aperture to allow the reflected light from the beam splitter to expose an individual frame, and then closes. The next frame is advanced to the window and the process is repeated until the procedure is complete.

After the procedure is finished the technologist can advance the film several more frames to produce a *leader*, turn the load/unload knob to unload position, cut the film free by moving the cutting blade handle underneath the receiver (Figure 228) and then remove the receiver and process the film. Once in the darkroom the receiver is opened and the leader pulled

out. The leader is then taped to a piece of ordinary radiographic film and fed into the processor. It should be noted that a special type of tape is needed for taping the leader to a piece of radiographic film. Do not use regular clear tape or staple the leader to the film both of these may damage the processor. The metallic taped needed for this can be obtained through any film supplier. Once processed, the rolled film can be cut into 3 or 4 frame segments for viewing. There are special adhesive holders made for this type of film which will hold 9 to 12 frames in a holder the size of a 14 x 17.

The spot film camera is growing in popularity due to speed and convenience. Spot film cameras are able to run at a rate up to 12 frames/second and provide an excellent system to record slower physiological studies such as an Esophagrams and Venograms. Another advantage is the very short delay time. The camera is fixed in position and does not need to move in and out of position like the cassette spot firmer.

Figure 228. Photospot camera, with frame advance button (black arrow *left*), and load/unload knob (black arrow *right*). Film cutting blade handle (white arrow, bottom) can be seen beneath the receiving magazine. Smaller knobs are latches to covers.

Figure 227. Diagram showing proper film threading path through rollers of the photospot camera in Figure 226, from supply spool (A) through shutter at top to take-up spool in receiver magazine (B). Light from the beam splitter is reflected down to the aperture by a mirror.

When compared to the cassette spot filmer, it has slightly lower resolution but also lowers the patient dose. When compared to the video disc, video tape and cine film, the spot film camera is superior in resolution but requires slightly higher patient dose. Spot film cameras are popular for many of the same reasons as regular spot films. There is no special processor needed, viewing is done on a standard view box and there are no special storage containers needed.

VIDEO RECORDING

Yet another means to record fluoro images is by way of a *video tape, video disc,* or *laser disc recorder.* The video recorders are much like the VCR or video disc player you have at home. The recorders are placed between the TV camera tube in the intensifier and the TV monitor. As the TV signal is sent to the monitor it is received by the read/write head of the recorder and converted to match the recording system. With video tape and video disc recorders electric current creates a changing magnetic field which is proportional to the signal it received. The video tapes and video discs are coated with iron oxide particles which act like tiny magnets and align with the magnetic field. The video tape functions just like the video tape in a VCR for recording and play back, while the magnetic disc functions much like a computer diskette. With the laser disc the signal is processed through a laser which in turn burns the signal onto the optical disc. Light is used to both record and play back the information. The optic disc in the past has been limited to a one time recording, with multiple play back, but newer models are available which allow for reuse of the disc.

The theory of operation for these systems is fully discussed in radiographic physics texts.

The video tape system comes in a variety of tape sizes, including 1/2", 3/4", 1" and 2" formats. The video tape resolution is the poorest of all recording systems, though it can be improved with the use of high resolution TV camera tubes, recorders, video tape, and TV monitors. The high resolution system will also add to the cost of the purchase. The high resolution systems attempt to overcome the loss of resolution by using a slow recording speed. The video tape recorder is best used for slower dynamic studies which do not require high resolution recording, such as venograms, esophagrams, and voiding urethrograms. The tape system provides dynamic replay but suffers a further loss of resolution when viewed at slow motion speeds or on freeze frame. The advantages to the tape system are its low cost, lower patient dose when compared to film recording, and immediate playback with no special processing needs. The video tape system is also very slow when moving from one study to another since the entire study must be fast-forwarded until the next one begins.

The magnetic and laser disc systems are becoming more popular for several reasons. They provide excellent freeze frame resolution and can be viewed under slow motion conditions. They also have immediate play back ability and no special processing needs. The disc is set up with a system of numbered curves or sections, this allows for a very fast change from one image to another, or from one study to another. The disc also has a longer shelf life than the tape system. The video tape image will decay with time and use, while the disc remains in nearly the original recording condition. The major disadvantage to the disc system is its cost, which is much higher than the video tape.

Both systems lower patient dose since no beam splitting is needed and they receive almost 100 per cent of the signal sent out from the TV camera tube. Other disadvantages are the need for extra viewing systems in the reading room, and special storage considerations. The tape or disc is usually not kept in the patient's folder, and magnetic tape and discs must be stored free of magnetic fields.

CINEFLUOROGRAPHY

Cinefluorography can be used in routine diagnostic studies, but is more likely to be found in a cardiac catheterization lab. Cardiac catheterization procedures require a very high speed film system and cine fills this requirement. Cine cameras operate much like a movie camera. Cine film (16 mm or 35 mm in width and in 200 or 500 foot rolls) is advanced through a system of rollers and positioned in front of an aperture, similar to a photospot camera. The x-ray tube, aperture window and the motor drive for the camera are all synchronized. As an exposure is made the window opens to expose a frame on the film, then the window closes and the motor advances the film to the next unexposed frame. Based on the 60 cycle electrical power used in the U.S. cine is capable of frame rates of 60 frames/second (some units are capable of up to 120 frames/second), which makes it an excellent system for dynamic studies of the heart.

Since the image from the intensifier tube is round and cine film frames are square, part of the image or part of the film will always be wasted. The technologist must determine the radiologist's preference for framing format on each study. The two most used formats are *exact framing* and *total overframing*. With exact framing, the entire circular fluoro image is made to fit within the square frame area on the film. This wastes much of the film, but ensures that no anatomy will be missed. With total over-framing, the image is magnified until no portion of the film frame is unused. The square film frame fits completely inside the circular fluoro image. The magnification of the image may be desirable, but some of the anatomy is clipped as a result.

The physician needs to be able to view the filming on the monitor as it takes place, so a beam splitter is incorporated into the system. The beam splitter reflects about 90 percent of the light to the cine camera, and the remainder to the TV camera tube. Although a low amount of light is reaching the tube, it is enough for the physician to adequately monitor the filming.

On an individual frame basis exposure to the patient is low, but filming can involve several hundreds of individual frames making the overall exam a high dose procedure. The resolution of an indi-vidual frame is poor, mostly due to its small size, in comparison to cut film or 105 mm film, but the rapid filming rate provides an excellent dynamic study which is not avail-able with any other recording system.

The processing of the cine film is more complicated than that of 105 mm or other types of radiographic film. Cine processors are dedicated units, that is, they only devel-op cine film, and require special develop-ment chemistry. Cine film is a highly spe-cialized film, so a normal radiographic processor should not be used to develop the film.

After processing the film, it is loaded and viewed with on a projector/viewer. This projection system can be run at different speeds from high to slow-motion or at a sin-gle frame at a time. This enables the pro-cedure to be viewed as a dynamic study or on a individual frame rate for a static dis-play.

MOBILE C–ARM FLUOROSCOPY

The mobile c-arm is one of the most intimidating pieces of equipment that a technologist is called upon to operate. In appearance it is like no other piece of radi-ographic equipment. Add to this the fact that the mobile c-arm is used in such areas as surgery, intensive care unit, and the emergency room and the situation can be difficult to deal with. Confidence in the use of the c-arm comes with experience!

The c-arm is a portable fluorography unit. In the simplest form it is an x-ray tube and an image intensifier attached to a moveable c-arm carriage (Figure 229). Newer and more expensive models have computers, video disc recorders, digital subtraction capabilities, and the means to produce hard copies of stored images.

The principles of operation of the c-arm are the same as for a normal fluoro unit, except that much of the manipulation is done manually by the technologist. When the initial set of scout films is done proper-ly, the entire case will be easier to perform. The c-arm is positioned in a way that allows the physician as much room as possible to work. In some cases you may need to be able to pull the unit in and out as required. The unit can be set up with the image intensifier either above or below the patient. The type of exam and the need for lateral positioning during the case will determine the positioning of the intensifier. The TV monitor must be positioned to allow both the physician and technologist to view the screen. In most cases a lateral projection will be needed, and the intensifi-er is positioned *above* the patient. This will

Figure 229. Diagram of C-Arm mobile fluoroscopy unit, showing transverse movement of entire arm (A), longitudinal swivel (B), 360-degree rotation (C), and 180-degree AP to lateral sliding movement (D).

allow the c-arm to rotate under the patient into the lateral position (Figure 229), and not over the patient, which in surgical situations would compromise the sterile field.

The intensifier head and x-ray tube housing are usually covered in a sterile drape during surgical procedures to maintain the sterile field. Covering the portion under the patient also keeps it free of any blood or other fluids which may drip down. It is also a good idea to cover the foot switch to keep it free from fluids. Once the initial set up is complete, it is important for the technologist to test the unit to be sure of its operation and to orientate the screen so it is anatomically correct. This is sometimes very difficult due to the small field of view and limited anatomical information.

One easy way to orientate the screen is to use your *right and left markers* during the test or scout film. Use one marker to indicate the right or left side and the other to indicate the top. A coin and paper clip taped to the intensifier will also work. Once the image is on the screen the technologist can use the screen rotation buttons and the screen reverse button to properly display the image.

The screen rotation buttons turn the screen in a clockwise and counterclockwise motion. The rotation buttons are used when the image needs to be turned to match it with the position of the patient. It should be noted that most physicians (unlike radiologists) prefer the image on the screen to match the position of the patient. That is, the left side and the top of the patient is on the left side and top of the screen as they view it. Another button which aids in screen orientation is the image *reverse* button. This button serves to flip the image so what was on the left side of the screen will be on the right side, like a mirror image.

During the procedure the technologist may be called upon to manipulate the intensifier so to follow the positioning of a pacemaker wire or Swan Ganz catheter. It is important to know what locks allow for what type of c-arm movement. There are four basic locks on a *c-arm, transverse, longitudinal, 360 degree circular rotation, 180 degree AP to lateral rotation* (Figures 229 and 230). The transverse lock allows the c-arm to be extended and retracted across the table or patient. For example, it could be used to follow guide wire from the shoulder to the midline of a patient. The longitudinal lock allows the entire c-arm to swivel to the right or left, moving lengthwise in relation to the patient's body. In situations where substantial movement of the intensifier is required, such as a pacemaker or Swan Ganz catheter placement, it may be easier

Figure 230. Close-up of typical locks on a modern C-Arm unit. Arrowheads left to right: Transverse lock, longitudinal swivel lock, 360-degree rotation lock, and 180-degree AP to lateral lock. Compare with Figure 229.

for the technologist to unlock both these locks giving the intensifier nearly free movement in any direction whenever it is needed. The 360 degree lock rotates the c-arm so that the intensifier is above or below the patient. This lock is generally not used during a procedure, it is only used to initially set up the equipment in the proper configuration. The 180 degree lock allows the tube head and intensifier to move between AP and lateral projections. The c-arm will move either over or under the patient depending on where the intensifier is positioned. If the intensifier is over the patient the lateral movement will be below or under the patient. If the intensifier is under the patient then the lateral movement will be over the patient. Extreme care must be used when changing from AP to lateral positioning. In some cases the c-arm will need to be raised or lowered while rotating the arm over or under the patient.

It should also be noted that in many surgical, intensive care, and emergency room uses of the c-arm a special table extension or dedicated intensifier table will need to be used. Normal surgical tables, beds, and gurneys arc not built with image intensification in mind and have a lot of metal under them. Care should be taken when using a dedicated intensifier table because it may have a weight restriction due to the lack of support under the patient surface.

As for the other functions of the c-arm, such as recalling previous images, subtraction, and producing hard copies of images, you will need to be oriented to the particular type of equipment used in your department. Experience during an actual case is important, but experience can be gained during slow periods by practicing setting up the c-arm and and using the different locks and functions.

MINIMIZING PATIENT EXPOSURE

Much of the control of patient exposure during fluoro is up to the operator, usually the radiologist. But there are cases when the technologist is called upon to operate the fluoro unit, such as spotting a gall bladder or terminal ileum. To reduce the patient exposure, the best thing that can be done is to minimize the actual fluoro-on-time. Prior to spotting the part of interest, review any overhead radiographs to confirm its anatomical location. Also reduce the OID by keeping the fluoro tower as close to the body part a possible. Use the magnification factors only when required, locate the part under normal magnification and film under the needed amount of magnification. Fluoroscopy should *never* be used to locate an anatomical part or centering point for overhead radiographs. Use of the fluoro unit by the technologist is done only when instructed by the radiologist.

Another method reducing patient exposure, particularly with pediatric patients and thin anatomical parts, is to remove the grid from below the intensifier tube. A button on the fluoro tower is provided to insert and retract the grid from the path of the beam. Removing the grid when not needed can reduce the exposure to less than $1/3$ the exposure with the grid.

SUMMARY

1. *Fluorography* provides the radiologist a means to study anatomical parts in real time, and review recorded images under static or dynamic conditions.

2. The *image intensifier* electronically amplifies the information it receives in the form of x-ray photons to produce an image on the TV monitor which is from 1000 to 20,000 times brighter.

3. Recording the images can be done on conventional spot films, 70, 90, or 105 mm rolled spot films, 16 and 35 mm cine film, video disc or tape recorders.

4. The fluorography unit automatically adjusts the needed technique in order to maintain the brightness level on the monitor. Brightness is kept near constant as the density or thickness of the anatomical part changes. This system of control is called *automatic brightness control or automatic brightness gain.*

5. The image on the monitor can be described in terms of the *brightness, con-trast, noise, and resolution* displayed on the monitor. Another two factors which affect the displayed image are the amount of *lag and vignetting* appearing on the monitor.

6. *Magnification* in fluorography, as opposed to normal diagnostic radiology, is used to improve the resolution of the displayed image. As the magnification selection is increased, the resolution increases. This applies only the selected magnification on the fluoro tower and not the magnification which is produced due changes in the OID, SID, or SOD.

7. Between *optic mirror and TV monitor* viewing, the mirror system provides the highest resolution but slightly higher patient exposure. *Cassette spot films* provide the highest resolution and patient exposure of all the recording devices. *105, 90,* and *70 mm* cine cameras (in that order) are 2nd, 3rd, and 4th in res-

olution and patient exposure. *35 mm* and *16 mm* cine are 5th and 6th in resolution and patient exposure, while the *videotape* and *disc* provide the poorest resolution but also the lowest patient exposure.

REVIEW QUESTIONS

1. What are the advantages of image intensification over Edison's fluorography system?
2. What is the difference between automatic brightness control and automatic gain control?
3. What specific knob on the console serves as backup timer for spot filming?
4. What purpose do the input phosphor, photocathode, and output phosphor serve?
5. The _____ divides the light off the output phosphor between ancillary recording devices and the monitor system.
6. List in order of their resolution, with one (1) being the best, the different types of recording devices.
7. Name and describe the four major locks on a mobile c-arm?
8. In order to minimize unwanted magnification, the _____ should be kept at a minimum distance.
9. _____ is probably the best dynamic imaging system for studies of the heart.
10. What are the seven (7) factors which affect the image quality on the TV monitor?
11. How is a fluorography tube different from a standard x-ray tube?
12. Explain overframing and exact framing.
13. When contrast is turned up too high at the TV monitor, what undesirable image effect may become visible?

Chapter 34

SPECIAL IMAGING TECHNIQUES

Q. CARROLL AND E. SEERAM

PARALLACTIC IMAGING METHODS

Depth perception is created in an image by simulating the double vision of the human eyes. The brain is able to perceive depth or distance in an image because of the *parallactic shift* of the image which occurs between the two eyes. Parallactic shift or *parallax* is the apparent change in position of an object against a background reference point when seen from two different points of view. To demonstrate parallax, hold a pencil close to your nose and alternate closing one eye and then the other. The pencil appears to shift position in relation to the background you see. Although you are not consciously aware of this shift as you go about your daily business, your brain automatically and continually compares the parallax of objects seen by each eye to provide a sense of depth. When one eye is lost, there can be no more depth perception.

When the observer is moving, parallax can be thought of as the amount of apparent shift of objects against the background, or the speed at which they seem to pass by. For example, when driving, telephone poles or other objects that are near to the road seem to pass by quickly, while objects that are at some distance from the road seem to pass by more slowly. The speed or amount of shift is related to the distance from the object to the viewer. These principles are taken advantage of in radi-

ographic imaging in the areas of foreign body localization, stereoradiography, and tomography.

FOREIGN BODY LOCALIZATION

There are several approaches to maximizing the detection of foreign bodies including soft tissue technique (Chapter 11), routine fluoroscopy, and positioning methods such as tangential projections. Parallactic shift is utilized in the single-film triangulation method and the fluoroscopic parallax method.

Single-Film Triangulation

The single-film triangulation method is especially useful when the exact depth of the object must be determined without moving the patient. A double-exposure is made on one film using one-half the normal technique for each exposure. For the first exposure, the x-ray beam is centered to the suspected location of the foreign body. For the second exposure, the x-ray tube is shifted in a direction perpendicular to the long axis of the foreign object. It is recommended that the tube be off-centered from the first exposure by about ten per cent of the SID (4 or 5 inches for a 40-inch SID). The film is not moved. The collimator must be opened up so that the field does not cut off anatomy of interest when shifted. This produces a double-image of the foreign body on the radiograph.

Exact measurements must be taken and recorded for the following:

SFD: The skin-to-film distance, measured from the uppermost surface of the body part to the film.

SID: The source-image distance.

TSD: The tube shift distance.

ISD: The image shift distance, measured from the radiograph.

With the above data, the following formula will yield the *foreign body-film distance,* (FBFD):

$$\frac{SID \times ISD}{TSD + ISD} = FBFD$$

The FBFD is now subtracted from the SFD (the skin-to-film distance) to obtain the depth of the foreign object from the surface of the patient:

SFD - FBFD = Foreign Body Depth

Because of parallax, the deeper the object is from the surface of the body, the less its image will shift on the radiograph.

Fluoroscopic Parallax

A metallic object at the end of a stick may be held to the side of the patient's body during fluoroscopy. If the fluoro tower is then shifted side to side, both the foreign body and the metal indicator to the patient's side will appear to shift across the image. As this occurs, the indicator may be moved vertically up and down. When the image of the metal indicator shifts at exactly the same apparent speed and distance as the foreign body, the indicator is at the level of the foreign body. The level of the indicator may then be measured from the tabletop or from the surface of the body as a direct measurement of the depth of the foreign object.

TOMOGRAPHY

Some anatomical objects are not visible on routine radiographs because of overlapping, more contrasty anatomical structures such as bones which superimpose and obscure them. Tomography refers to the use of *motion* to blur out such overlying structures so that the anatomy of interest can be seen through them. The purpose of tomography is the *desuperimposition* of obstructing images (the reduction of noise). Tomography is known by a variety of names, including *laminography, planigraphy,* and *body-section radiography.*

The desuperimposition process achieved with tomography may be further divided into two specific objectives: *Analysis* is the dividing of complex anatomy into small parts, so that each part may be diagnosed individually. Typical tomograms use large movements of the x-ray tube to focus in on very thin sections of anatomy for analysis. An example of analysis is tomography of the inner ear, where the ossicles, the cochlea, the vestibular area and the auditory nerve canal are each individually focused upon for diagnosis. *Localization* is the purpose of *zonography*–a type of tomography which employs only very small movements of the tube. These small movements result in thick sections of anatomy being in focus on the zonogram, so that a part of the body may be scanned through with a limited number of exposures in search of suspected pathology. An exam-

Figure 231. Diagram illustrating the displacement and blurring of images of objects above and below the fulcrum point of a tomographic tube movement. Note that during the course of the tube movement, the images of the triangle and square have moved across the film surface.

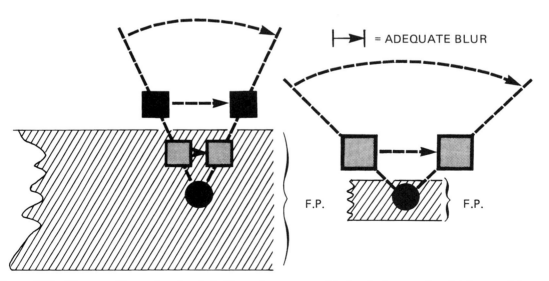

Figure 232. Diagram illustrating the definition of a tomographic focal plane as that thickness of tissue within which objects are not displaced enough to be visibly blurred. (*Left*) the gray box is not visibly blurred, will appear sharp in the image and is considered to lie within the focal plane. (*Right*) Increased tube movement now visibly blurs the gray box, and it is considered to lie outside the thinner focal plane.

ple of zonographic localization is the pinpointing of pulmonary lesions of low contrast, which may be highly suspected but difficult to visualize on a routine chest radiograph. Using zonography, the lungs may be scanned in sections from front to back, employing only 8-12 exposures.

Although most tomography is performed by moving the x-ray tube and the film in concert during the exposure, it is also possible to obtain tomographic images by having the patient move a body part during the exposure, while the x-ray tube and film remain stationary. This method is called *autotomography* and is commonly used in such procedures as the thoracic spine (breathing technique) and the upper cervical spine (wagging-jaw technique).

The way that tomography works is illustrated in Figure 231. The central ray of the x-ray beam is centered through the anatomy of interest to the film. As the x-ray tube moves in one direction, it also rotates on its axis so that the central ray remains centered through the anatomy of interest, forming a *fulcrum point*. The film moves in the opposite direction to maintain its centering to the CR. Note in Figure 231 that in doing so, the anatomy of interest (the circle) is always projected to the center of the film and is therefore not blurred. However, anatomy above and below the part of interest is projected by changing peripheral rays throughout the exposure, so that its image moves across the film and is blurred. Note in Figure 231 that the triangle and the square exchange places on the film from one extreme of the tube movement to the

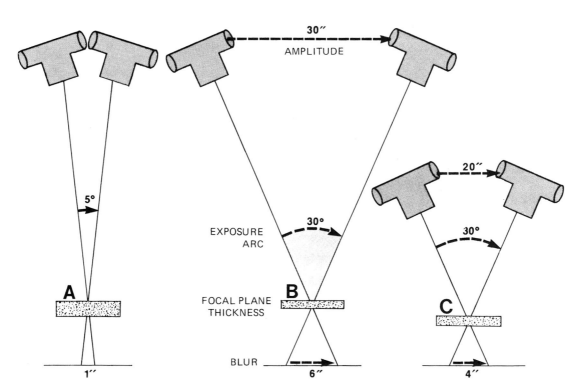

Figure 233. Diagram of two methods of obtaining thinner tomographic focal planes. Plane B is thinner than plane A because of increased exposure arc (30 degrees versus 5 degrees). Plane B is thinner than plane C because, even though the exposure arcs are equal, amplitude is greater for B (30 inches versus 20 inches) due to the longer SID.

other. They have both been blurred across the length of the film. The circle will be visibly in focus on the resulting radiograph, while the objects above and below it will be blurred out of visibility.

THE FOCAL PLANE

The further an object is above or below the fulcrum point, the more distance it will be blurred across on the film. Actually, everything is blurred on the tomogram to a greater or lesser degree. But there is a limit to the capacity of the human eye to see microscopic levels of blurring, so that an object must be blurred by a certain minimum amount before the blurring becomes visible to the eye. The practical effect of this is that a *focal plane*, a layer of anatomy with a distinct thickness which will be visibly recorded on the film, is produced during tomography (Figure 232). Within the focal plane thickness, no anatomy has been blurred enough for the eye to detect the blur, so it all appears reasonably focused. Anatomy which has been visibly blurred is considered to be outside the focal plane. In Figure 232, an imaginary minimum distance to cause visible blurring is diagrammed. This distance represents the limit of the human eye to detect blur. On the *left* side of the diagram, note that the solid box has been blurred across a distance greater than this minimum. It will be blurred on the image and not considered to be within the focal plane. The hollow box, however, is close enough to the plane of the fulcrum point that it has not been blurred across the minimum distance. It will appear focused on the image and is considered to be within the focal plane. To blur out this hollow box, the distance of the x-ray tube movement must be increased. As shown on the *right* side of Figure 232, where the tube movement is increased, the

hollow box would no longer be considered to be within the focal plane since it is now blurred from visibility. In effect, the focal plane has been made *thinner*. That is, there is a thinner layer of tissue which is shown in focus on the resulting radiograph.

Greater blurring effectiveness obtained through the tube movement always results in thinner focal planes. Two aspects of the tube movement bear upon its blurring effectiveness: the exposure arc and the amplitude (Figure 233). *Exposure arc* refers to the angle between the extremes of the tube movement formed by the central ray, measured in degrees. The greater the exposure arc, the thinner the focal plane and the more effective the blurring. *Amplitude* refers to the actual distance traversed by the x-ray tube during the tomographic movement. The amplitude may be increased without changing the exposure arc by changing the pattern which the tube makes in moving. For example, the tube may trace out a 30-degree circle (15 degrees to each side of vertical) rather than a 30-degree line. In doing so, it travels more than three times the total amplitude distance. The blurring of unwanted structures in the image is slightly more effective for circular movements than for linear ones of the same exposure arc for this reason.

MOVEMENT PATTERNS

In an attempt to obtain greater amplitudes, a number of different tomographic movement patterns have been developed over the years. Since all of the variations involve changing direction during the exposure, they are collectively referred to as pluridirectional movements. Pluridirectional tomography equipment is much more expensive than the unidirectional, linear tomograph, but *pluridirectional* movements have two distinct advantages over linear movements. The first advantage is the increased blurring effectiveness, or *selectivity*, by which thinner focal planes may be obtained for detailed analysis. The second is the elimination of *false images*.

False Images

False images are images *created* by the geometrical relationship between the tomographic tube movement and the anatomical structures within the patient. These images must not be considered to represent any real objects in the patient. They are *not* a form of distortion (a common misconception) but rather a form of *noise*. A distorted image, although it is changed in shape, still represents a real object within the patient. A false image, however, is an illusion created by movement. False images are a form of noise because they are completely useless and they obscure the desirable image.

The most common type of false image is *streaking* (Figure 234). Streaks of density are produced on linear tomographs when long structures lying roughly parallel to the tube movement are not sufficiently blurred (Figure 235). An area is left on the film over which some portion of the object was projected throughout the exposure. Nonetheless, since the portion of the object over that area was constantly changing during the exposure, its appearance does not accurately represent any real anatomy. To reduce streaking artifacts, it is recommended that whenever possible the anatomy to be blurred (not necessarily the anatomy of interest) be placed perpendicular to the long axis of the tube movement, so that the blurring distance required to completely blur out its image is reduced to its own width (Figure 235). For example, most linear and eliptical movements are oriented with their long axis along the length of the

Figure 234. Linear tomograph (30 degrees) of skull exhibiting linear streaks.

Figure 235. Diagram showing how streaking is produced when tomographic movement is insufficient to completely displace an image lengthwise. Placing obstructing anatomy to be blurred width-wise to the direction of tube movement is effective in eliminating streaking.

x-ray table. During lung tomography, the ribs lie perpendicular to this movement and are well blurred. During an IVP, however, the ureters which lie parallel to the tube movements are likely to produce streaking artifacts.

Annular (circular) artifacts may also be created when a circular x-ray tube movement cuts through a tube or vessel at a semi-axial angle. In order to eliminate linear and circular false images, more complex tube movements in which the pattern crosses over itself (the circle-eight, the cruciate and the hypocycloidal movements), and the spiral movement, were developed. By far, the spiral and the hypocycloidal tube movements are the most effective and produce the thinnest focal planes available.

APPLICATIONS

Table XXXIV lists the various tube movement patterns with degrees of exposure arc, the typical thicknesses of focal planes obtained with those movements and the anatomy for which each movement type is recommended.

For the tube movement to be effective, the exposure must be *spread out* across the entire tube movement. If the exposure terminates before the movement is completed, the full effect of the blurring will not be obtained. Table XXXIV also presents the typical minimum times required for each type of movement to complete its cycle. The exposure time used in setting the electrical technique must be exactly as the manufacturer of the equipment recommends for each tube movement. The milliamperage will then need to be decreased substantially to maintain the proper total mAs.

To avoid creating double images and uneven density, the x-ray tube must be moving at a constant rate of speed throughout the exposure. It cannot be accelerating or stopped during the exposure. Therefore, the tube must be in motion before and after the exposure to allow for acceleration and deceleration. As an example, for a 30-degree linear tomogram, the tube would be angled more than 15 degrees to one side of vertical before starting. When the exposure button is depressed, the tube accelerates. The exposure itself does not start until the tube reaches the

TABLE XXXIV

Tomographic Tube Movements: Resulting Focal Plane Thicknesses,
Typical Exposure Times, and Recommended Applications

Tube Movement	Focal Plane Thickness	Exposure Times	Recommended Applications
10-degree Linear Zonography	1 cm	1 Sec.	Biliary, Urinary, Pulmonary and Mediastinal Localization
30-degree Linear Tomography	4 mm	2 Sec.	Biliary, Urinary, Pulmonary and Mediastinal Analysis
25-degree Eliptical or Circular	3 mm	3 Sec.	Extremities (including casts), Spines, Brain Ventricles
Hypocycloidal, Spiral or Circle-Eight	1–1.5 mm	6 Sec.	Inner Ear, Petrous, Facial, Orbital, Sella Turcica, Lymph Nodes, Cervical, and Vertebral Analysis
Autotomography			C1–C2 (wagging jaw), Brain Ventricles (head rotation), Sternum and T–Spine (breathing)
Pantomography			Dental

15-degree mark. When the tube reaches 15 degrees to the opposite side of vertical, the exposure terminates and the tube begins to slow down to a halt. The exposure switch must be kept depressed until the entire exposure is completed.

TECHNIQUE

In addition to the reduction of the mA station to compensate for the longer exposure time previously described, there is one other important technique consideration. Most tomographs move the tube and film in a plane parallel to the tabletop. On these machines, the *average* target-film distance during the movement is increased above the usual 40 inches, with 40 inches at vertical being the minimum and the extremes being as much as 55-60 inches. A loss of density results. A practical rule of thumb for such machines is to roughly double the total technique from a standard technique chart to maintain image density.

To reiterate the necessary technique adjustments for tomography, first find the technique on a routine chart for that anatomy and double the listed mAs. Set the exposure timer as required by the manufacturer for the tube movement being used. At that time, reduce the mA station as needed to achieve the desired (doubled) mAs. On occasion, this mAs value will not be obtainable and a reduction in kVp will be necessary, using the 15 per cent rule.

FOCAL DEPTH, INTERVALS AND SCOUT FILMS

The *focal depth* refers to the location of the focal plane in centimeters from the *back* or *down-side* of the patient *upward.* Usually several exposures are taken at different levels within the patient, commonly called cuts or *sections.* The focal depth is the location of the focal plane for each cut. It is

determined by the location of the fulcrum point in the patient. Different tomographs will automatically move the table, the entire tube-Bucky linkage arm assembly, or the rotational axis of the tube to change the level of the fulcrum point within the patient. It is important to remember that the focal depth indicated by the machine is measured upward from the *tabletop.* Therefore, if a sponge or pad is placed under the patient, the thickness of that object must be subtracted from the indicated focal depth to obtain the actual focal depth from the patient's down-side. Tomographic films must be marked accurately as measured with reference to the patient and not to the tabletop for focal depth.

Before proceeding, the radiographer must determine the interval of distance to be used between the cuts that will be taken. This interval should be based directly upon the thickness of cut obtained by the tube movement as listed in Table XXXIV. If the intervals between the focal depths of the cuts taken are too small, unnecessary patient dose results. If they are too great, then important anatomy or pathology may be actually missed between cuts and lead to a misdiagnosis. As a rule, the interval used should be slightly less than the thickness of the focal plane obtained. Consulting Table XXXIV, for example, hypocycloidal cuts should be taken about every millimeter of depth, whereas 30-degree linear cuts may be taken every 3 millimeters.

Having determined the intervals to be used, *two* scout films should be taken for a tomographic procedure at two different but adjacent focal depths. Providing the radiologist with two scouts allows him to be certain of how many cuts to take in each direction, because he is able to see which scout is approaching the middle of the anatomy of interest. This procedure will spare much unnecessary patient dose, which results from taking the same number of cuts in both directions from one scout, only to find that several to one side were completely out of the anatomy of interest. The radiographer can also save patient dose by having a thorough knowledge of anatomy to localize a starting depth for scout films. For example, the kidneys typically lie about one-third of the way from the patient's back to his front. Thus, a good starting point on a 22-cm patient would be to take one scout radiograph at 7 cm and one at 8 cm. Because of all of the additional considerations and thorough knowledge of anatomy required of tomographic radiographers, this area may be considered as an advanced subspecialty of radiography.

XERORADIOGRAPHY

Xeroradiography is an electrostatic imaging process whereby x-rays are converted into a latent charged image. Specifically, xeroradiography is a dry nonsilver electrostatic imaging technique based on the use of a photoconductive material, usually selenium, deposited onto an aluminum base. Together they form the xeroradiographic image receptor (plate), which measures about 23cm x 36cm.

Xeroradiography is accomplished in three steps: First, the plate must be charged, that is, positive electrostatic charges are placed on the photoconductive surface, after which the plate is placed in a cassette, so that the charge can be maintained. This is all done in a machine referred to as the *conditioner*. After the plate has been used, it is returned to the conditioner so that any latent residual image can be removed before the plate is charged again.

In the second step, the charged plate is then exposed to x-rays which discharge the plate to produce a latent electrostatic image. In the final step, the latent image must be processed to render it visible. This is accomplished in the *processor* which develops the latent image, transfers and fuses the image onto a sheet of paper. The plate is subsequently cleaned in the conditioner so that it is ready for another examination.

The processing of the latent image is such that, while in the processor, the plate is removed from the cassette and placed into a special chamber where it is sprayed with charged blue powder particles called the *toner*. The charged powder particles distribute themselves according to the charge distribution on the plate rendering the latent image visible. The image is then transferred to a sheet of paper which now undergoes a fixing process by the application of heat to the sheet of paper, fusing the powder to it.

The xeroradiographic image appears bluish because of the blue powdered particles. Normally, regions in which the anatomy is thick appear deep blue while less thick regions appear less blue. This image may be reversed during processing.

One of the advantages of the xeroradiographic process is that it has a wide exposure latitude. As such, it has been used to image not only the extremities but also the breast. Imaging the breast using xeroradiography is referred to as *xeromammography*. This still remains an optional application of xeroradiography.

The contrast of the xeroradiographic image is low, however, details can be enhanced by a process referred to as *edge enhancement*, in which more powder is attracted to the edge region of the anatomy, a region where thick and thin parts meet.

The technologist performs the following essential tasks in xeroradiographic imaging:

   (a) The plate is placed in the conditioner for clearing and charging.

   (b) The cassette is then exposed to x-rays. During this procedure, the cassette must be carefully handled so that the plate does not lose charge.

   (c) The exposed plate is now inserted into the processor.

   (d) The xeroradiograph is then collected for viewing by the radiologist.

LASER IMAGING SYSTEMS

The word "laser" is not a new word since it has become commonplace in several facets of human activity. For example, lasers are now used the military, communications, surveying, industry, space studies and in medicine. In medicine, lasers are used in surgery (as a scalpel) gastroenterology, dermatology, otolaryngology, urology, pulmonary medicine, and finally in radiology.

WHAT IS A LASER?

The term *Laser* is an acronym for *Light Amplification by Stimulated Emission of Radiation.* It was invented in 1960 by T.H. Maiman, who worked on what was called a Ruby Laser as shown in Figure 236. Three essential components comprise the laser:

1. The *medium,* which in this case is the Ruby rod, which gives rise to the laser beam and also indicates the operating wavelength of the laser.

2. A *source of power* which provides energy to the medium. This is also referred to as the *pumping source.*

3. A *resonant cavity* which may assume a cylindrical shape or that of a prism.

Figure 236. The essential components of a ruby laser.

The production of a laser beam is such that when atoms in the medium (solid, liquid or gas) are excited by a certain amount of energy (supplied by the power source). Their electrons are raised to an excited energy state and this process results in the emission of light. This light is confined to the cavity which begins to resonate at one of the emission frequencies. As a result, the light energy is amplified at this specific frequency resulting in the production of a coherent beam of light (light in which the waves are in phase and have the same frequency). This is the laser beam.

TYPES OF LASERS

Lasers differ according to the medium which is used to produce the laser beam. This medium can be a solid, liquid or gas. The ruby laser described earlier is an example of a laser which used a solid.

Other types of lasers include semiconductor lasers as well as those which use gas, such-as the argon ion laser, the nitrogen, carbon dioxide and helium laser, and the helium-neon laser, one which is commonly used in radiology.

The helium-neon laser emits red light with an output power of 10 to 100 milliwatts (mW).

LASERS IN RADIOLOGY

There are four ways in which lasers are presently being used in the radiology department:

1. In digitizing x-ray films. These are referred to as Laser Film Digitizers.
2. In Scanning Laser-Stimulated Luminescence X-Ray Imaging Systems.
3. In Laser Film Printers.
4. In Laser Optical Disk Storage.

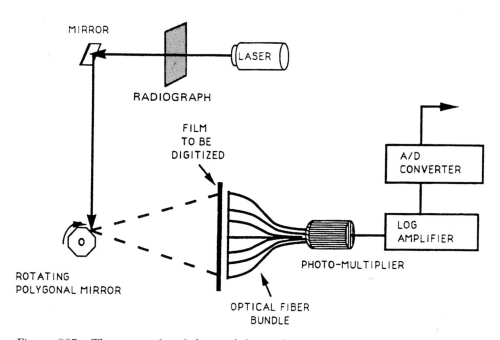

Figure 237. The principle of digitized fim radiography using a laser beam (from Greene, RE and Oestmann, JW (1992). *Computed Digital Radiography in Clinical Practice.* Thieme Medical Publishers, Inc. Reproduced by permission.)

Laser Film Digitizers

A Laser Film Digitizer converts x-ray films into digital images. This process is referred to as *Digitized Film Radiography* (DFR). Such a system is illustrated in Figure 237. The film to be digitized is scanned line by line by the laser beam. The laser light which is transmitted through the film is detected by special detectors which generate an output signal. These detector signals are then digitized and subsequently fed into a digital computer for processing and storage.

Digitized Film Radiography is used not only for archival storage of digitized x-ray films but also for transmission of images from the radiology department to other parts of the hospital such as intensive care and cardiac care units. In addition, not only is the image sent but also a copy of the radiologist's report is transmitted as well.

Scanning Laser-Stimulated Luminescence X-Ray Imaging Systems

These systems make use of a special *storage phosphor imaging plate* which is *photostimulable*. When the plate is exposed to x-rays, the phosphor electrons are raised to a higher energy level and remain trapped there until the plate is scanned by a laser beam. As the beam scans the plate, it luminesces and this light is detected and converted into electrical signals which are then converted into digital data. These data are processed by the computer which generates images that can be recorded on film or stored on magnetic tapes and disks as well as on optical disks. This process is shown in Figure 238. This technique will be described further in the next chapter.

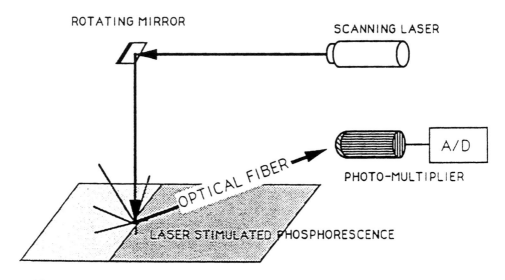

Figure 238. The basic principle of storage phosphor imaging. A laser beam is used to read the storage phosphor imaging plate which holds the latent x-ray image. The image data from the plate are detected with a photomultiplier tube and the data is subsequently digitized for input into the computer. (From Greene, RE and Oestmann, JW (1992). *Computed Digital Radiography in Clinical Practice.* Thieme Medical Publishers, Inc. Reproduced by permission.)

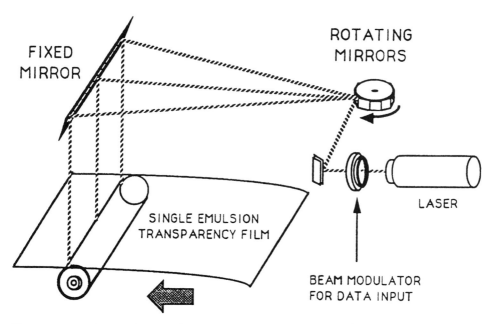

FIXED MIRROR

ROTATING MIRRORS

LASER

SINGLE EMULSION TRANSPARENCY FILM

BEAM MODULATOR FOR DATA INPUT

Figure 239. The fundamental principle of a laser printer. (From Greene, RE and Oestmann, JW (1992). *Computed Digital Radiography in Clinical Practice.* Thieme Medical Publishers, Inc. Reproduced by permission.)

Laser Film Printers

Laser Film Printers are becoming commonplace in radiology departments which have digital imaging equipment such as CT, MRI, and Digital Fluoroscopy and Radiography.

These printers typically use a helium-neon (or solid state diode) laser to write digital data onto special film. The digital data from the computer is sent to the printer, which, through a series of operations convert the data into a signal which is sent to the laser. The laser then scans the film to produce the image as can be seen in Figure 239. Heat from the laser develops an image in a carbon-based emulsion. This technology eliminates the need for *chemical* processing.

Optical Disk Storage

Another way lasers are used in radiology is in the storage of information, particularly image data. The storage device is the optical disk. The optical disk makes use of a high intensity laser beam to write data onto the disk and a low intensity laser to read the information from the disk.

Optical disks are now being used in conjunction with CT units. A 5.25-inch optical disk can store about 1 gigabyte of data.

SUMMARY

1. *Tomography* desuperimposes obstructing structures from the anatomy of interest by blurring all objects which lie above or below the focal plane. The greater the amplitude or exposure arc, the thinner the *focal plane*.

2. More complex tomographic tube movements help eliminate *false images* such as streaking, which are created by the geometrical relationship of the movement to the anatomy. Movements with a long axis are best used when aligned perpendicular to the long axis of the anatomy to be blurred.

3. On most tomographs, the total *technique* used should be roughly double that for the same anatomy in conventional radiography. Exposure times must be long enough for the tube movement to complete its cycle.

4. Two tomographic *scout films* at different focal depths should be taken so that the radiologist can orient himself. *Intervals* between cuts should be slightly less than the focal plane thickness being obtained, so that no anatomy is missed and patient dose is minimized.

5. Single-film triangulation and the fluoroscopic parallax method for foreign body localization use the apparent shift of images when the observer's viewpoint is changed to determine the depth of foreign bodies.

6. *Xerography* uses electrically charged plates to record an image. Its main advantage is edge enhancement.

7. *Laser* printers eliminate the need for chemical processing. Lasers are also used in digitizing film images, optical disc storage, and to expose photostimulable plates.

REVIEW QUESTIONS

1. Define parallax:
2. Explain the two diagnostic purposes for the use of tomography to desuperimpose anatomical parts:
3. Define autotomography and give an example of a procedure which uses it:
4. Define focal plane:
5. Define tomographic amplitude:
6. The longer the exposure arc, the _____ the focal plane produced.
7. Define false image and give an example:
8. Describe the advantage of pluridirectional tube movements over unidirectional (linear) ones in regard to image qualities:
9. For inner ear anatomy, which tomographic tube movements would be recommended:
10. What is the typical focal plane thickness obtained with 30-degree linear tomography:
11. Most tomographs use movements which result in varying tube-film distances throughout the sweep of the tube. As a rule of thumb, to compensate for this, the mAs value from a routine chart must be _____.
12. If a hypocycloidal movement produces focal planes 1.2 mm thick, the proper interval to change each focal depth (cut) is:
13. For a 25 cm-thick patient, at what focal depths should the first two "cuts" be taken for an IVP series:
14. List the four measurements that must be known in order to calculate the depth of a foreign body using the single-film triangulation method.
15. In xerographic processing, what attracts the toner powder to the areas of the plate that received less exposure?
16. What two machines are required for xerography in addition to an x-ray machine?
17. Although xerograms have inherently

low contrast, what special image characteristic results in enhanced visibility of detail ?

18. What is the meaning of the acronym LASER ?
19. List three components of a laser.
20. List four ways in which lasers are used in radiology.
21. What type of laser is commonly used in radiology?
22. What is the purpose of a laser film digitizer?
23. How is a laser used in storage phosphor plate imaging?
24. A laser film printer writes digital data onto what recording medium?
25. What is a laser optical disk used for in radiology ?

Chapter 35

DIGITAL IMAGING

EUCLID SEERAM

The application of computer processing of images (digital image processing) in the Radiology department has come to be known as *Digital Imaging*.

Digital image processing has its roots in the space program where various techniques were used not only to enhance images sent back from space but to restore them as well. Today the space program continues to utilize digital image processing and it has become the field which generates and uses the largest amount of digital data.

The success of image processing in the space program has had significant impact on applications in other fields. In Radiology, for example, digital imaging techniques are the basis for Computed Tomography, Magnetic Resonance Imaging and Digital Radiography and Fluoroscopy. In fact, Radiology has become the field which generates and uses the second largest amount of digital data.

THE NATURE OF IMAGES

Images can be represented in several ways. In photography for example, images are formed by focusing light onto photographic film. In conventional radiography, images are projected onto x-ray film. In addition, images can be paintings, drawings, or they can be formed by photo-electronic means as well as be represented as mathematical functions. These images are referred to as *analog images*, which means that the information they represent is changing continuously with time, compared to information available in discrete units. The sine wave is a popular representation of an analog signal.

Images obtained in the conventional radiographic mode are analog images. In digital imaging these analog images must be changed into digital data so that they can be processed by a digital computer. In effect, the analog information is "rounded out" to discrete numbers so the computer can handle it (Figure 240). Once the computer processes this information, it produces an output image in digital form as shown in Figure 241.

THE DIGITAL COMPUTER

Digital Imaging requires a digital computer. It is mandatory that the technologist understand the fundamentals of the computer in order to fully appreciate digital imaging applications in Radiology.

Hardware

The hardware refers to the physical units of the computer: the input devices, the processing system, the storage devices and

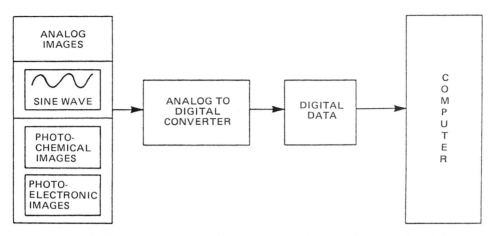

Figure 240. Block diagram showing the conversion of analog data into digital data for input into a digital computer. (From Seeram, E. *X-Ray Imaging Equipment–An Introduction.* Charles C Thomas. 1985. Reproduced by permission.)

the output devices connected as shown in Figure 242. Input devices are physical devices such as keyboards, for example, which are used to send information to the processing system. The processing system is usually referred to as they *central processing unit (CPU)* and it serves to convert the input data through a series of processing operations, into output data.

The CPU consists of two major units, the

0	0	0	0	0	0	0	0	0	0
0	0	0	11	11	11	11	0	0	0
0	0	11	11	11	11	11	11	0	0
0	11	11	11	555	555	11	11	11	0
0	11	11	555	555	555	555	11	11	0
0	11	11	555	555	555	555	11	11	0
0	11	11	11	555	555	11	11	11	0
0	0	11	11	11	11	11	11	0	0
0	0	0	11	11	11	11	0	0	0
0	0	0	0	0	0	0	0	0	0

Figure 241. Computer processing of digital input data results in information which can be displayed in digital form. In this oversimplified example, the background is assigned a numerical value of zero, soft tissue has a pixel value of 11, and the bone in the middle is assigned a value of 555.

arithmetic/logic unit (ALU) and the *control unit.* While the ALU performs arithmetic and logical operations on data, the control unit directs the flow of data between what is referred to as *primary memory* and the ALU as well as between the CPU and the input/output devices.

Primary memory is also referred to as *main memory, internal memory* and *random access memory (RAM).* These are used to store the programs and data on which the computer is presently executing. These programs and data are erasable and RAM is said to be *volatile,* which means that the information in memory is lost when the computer is turned off. In contrast to this, the computer has memory chips which contain nonerasable programs. These chips are referred to as *read only memory (ROM).*

Once the data has been processed it is now ready to be sent to an output device so that it can be of use to people. Output devices generate either *hard copy* or *soft copy* of the data. While hard copy implies that the data has been recorded in a permanent form on film, soft copy refers to a temporary display of the information on a moni-

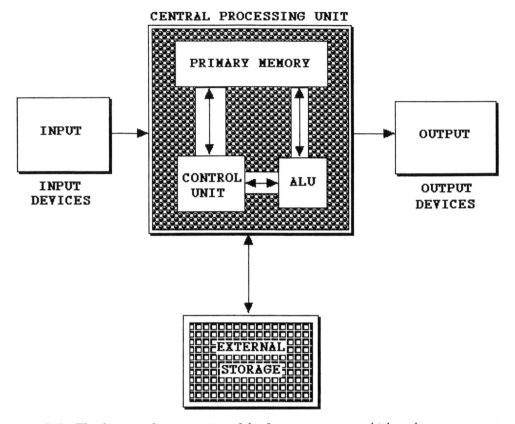

Figure 242. The functional organization of the four components which make up a computer.

tor, for example. Output devices include magnetic tapes, disks and optical disks, as well as printers, plotters and the cathode ray tube (TV monitor).

It is clear from Figure 242 that there is a flow of information from input/output devices (I/O devices) and memory to the CPU. Such flow of data is facilitated through the use of a multiwire line called a *bus.*

The final component of hardware is that of storage of information external to the computer. Such storage is referred to as *secondary storage.* Secondary storage is intended to hold large quantities of programs and data on line to the CPU. This is accomplished through the use of such devices as magnetic tapes and disks. An emerging technology to store information in

Radiology is the optical disk which uses a laser beam to write and read data. *Optical disks* make use of either a compact disk read-only memory (CD ROM), WORM (write once, read many) or fully erasable technology.

The digital computer is based on the *binary system.* This system is a two-state system; a 0-state and a 1-state. A zero or a one is referred to as *bit* (binary digit). Computers therefore use a variety of binary-based codes to represent data and programs. A series of 8-bits is referred to as a *byte* and this is used to express the storage capacity of the computer. The size of the storage is often expressed in kilobytes (thousands of bytes); Megabytes (millions of bytes); Gigabytes (billions of bytes); or in Terabytes (trillions of bytes).

Software

Software refers to computer programs. These are not physical devices but rather instructions which make the hardware components perform specific functions. There are two categories of software, *system software* and *applications software.*

In general, systems software refers to the *operating systems* which are a primary set of computer programs that coordinate the activities of the computer system. These programs perform the background tasks for people who are not only using the computer but those who are programming it as well. Popular operating systems are MS-DOS, PC-DOS, UNIX, OS/2 and Macintosh System Software. These enable applications software to be executed.

Applications software are programs that do useful work, such as scheduling, payroll and accounting, inventory control, preparing bills and budgets, managing files and databases and playing games, of course. Out of applications software has come *productivity software* which are easy-to-use program packages such as word processing, spreadsheets, graphics, database management, and communications packages.

DIGITAL IMAGE PROCESSING CONCEPTS

The processing of the digital information by the computer which performs specific operations on the data to produce images which may serve a more useful purpose is called *digital image processing*. The computer-processed information can be manipulated in a number of ways to provide benefits such as image enhancement and restoration.

DIGITIZING IMAGES

How can analog images be converted into digital information? In Figure 243 the steps in digitizing an image are shown. In the first step the image is divided up into an array of small regions by a process known as *scanning*. Each small region is referred to as a *pixel* or picture element. Scanning results in a *matrix* of numbers consisting of rows and columns. In Figure 243, the matrix formed as a result of scanning is a 9 x 11 matrix which contains 99 pixels.

The next step involves a process called *sampling*. In sampling, the brightness of each pixel is measured by using special devices such as a photomultiplier tube (PM Tube) to detect the transmitted light and convert it into an electrical signal (analog signal).

The final step in digitizing an image is *quantization*. The analog signals obtained from sampling must be converted into digital information before they can be sent to the computer. In quantization, each brightness value is assigned a discrete number (0, a positive or a negative number) called a *gray level*. An image would therefore be made up of a range of numbers or gray levels. The total number of gray levels is called the *gray scale*. Figure 243 shows a four-level gray scale as a result of quantization. An image can thus be represented in 2, 4, 8, 16, 32, 64, 128, 256, 512, or 1024 gray levels. This range of numbers is referred to as the *dynamic range* and relates to the range of numbers that each pixel can represent. For example, if a pixel can represent four shades of gray, its (pixel) dynamic range is 2-bits deep ($2^2 = 4$).

Another concept which is important to digital image processing is the conversion

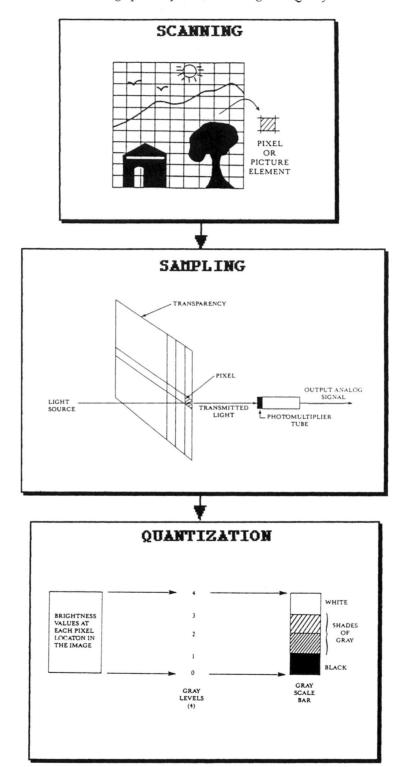

Figure 243. Three steps in digitizing any image: Scanning, sampling and quantization. (From Seeram, E. *X-Ray Imaging Equipment–An Introduction.* Charles C Thomas. (1985) Reproduced by permission.)

of analog data to digital data. This is achieved through the use of an *analog-to-digital converter (ADC)*. An important characteristic of the ADC is *accuracy* which refers to how close the digital data represents the analog signal. The range of the signal is divided up in to a number of parts of which the unit is the *bit* (binary digit). The more bits, the more accurate is the conversion. For example a 1-bit ADC divides up the analog signal into two equal parts; a 2-bit ADC will generate four equal parts (2^2); and 8-bit ADC will result in 256 parts (2^8) or 256 numbers ranging from 0-255 and representing 256 shades of gray.

Now that the computer has digital data to work with, it performs certain operations on the data to generate a numerical image. This image can be recorded on tape or disc or it can be displayed on a television monitor for viewing. For it to be displayed on the monitor, the digital image must be converted to an analog signal since the monitor works only with these signals and not digital data. For this conversion, a *digital-to-analog (DAC)* converter is required. The arrangement of the ADC and DAC are shown in Figure 244.

IMAGE PROCESSING OPERATIONS

The major advantage of digital imaging is that the computer provides the opportunity to manipulate images and convert them into a more useful form by operating on the pixel array of data (which is already in digital form). Various computer programs are available for image processing operations such as *manipulation, restoration, enhancement,* and *analysis.*

In image manipulation, the digital data can be magnified and the range of numerical data allows one to roam up and down with a display window (windowing) to change the picture contrast. In image restoration, noise and blurring can be corrected, while image enhancement improves the visual appearance of the image. Finally, image analysis allows the operator to perform measurements and other quantitative analysis on the data.

These four fundamental processes are made possible by the following image processing operations.

1. *Point Processing Operations*–These work on individual pixels in the input image to change the identical gray scale pixel in the output image. These operations make use of the histogram of the input image. A *histogram* is a bar graph plot of the number of pixels in the image that have the same gray level. By scaling the histogram appropriately, the appearance of the output image can be changed.

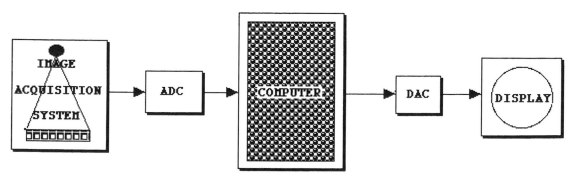

Figure 244. The general positions of the ADC and DAC in a digital imaging system.

2. *Area Processing Operations*–These work on a group of pixels in the input image rather than individual pixels, to generate an individual pixel in the output image. These processing operations are also referred to as spatial processing operations. *Convolution* is the most common form of spatial processing. These operations can also be referred to as *digital spatial filtering*, since an image can also be represented as frequencies (number of cycles per second). These frequencies can be changed to modify the output image. Two common filtering techniques are *low-pass filtering* and *high-pass filtering.*

While low-pass filtering operates on low frequencies to change them to alter the appearance of the output image (one such low-pass filter results in smoothing the image) high-pass filtering operates on high frequencies (one such filter results in *edge enhancement*).

3. *Geometric Processing Operations*–These allow the operator to magnify, minify, rotate, translate and wrap the image.

4. *Information extraction*–These allow the operator to perform quantitative analysis on the image, edge detection and image segmentation techniques.

COMPONENTS OF AN IMAGE PROCESSING SYSTEM

An image processing system consists of a minimum of three components arranged as shown in Figure 245. In a radiology image processing system, *image acquisition* consists of several different methods whereby data can be collected from the patient. Once this data is collected, it is then sent to the *image processing system.* In a digital imaging system, the processing is accomplished by computers. After processing, the output from the computer can be:

a. *displayed* on to a monitor for viewing by the technologist and radiologist
b. *stored* onto magnetic tapes, disk and/or optical disks
c. *recorded* onto film for subsequent reading by the radiologist

In some instances, images can be sent to a remote location through the marvels of communications technology. In this case, *picture archiving and communications systems (PACS)* play a vital role in transmitting images. These components will be described in the remainder of this chapter.

A DIGITAL RADIOGRAPHY SYSTEM

While Figure 245 shows a generalized

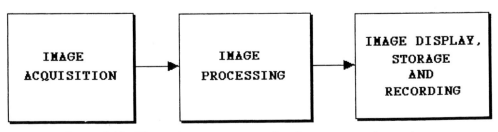

Figure 245. The major components of an image processing system.

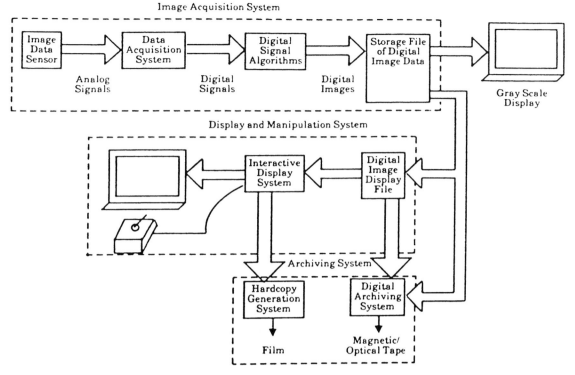

Figure 246. Elements of a digital radiography system. (From MacMillan et al. (1989) Digital Radiography. *Investigative Radiology*, 24:735-741. Reproduced by permission.)

image processing of system, Figure 246 illustrates a digital radiography system. The major components include the image acquisition system, display and manipulation system and the archiving system. Each of these will be described subsequently.

DIGITAL IMAGING APPLICATIONS IN RADIOLOGY

In imaging, the computer is used to generate images based on data collected from the patient. These applications range from Digitized Film Radiography (DFR), Digital Radiography and Fluoroscopy, Computed Tomography (CT) and Magnetic Resonance Imaging (MRI) to three dimensional imaging and PACS.

DIGITIZED FILM RADIOGRAPHY

Digitized Film Radiography (DFR) is the conversion of radiographic films into digital images. The process is shown in Figure 247. A laser beam scans the film to be digitized. The light intensity passing through the film is detected and the signal is sent to the ADC and subsequently to the computer which generates a digital image.

These images can be stored on magnetic tapes and disks and they can be enhanced and transmitted over networks. The advantages of this technology are obvious and include assisting the radiologist in making a diagnosis because the images can be digitally manipulated and they can be easi-

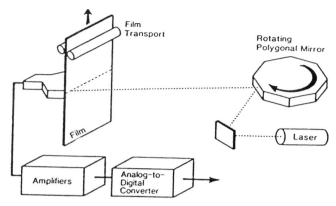

Figure 247. Digitized film radiography. See text for explanation. (From Cook et al. (1989) Digitized Film Radiography. *Investigative Radiology*, 24:910-916. Reproduced by permission.)

ly sorted, handled, and transferred.

DIGITAL PROJECTION RADIOGRAPHY SYSTEMS

Spot and Slot-Beam Systems

A digital projection radiographic system implies that the X-ray beam passes through the patient to project the anatomy on to some form of detector; as is the case with conventional film-screen radiography. Several forms of digital projection systems have been implemented. These include spot-beam imaging, slot-beam imaging, digital fluoroscopy, and photostimulable storage phosphor digital radiography.

Figure 248 shows a spot-beam configuration. These scanners utilize a point or a pencil-shaped beam to scan the patient. In

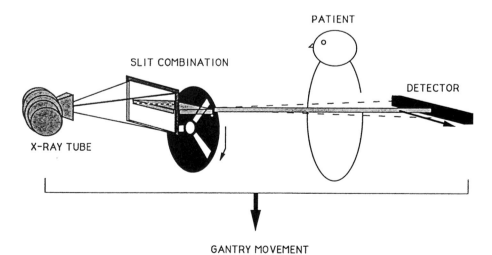

Figure 248. A "spot" beam or "pencil" beam scanner configuration. (From Greene, RE and Oestmann, JW (1992). *Computed Digital Radiography in Clinical Practice.* Thieme Medical Publishers, Inc. Reproduced by permission.)

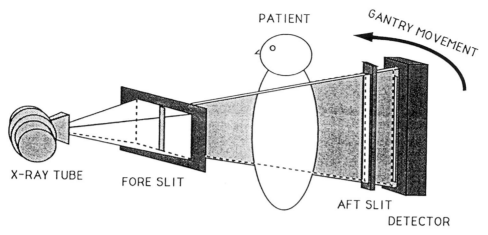

Figure 249. A "slot" beam or "fan" beam scanner configuration. (From Greene, RE and Oestmann, JW (1992). *Computed Digital Radiography in Clinical Practice.* Thieme Medical Publishers, Inc. Reproduced by permission.)

Figure 249, a slot-beam system is illustrated. Both these systems take a long time to acquire images due to the scanning nature of the beams, however, they both result in very little scattered radiation because the beams are highly collimated. In addition, the spatial resolution in these systems is low while the radiation detection efficiency is high.

DIGITAL FLUOROSCOPY

The ideas relating to Digital Fluoroscopy may be traced back to the 1970s when image intensifiers were used in a technique called *digital subtraction angiography (DSA)* which will not be discussed in this chapter. Later, with refinements in video digitizer technology, systems using image intensifiers were developed for routine use in the radiology department.

A typical digital fluoroscopy system for use in gastrointestinal and genitourinary work is shown in Figure 250 The essential components include the imaging system (X-ray tube, image intensifier, light coupling optics and the TV camera tube) data acquisition electronics (video preamplifier and A/D converter), TV digitizer, and image display and recording.

The imaging system captures the data from the patient. The TV camera tube is a high resolution tube (1023 scan lines at 60 Hz) which can operate in the interlaced and progressive scanning modes, however, the progressive scanning mode provides a higher signal-to-noise ratio which means that the image is a much sharper image compared to the image produced by interlaced scanning.

The signal leaving the TV camera is the video analog signal and it is this signal that is sent to the TV digitizer which converts it into a digital image. This digital image can be stored in the image memory and by using a computer system the image can be manipulated further. The digital data is then converted into analog signals by the D/A converter for display on a high resolution TV monitor. In addition, the digital data is then sent to a laser printer to be recorded onto X-ray film, or it can be transmitted to another location through a PACS (to be described subsequently).

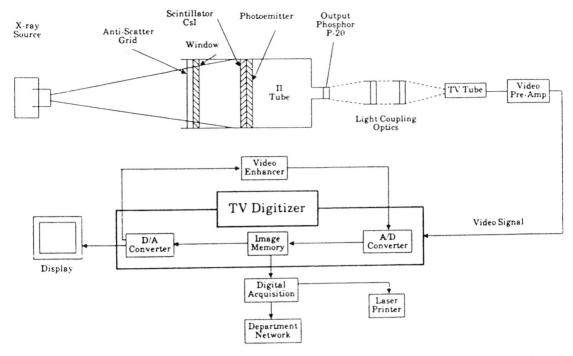

Figure 250. A digital fluoroscopic imaging system. See text for further explanation. (From MacMillan et al. (1989) Digital Radiography. *Investigative Radiology,* 24:735-741. Reproduced by permission.)

PHOTOSTIMULABLE STORAGE PHOSPHOR DIGITAL RADIOGRAPHY

Photostimulable Storage Phosphor Digital Radiography (PSPDR) was introduced as a means of replacing film/screen imaging. PSPDR is also referred to as *Scanning Laser-Stimulated Luminescence or Storage Phosphor-Based Digital Radiography.*

A Storage Phosphor-Based Digital Radiography system is illustrated in Figure 251. There are four essential components:

1. X-ray detection by an Imaging Plate (IP)
2. Laser scanning of the IP
3. Computer processing of the data from the laser scanner
4. Image recording by a laser printer and storage of the information.

The imaging plate is a flexible plate about less than 1 mm in thickness and it is coated with *barium fluorohalide* phosphor which is photostimulable, that is, during exposure electrons in the phosphor crystals are raised to a higher energy state and there they remain trapped. The plate is then scanned by a He-Ne laser which causes the trapped electrons to return to their stable state and in the process emit light. The light is converted into electrical signals which are subsequently converted into digital data fed into the computer for processing.

After processing, the digital output image can be laser-printed onto film and subsequently displayed on a gray scale display device, or it can be stored in a large volume memory such as optical disks.

Storage Phosphor-Based Systems are becoming commonplace and they are gaining widespread use in several areas in radiolo-

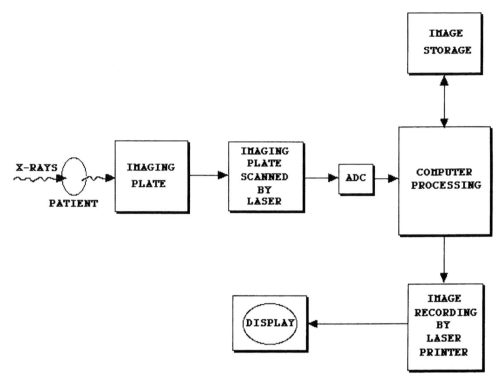

Figure 251. The general configuration of a scanning laser-stimulated luminescence x-ray system.

gy including chest and extremity imaging, mobile radiography, excretory urography and GI tract imaging.

DIGITAL IMAGE RECONSTRUCTION FROM MULTIPLE PROJECTIONS

The idea of collecting a set of X-ray transmission (attenuation) measurements from a patient and using special mathematical techniques (Fourier transformation, for example) to build up an image of a selected slice in the patient is referred to as *image reconstruction from multiple projections.* A computer is central to this process for it is used to reconstruct the image and therefore the technique is digital in nature.

Two techniques to reconstruct an image from a set of projection data are *Computed Tomography (CT)* and *Magnetic Resonance Imaging (MRI).*

Computed Tomography

CT involves at least three processes: *data collection, data processing* and *image display, recording* and *storage.*

Figure 251 illustrates these processes. First data is collected from the patient. This involves a very systematic way of having the X-ray tube scan the patient. The tube is coupled to a set of detectors which measure the relative transmission of X-rays. The analog signals from the detectors and are sent to ADCs where they are sampled and digitized.

The data is then sent to a computer which performs a mathematical technique for reconstructing the image. The image can be displayed on to a television monitor or it can be stored on magnetic tapes, disks, or optical disks. It can also be sent to a video or laser multiformat camera to be recorded on film.

The transmission measurements are converted into attenuation and thickness data and are used to calculate *CT numbers* or *Hounsfield numbers* (after the inventor).

The computed CT numbers are arranged to form an image *matrix* usually a 512 x 512 x 12-bits in which the numbers in each pixel correspond to the voxel (volume element) of the anatomy of interest in the original (scanned) slice. Each number is assigned a gray level and hence a gray scale image can be generated. The range of the CT numbers is referred to as the *window width (WW)* and the center of the range is called the *window level (WL)*. Window width and level can both be manipulated by the operator to alter the contrast and brightness or "density" of the image.

Magnetic Resonance Imaging

Magnetic Resonance Imaging (MRI) is a digital imaging technique based on Image Reconstruction principles similar to those used in CT.

Magnetic resonance, (MR) is based on the fact that when protons (magnetic dipoles) are placed in a strong magnetic field, they move from their normal random distribution and align with the magnetic field. At the same time, because they are spinning on their own axes, they begin to wobble (like a spinning top wobbles) or *precess* at a particular frequency because of the influence of the magnetic field.

This precessional frequency is the *Larmor frequency*. When exposed to radiowaves (RF) of the same frequency, the Larmor frequency, the protons absorb energy. When the the RF is turned off, the protons emit radiowaves which can be collected by a detector (antenna) and used by a computer to produce an image of the dis-

tribution of the protons in the body. Because the body is made up of mostly water, the principles of MR are used to produce images of the hydrogen nuclei (protons) in the water. This technique is Magnetic Resonance Imaging (MRI).

A block diagram of an MRI system is shown in Figure 252. The imaging process is as follows:

1. The patient is placed in the magnet. The coils in the magnet surrounds the patient.
2. The patient becomes magnetized (protons align with the magnetic field).
3. The patient is exposed to radio waves generated by the radio frequency transmitter for a short period of time.
4. The radio waves are turned off.
5. The patient emits radio waves which are detected by the receiver.
6. The receiver sends the analog signals to the ADC. Digital data is sent to the computer for processing.
7. The output from the computer is the MR image which can be stored magnetically or optically, recorded on film or displayed on a TV monitor for viewing.

As can be seen in Figure 252, the input refers to the MRI control console which allows the technologist to input all relevant parameters needed to produce, store, record and display images. Image qualities, manipulation and terminology are similar to those of CT, with *window width* representing gray scale and *window level* representing the average density or brightness.

A full discussion of CT and MRI is outside the scope of this text, and may be found in most radiologic physics books.

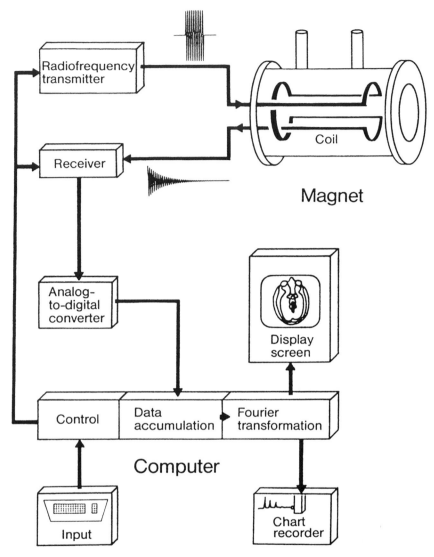

Figure 252. Block diagram of a magnetic resonance imaging system. See text for further explanation. (From Roth, K. (1984) *NMR Tomography and Spectroscopy*. Springer Verlag. Reproduced by permission.)

IMAGE TERMINOLOGY

Perhaps the most confusing aspect of computerized imaging methods for a radiographer to learn is the difference in terms used to describe the image and the equipment functions. It is particularly useful to be able to translate the terms used to describe computerized images into the more common terms used in radiography–density, contrast, noise, etc.

The primary reason that different terms are used in these computerized modalities is that these image qualities are not final but are able to be manipulated, so that there are controls on the machine to change them if desired after the image is displayed on the CRT screen. After one exposure is made, several different images may be derived, observed and permanently recorded by adjusting the center of the gray scale up or down and by adjusting the range of densities displayed to broaden or restrict it.

In digital fluoroscopy, the *center* refers to the mid-point of the gray scale displayed in the image. It might be considered as the *average* brightness level or density level and is therefore the equivalent of *density* in radiography. In computerized tomography, the same mid-density level is referred to as *window level.* Moving the center or window level adjusts all of the densities displayed up or down by an equal amount, just as changing mAs does in radiography.

The total number of different brightness levels or density levels may also be broadened or restricted, which in turn changes the ratio of difference from one density to the next. This range of brightness levels is equivalent to *gray scale* in radiography (the opposite of *contrast*). In digital fluoroscopy, it is referred to as the *window.* In computerized tomography, it is called *window width.*

APPLICATION OF TECHNIQUE

Technologists specializing in any of these areas must become familiar with the typical computer keyboard and the basic language used on computer terminals, which has several variations from a typing keyboard. To initiate a procedure, a new frame or file must be acquired from the computer, into which the technologist enters all of the pertinent demographic patient data as well as basic format and technique data for the procedure.

Electrical technique factors are entered into the computer on CT scanners but are usually set at the regular x-ray generator console for digital imaging. Digital imaging techniques are typically equal to normal radiographic techniques for the generator used. For a given anatomical part, an overhead radiographic technique may be taken from the routine technique chart for use in digital fluoroscopy rapid sequence spot exposures. All of the guidelines for optimum kilovoltage, adequate penetration for the anatomy and intensity control by milliampere-seconds discussed in Chapters 4-6 apply to digital imaging. Occasionally, higher kVp levels are required to ensure adequate flux or intensity at the detectors, in which case mAs may be adjusted downward by the 15 per cent rule, so that the *total* technique is still roughly equivalent to that of an overhead exposure. Computerized tomography scanners use equivalent techniques to radiography also but typically employ much higher kVp levels with the mAs adjusted downward according to the 15 per cent rule.

In addition to electrical technique factors, several other image variables may be predetermined in computerized imaging. The *matrix size* refers to the number of pixels, lengthwise and crosswise, which will be displayed on the CRT screen. Matrix size bears primarily upon the resolution of sharpness in the image. The greater the number of pixels to be displayed, the smaller the pixels must be to fit into the matrix. Smaller pixels result in sharper image edges, just as smaller crystals in intensifying screens and film lead to sharper edges. Each pixel is *filled* with one density level. A small matrix size with large pixels will result in a checkerboard image with very poor resolution. Therefore, the largest feasible matrix sizes, with the smallest pixels, are always the most desirable.

Magnification modes may also be selected in order to focus in on specific regions of anatomy. These usually work by changing the effective size of the input phosphor on the image intensifier tube. In other words, the useful beam is effectively collimated to the specific anatomical region, but, since the image will be displayed on the same CRT screen, it will appear magnified to fill that screen.

For digital fluorography, the camera time or *C-time* must be set to include the exposure time being used, *in addition* to a 33-millisecond lag time which the camera needs to interrogate the next frame before the next sequential exposure begins.

After the patient has been positioned for digital fluoroscopy or digital subtraction angiography, a scout frame must be taken to evaluate the adequacy of the electrical technique factors. With the *window* (gray scale) set at 1.0, an exposure is acquired into the computer memory. The *center* knob is then adjusted up and down to determine the point at which the image becomes completely blacked out. Image *blackout* should occur close to a center number specified by the equipment manufacturer. If blackout occurs at a center above this number, an increase in electrical technique is needed. If blackout occurs below this number, the kVp or mAs must be reduced. A recommended center for *white-out* is also specified by the manufacturer and may be checked.

Having evaluated the scout frame and made any necessary adjustments, the machine may be set for rapid serial framing and any injection readied. The exposure switch (many machines have a foot switch) is depressed first and then the *begin* button on the computer console is depressed to initiate the procedure. The exposure switch must be kept depressed until the exposure sequence is completed and the end button pressed. *Cine forward* or *cine reverse* buttons are used to review the exposures.

At this point, each image may be manipulated by further adjustments to the center, window, orientation (inverting or rotating), or the subtraction of any other chosen frame (see Chapter 32 for an explanation of subtraction technique). Subtraction images may be *pixel-shifted* to align the two images if slight motion has occurred. The computer can then be directed to save any of these manipulated images onto computer disks for permanent storage.

THREE DIMENSIONAL IMAGING (3-D IMAGING)

Another exciting avenue of digital imaging techniques such as CT and MRI is that of 3-D imaging. At the heart of 3-D imaging is the computer. 3-D imaging involves the use of computer programs to transform the conventional CT or MR transaxial slice data into simulated 3-D images. This is referred to as *rendering techniques*.

There are two classes of 3-D Rendering Techniques. These are:

1. Surface-based Rendering Techniques
2. Volume-based Rendering Techniques

Essentially 3-D imaging consists of:

a. *Volume formation*, where initially-acquired images are stacked to form a volume.
b. *Classification*, which determines the various tissue types present in individual voxels.
c. *Image projection*. This is the last step and it involves projecting the classified data into a 2-D or 3-D image.

It is beyond the scope of this chapter to discuss the details of 3-D imaging, however, a brief description of the two classes of rendering techniques is in order. In *surface-based rendering*, only the surface of the patient or object is demonstrated. For example, the computer program is such that given a set of numbers (digital image) it takes only the numbers corresponding to the anatomy intended to be displayed and then it carries out the 3-D reconstruction. Subsequent shading of specific pixels is done to give the illusion of depth. This perception of depth allows the image to appear in 3-D. In *volume-based rendering techniques*

not only is the surface of objects displayed but also other portions of a specified volume within the patient or object. The computer programs must also look at the numbers (values) for the other parts of the anatomy to be displayed such as bone and muscles for example. This volume is then classified and the pixels are displayed as though they are translucent, so that it is now possible to see in front and behind various tissues. 3-D imaging has found applications in radiation therapy, cranio-facial surgery, and orthopedics.

PICTURE ARCHIVING AND COMMUNICATIONS SYSTEMS (PACS)

In this chapter, several digital imaging techniques were described. The images produced by these systems can be stored on magnetic tapes and disks as well as on optical disks. This means that a system could be developed to retrieve these stored

images, display them for viewing and interpretation on a television monitor, transmit them to remote locations as well as provide archival storage. Such a system is a *Picture Archiving and Communications System (PACS)*.

The major components of a PACS is

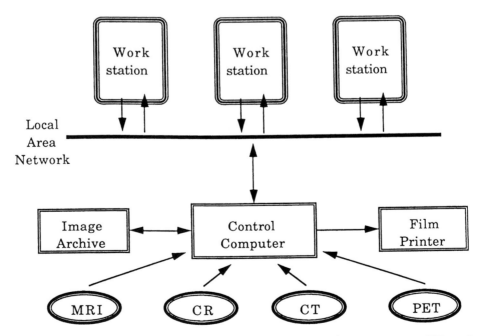

Figure 253. The essential components of a PACS. (From Greene, RE and Oestmann, JW (1992). *Computed Digital Radiography in Clinical Practice.* Thieme Medical Publishers, Inc. Reproduced by permission.)

shown in Figure 253. These include image acquisition systems, image archive, the image display work station, a control computer, and a local area network (LAN).

First, the *image acquisition devices* (MR Scanner, CT Scanner, Computed Radiographic Unit and PET Scanner) send their images to a *control computer* which stores the images (for later retrieval) onto magnetic disks, tapes and optical disks, several of which (about 100 or more) can be found stacked together in a device called an *optical jukebox.* These images can also be printed onto film by a laser printer, for example.

The important point about the control computer is that it should interface with both the Radiology Information System, (RIS) as well as the Hospital Information System (HIS).

In addition to interfacing is another important component of PACS, that is, the *image display work station.* These work stations feature a keyboard, a pointing device (mouse or trackball) and one or more display devices such as monitors. A vital function of a display monitor is that it must be a high resolution monitor (2048 x 2048 is the minimum matrix size) which would enable a radiologist to make a diagnosis. A PACS should also allow the operator/viewer to manipulate these images using such image processing operations as edge enhancement, windowing, highlighting, scrolling, zooming, and so on.

A PACS can also facilitate the transmission of images to various parts of the Hospital or within the Radiology Department. Such transmission is accomplished using *local area networks (LANS)* in which case, work stations are connected by a cable. New technologies employ fiber optic LANS. If the data is to be transferred to another building or a remote facility located in another city, for example, then *wide area networks (WANS)* will be used.

DIGITAL TELERADIOLOGY

The transmission of images at a distance has been referred to as *teleradiology.* The technology dates back to 1954 in Montreal, Canada, where two hospitals were linked together with a coaxial cable.

A typical teleradiology system is shown in Figure 254. The major components include equipment to transmit (send)

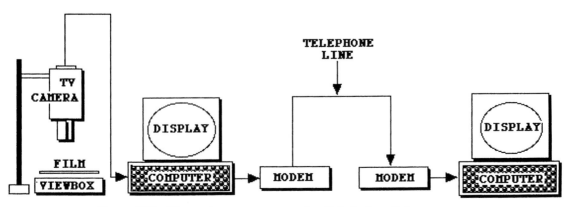

Figure 254. The major components of a digital teleradiology system.

images and equipment to receive and display these images. The transmission components include a film illuminator box with film, a video camera to capture the image on the box and a personal computer with a modem which is used to send the images through a phone line. The analog signal from the camera tube is digitized using an ADC and the digital image is stored in the computer.

The stored image is then sent to the modem (modulator-demodulator) and subsequently through the phone line at a certain speed (bits per second).

The signal from the phone line is received by another modem located at the remote site. This modem then sends the information to a microcomputer which is coupled to a monitor. The image is now ready for viewing.

Teleradiology systems have become affordable and more and more departments are beginning to acquire these systems.

CONCLUSION

Digital imaging is becoming commonplace in radiology. Already conventional radiographic equipment is being converted to digital equipment. This is evident in areas such as chest, genitourinary, gastrointestinal and even breast imaging and including CT, MRI and Digital Angiography.

The technologist must therefore make every effort now to understand these principles which will become increasingly important in the near future.

REVIEW QUESTIONS

1. What is meant by the term "digital imaging"?
2. What is an analog image and give examples of analog images.
3. Identify four devices which make up a digital computer.
4. Define the term "digital image processing"
5. What are the three steps involved in digitizing images?
6. What is the radiographic equivalent of gray level?
7. What is the radiographic equivalent of gray scale?
8. What is the difference between the ADC and the DAC?
9. Digitizing the image in a computer allows us to manipulate the image qualities _____ recording the image
   (before or after)
   permanently.
10. In digital fluoroscopy, the gray scale (contrast) range is called the:
11. In computerized tomography, the average density level is called the:
12. An image displayed on a CRT (TV) using a *small* matrix size will have _____ resolution of details.
13. Cine forward and cine reverse buttons are used to:
14. Is it possible on CT scanners to produce radiographs from different viewpoints *without* further radiation exposure, once an original series of "cuts" has been obtained?
15. How many gray levels would be generated by a 10-bit ADC?

16. Identify four image processing operations.
17. Explain the meaning of the term "digital spatial filtering."
18. How does high pass digital filtering affect the appearance of the image?
19. What are the three major components of a digital image processing system?
20. Why are films digitized in radiology?
21. List the steps involved in digitizing images in Fluoroscopy.
22. What is meant by Image Reconstruction from Projections? List two applications in the radiology department.
23. Identify two three-dimensional techniques used in radiology.
24. Explain the difference between surface-based 3-D and volume-based 3-D techniques.
25. What is PACS? Describe the major components of a PACS in radiology.
26. Define Teleradiology:
27. A digital imaging system with a dynamic range that is 4 bits deep can produce how many different shades of gray?

Part VI

PROCESSING THE RADIOGRAPH

Figure 255. Arteriogram of a 5-month-old expired fetus. Injection was made with barium sulfate.

Chapter 36

PROCESSING STEPS AND CHEMISTRY

EVEN THOUGH the efficiency of the x-ray apparatus may be high and the best exposure practice employed, the radiograph will be of inferior quality if the processing of the exposed x-ray film is carelessly or slovenly executed. The greatest error in the production of a radiograph often may be a flagrant disregard of the simplest of processing rules. Hence, one of the important operations is the processing procedure that brings about the physical and chemical changes to render visible the latent image created by the x-rays. This procedure requires the assistance of photographic chemistry.

STEPS IN PROCESSING PROCEDURE

Processing x-ray film to a radiograph involves at least six procedures:

1. Storing and Handling X-ray Film

The proper storage and handling of x-ray film is an important aspect of radiography. Since film is a delicate material, the manner in which it is stored and handled determines whether the radiograph will be free of artifacts.

2. Mixing and Replenishing Solutions

The manner in which the various chemical solutions used in processing are mixed and replenished (replaced) is important, since good quality radiographs are only produced when these solutions operate efficiently. Recommended methods for mixing and rates of replenishment should be carefully followed.

3. Development Process

Development of the x-ray film changes the silver bromide crystals containing the latent image to black metallic silver that constitutes the visible image. The solution used to effect this change is called a developer.

4. Fixing Process

The fixing process involves two activities and is the procedure for removing the unexposed and undeveloped silver bromide from the emulsion and for hardening the soft gelatin emulsion containing the metallic silver image. The chemical solution employed for these purposes is known as the fixing solution.

5. Washing Process

Washing is the process whereby the soluble fixing bath and silver salts are removed from the film emulsion by means of clean, flowing water.

6. Drying Process

Drying is the treatment of drying the wet radiographs for permanency and for use by the radiologist.

All of these processes must be completed in some fashion, whether using automatic processors or manual processing technique, to fully develop a radiographic image which may be preserved in a relatively permanent manner. Processing centers around the chemical interactions of the developing and fixing processes. Before discussing the specific procedures for automatic and manual processing, a basic understanding of the chemical constituents and functions of the developing and fixing solutions is necessary.

DEVELOPER CONSTITUENTS

Conversion of the silver bromide to metallic silver must be accomplished by the many chemicals contained in the developing solution and it is necessary that the developer formula be standardized with all chemicals in balance so that the results will always be the same. Each film manufacturer recommends formulae that produce the best results with that manufacturer's film.

An x-ray developer usually contains six types of ingredients (Table XXXV).

1. Solvent. Chemical reactions that occur in development require that all chemicals be dissolved in water. Besides acting as a solvent for the chemicals and as a means for their ionization, water aids in softening the gelatin emulsion.

2. Reducers. The purpose of a reducing agent is to convert the exposed silver bromide crystals to black metallic silver. A reducing agent cannot be a developer unless it reacts more rapidly with *exposed* silver bromide crystals than those that are unexposed. However, the exposure must be of a degree that will cause a satisfactory image to be formed in a given development period at a given temperature. In a properly exposed radiograph, this action is usually completed upon full development and *before* the unexposed crystals have an opportunity to develop to any perceptible degree. Reducing agents commonly employed are elon, metol, phenidone and hydroquinone.

Elon or *metol* is used only in manual developer solution. Their function is to develop the medium-range gray tones of the image, providing image scale. These gray densities are developed quickly, in the first one-half of the developing time. Manual developer is often called *MQ developer*. The abbreviation refers to the metol (M) and the hydroquinone (Q) which typically make up manual developer. Both metol and elon are unpredictable in their chemical action at temperatures above 75° Fahrenheit (24° C). Since automatic processing utilizes high temperatures to shorten processing time, a more reliable chemical had to be found for use at these temperatures.

Phenidone replaces elon or metol as the functional agent for developing the gray tones and radiographic scale of the image in automatic processing. For this reason, automatic developer solution is often referred to as *PQ developer* (phenidone-hydroquinone). Phenidone is designed for reliable and predictable functioning at the high temperatures (84-98°) used in auto-

TABLE XXXV

Constituents of an X-ray Developing Solution and Their Functions

Chemical	General Function	Specific Function	
Phenidone (automatic), Elon or Metol (manual)	Developing or reducing agents.	Builds up gray densities quickly in first half of development period.	Developing agents reduce exposed silver bromide crystals in emulsion to black metallic silver constituting the image.
Hydroquinone		Builds up contrast slowly during development period.	
Sodium sulfite	Preservative	Prevents rapid oxidation of developer.	
Sodium carbonate	Alkali or activator	Governs reducing activities of developing agents; provides necessary alkaline medium and swells gelatin emulsion so that reducing agents can attack exposed silver bromide crystals.	
Potassium bromide	Restrainer	Controls activity of reducing agents and tends to prevent fog.	
Glutaraldehyde (automatic only)	Hardener	Controls the swelling and softening activity of the alkali, so that the emulsion is not torn off by sticking to automatic rollers.	
Water	Solvent	Provides medium into which the other chemicals may be dissolved in solution.	

matic processors.

Hydroquinone is employed in both automatic PQ and manual MQ developing solutions. Its function is to develop the maximum densities in the image, bringing out the *blacks* of the image. Thus, it is responsible for the full development of the image contrast. Hydroquinone acts upon the silver bromide crystals in the emulsion at a very slow rate, requiring the full development time to complete its function. For this reason, films which are immersed in the developer solution for too short a time demonstrate a loss of contrast and a *washed-out* appearance. The activity of these chemicals requires their presence in an alkaline* solution. Together, the reduc-

ers produce an image with satisfactory contrast in a minimum of time provided the temperature of the solution remains in the optimum range. Reducers are not stable in the presence of oxygen, for they can readily absorb it from the air or the water.

3. Activator. The *activator* or alkali *softens* the gelatin of the emulsion and provides the necessary alkaline medium to the solution, so that the developing agents can diffuse into the gelatin emulsion and attack the exposed silver bromide crystals. In general, the more alkaline the developer the more powerful and rapid is its action. The chemicals most frequently used are sodium carbonate and kodalk.

Sodium Carbonate. Sodium carbonate is the alkali usually found in regular x-ray developer. It has been used for many years but there are some disadvantages to be recognized in its use. When a film is

---

*In chemistry, there are two types of solutions—alkaline and acid. Developers are usually alkaline in solution: and fixers , acid in solution.

processed in a warm x-ray developer containing sodium carbonate and then transferred to a cool acid fixing bath, tiny bubbles of carbon dioxide gas may form in the soft gelatin. As the bubbles escape, they form tiny craters or pits in the emulsion thereby breaking up the normal character of the silver image. The finished film or radiograph then is said to have been blistered. To overcome this occurrence when sodium carbonate developers are employed, the temperatures of developer, rinse, and fixer solutions should be approximately the same.

Kodalk. Kodalk is a highly alkaline chemical activator (sodium metaborate) found in rapid x-ray developer. It has the same function as sodium carbonate. It is more capable of being used when high temperatures are encountered since it does not cause gas formation in the emulsion when the film is immersed in a cooler fixer. It is the most efficient activator available today.

4. Preservative. The function of the preservative is to retard the activity of the reducing agents to within controlled limits so that the "life" of the developing solution is maintained over a reasonable period of time. As mentioned previously, the reducing agents react quickly with oxygen and if this reaction is not controlled, the developing solution would not last very long. The chemical, *sodium sulfite*, is used as a preservative since it serves to retard oxidation of the reducing agents and prevents the formation of stain on the film. It has an affinity for oxygen and reacts with the oxygen of the air or solution forming sodium sulfate thereby extending the life of the reducing agents.

5. Restrainer. The restrainer is employed to limit the action of the reducing agents to the breaking up of the *exposed* silver bromide crystals only, without attacking the unexposed crystals in the emulsion

during the normal course of development. This function is quite important if a satisfactory image is to be produced, for if the restrainer is omitted the unexposed crystals would also develop, and a veil of "fog" (silver deposit) would be deposited over the image. *Potassium bromide* is, therefore, added to the developing solution as a restrainer.

However, the restrainer need only be added when mixing the *initial* batch of developer solution from which the deep tanks in the processor or manual tank will be filled. The restrainer is not included in the replenishment solution. The active restraining ingredient is the bromine. Each time a film is developed, bromine from the silver bromide in the emulsion is deposited into the developer solution, leaving only silver on the film. Therefore, the active restraining ingredient is automatically replenished as films are developed, and bromine is not needed in replenishment solutions. Because it is only used when mixing the initial batch of developer, the restrainer is often referred to as *starting solution* or *starter.*

6. Hardener. A hardener must be added to automatic PQ developer solution in order to control the action of the alkali and water, which soften and swell the emulsion so that the developing agents can penetrate into it and act on the crystals. Without the hardener, the emulsion becomes so soft that it will stick to the automatic processor rollers, peeling off and damaging the film. Gluteraldehyde is the chemical commonly used as the hardener for automatic developer solutions. It is not necessary for manual development because the films do not touch any surfaces during manual processing.

Table XXXV summarizes the functions of the various chemicals in developer solution.

REDUCTION AND OXIDATION

The "active ingredients" for developer solution are called *reducers* because this word describes the chemical action they have upon the silver atoms in the film emulsion. While these chemicals *reduce* the silver bromide in the film, the film *oxidizes* the developer solution.

A chemical compound is reduced when another chemical *donates electrons* to it. A compound is oxidized when electrons are *removed* from it by another chemical. So, reduction and oxidation are really mirror images of each other, and always occur together.

In the process of chemical development, the reducing agents donate electrons to the silver bromide crystals in the film emulsion. Silver ions (Ag^+) are thus electrically neutralized to form silver atoms, as shown in the following basic chemical equation:

$$Ag+ \quad + electron \quad \rightarrow \quad Ag$$

Silver   Silver
ion   atom

It is said that the silver ions have been *reduced* into black metallic silver. The same interaction may be thought of as the silver ions *removing* electrons from the solution. The developer solution is *oxidized* by the film, and thus becomes chemically weaker as it is used. The oxygen in normal room air also tends to "steal" electrons from the developer solution over a period of time, and processing chemicals must be protected from exposure to air as much as possible in order to preserve their effectiveness. Thus, developer solution becomes oxidized and weakened *both* by room air and by the films passing through it, and it must be chemically replenished to maintain its useful strength.

Since reducing agents in the developer solution contribute electrons to the silver ions in each exposed silver bromide crystal, these silver ions become neutral and are no longer tonically attracted to the bromine atoms in the crystal (see Figure 127 in Chapter 15). The chemical bonds between the silver and the bromine are broken by the reducing agents. The bromine atoms are attracted by other chemicals in the developer solution and they migrate out of the film emulsion into the solution.

The silver atoms, remaining in the emulsion, coagulate or "clump" together with the partial silver deposit already formed by radiation exposure at the sensitivity speck site, as described in Chapter 15. Continued build-up of silver at exposure centers produces the final visible or manifest image.

FIXER CONSTITUENTS

The constituents of a fixing solution and their functions in the fixation process are as follows, Table XXXVI:

1. **Solvent.** The solvent employed in mixing the chemicals of a fixing solution is *water*.

2. **Acidifier.** *Acid* serves a double purpose for it permits the use of potassium alum as a hardening agent and neutralizes any alkaline developer that may be carried over from the developing solution.

This latter action quickly stops development and prevents the formation of stain. The acid usually employed is *acetic acid*.

3. **Clearing Agent.** The function of the *clearing agent* is to change the residual unexposed and undeveloped silver bromide crystals in the emulsion to soluble silver

TABLE XXXVI

Constituents of an X-ray Fixing Bath and Their Functions

Chemical	General Function	Specific Function
Ammonium thiosulfate (hypo)	Clearing Agent	Dissolves unexposed silver bromide crystals. Does not affect reduced metallic silver of image.
Sodium sulfite	Preservative	Maintains equilibrium of chemicals in solution.
Aluminum chloride or potassium Alum	Hardening Agent	Shrinks and hardens emulsion.
Acetic Acid	Acidifier	Provides acid medium and neutralizes developer carried over in film.
Water	Solvent	Provides medium into which the other chemicals may be dissolved in solution.

Figure 256. Radiograph exhibiting areas of translucence caused by fixer splash on film prior to development. The fixer dissolved out the silver emulsion.

salts that are readily removed by washing the film in water. This is accomplished without damage to the silver image. If the film is not properly cleared, the remaining silver bromide crystals will darken on exposure to light and obscure the radiographic image. The usual chemical employed for this purpose is *ammonium thiosulfate* or sodium thiosulfate—commonly known as "hypo." The clearing action involves a chemical reaction between the sodium or ammonium thiosulfate and silver bromide in the emulsion wherein silver thiosulfate is formed and remains in solution.

4. Hardening Agent. The *hardening agent* is used to decrease the possibility of physical injury to the gelatin emulsion. A swollen emulsion is easily scratched or distorted by physical means during the washing and drying processes. The hardener restrains swelling of the gelatin and hardens it so that it can withstand the normal effects of processing. The hardener also helps reshrink the emulsion to its original thickness. The hardened emulsion is protected from injury after development is completed, as a small portion of the hardener is retained by the emulsion. The two most common chemicals used as hardeners in the fixing solution are aluminum chloride and potassium alum. Chrome alum or aluminum sulfide may also be used.

5. Preservative. The *preservative* prevents decomposition of the clearing agent by the acid with a resultant precipitation of sulfur at normal temperatures. It assists in clearing the film and prevents the residual developer carrier over in the film from oxidizing and discoloring the fixing bath. The chemical used is *sodium sulfite*.

The constituents of fixer are the same for both automatic and manual solutions. They are summarized in Table XXXVI.

Developer solution is a relatively strong alkaline chemical, while fixer solution is a fairly weak acid, which accounts for their strong odors. Alkalis and acids are chemical opposites. When mixed together, they neutralize each other's chemical activity. When handling them, care must be taken not to splash fixer solution into developer tanks or containers and vice versa. Figure 256 demonstrates how splashing fixer solution (or any other chemical, including water) onto a film prior to processing can have a deleterious effect.

SUMMARY

1. The *development* process is designed to reduce exposed areas on the radiograph to black metallic silver, clear off of the film the unexposed silver bromide crystals, and harden and fix the permanent image for preservation.
2. *Developer* solution consists of solvent, reducers, an activator, a preservative, restrainer if it is a fresh batch, and a hardener if it is automatic solution.
3. *Fixer* solution consists of solvent, a clearing agent, an acidifier, a hardener and a preservative.
4. *PQ developer* is used in automatic processing. Its reducers are phenidone and hydroquinone, and it includes a hardening agent, gluteraldehyde, to prevent film from sticking to rollers. *MQ developer*, usually containing metol and hydroquinone as reducers, is used for manual processing.
5. Chemical *reduction* occurs when a compound gains electrons from some other compound. *Oxidation* is the loss of electrons. Developer solution is oxidized as it reduces the film emulsion.

REVIEW QUESTIONS

1. What is the function gluteraldehyde and why is it used in automatic developer solution?
2. When is "PQ" developer used?
3. Why isn't potassium bromide included in *replenisher* solution for the developer? What are the two purposes of the "fixing" process?
4. What is the solvent for *both* developer and fixer solution?
5. Which solution, developer or fixer, is a relatively weak acid?
7. Which densities become visible in the first few seconds of development, the grays (gray scale) or the blacks (D-max) (maximum densities)?
8. Define "clearing" *and* state which chemical performs this function.
9. As developer solution reduces the film, what does the film do to the solution?
10. When a compound *gains* electrons from some other chemical, it undergoes _____.

Chapter 37

DEVELOPMENT VARIABLES

THE PURPOSE of development is to convert chemically the invisible latent image to the visible silver image by means of a developer solution. In the conversion of the exposed silver bromide crystals to metallic silver, the film is immersed in an alkaline developer solution that softens and swells the gelatin so that ionization of the exposed silver bromide crystals occurs and the reducing agents transform the silver ions into clumps of black metallic silver. The unexposed silver bromide is unaffected by this treatment during the development period required by the exposed crystals.

INFLUENCE OF DEVELOPMENT TIME

The time of development given to an exposed x-ray film materially affects the amount of silver deposited on the radiograph. As the time of development increases up to a certain point, the amount of silver deposit increases; as the time decreases, the quantity decreases. In general, the time required to develop a film in a given developer depends upon the emulsion and its thickness. The influence of the *time* of development on the latent image at a given temperature is illustrated in Figure 257. A series of ten (10) correctly exposed hand radiographs was made employing identical x-ray exposure factors. Films were developed manually at one-minute intervals at a constant temperature of 68°F. in *regular* x-ray developer, Figure 257.

1. Radiograph 1, developed for 1 minute, shows only slight traces of silver deposit. Image detail is lacking and the contrast is low. Note the streaked background density which is characteristic of the underdeveloped radiograph.

2. No. 2, developed for 2 minutes, shows some of the important features of the image and a greater overall deposit of silver may be noted. Image detail and contrast are somewhat improved.

3. No. 3, developed for 3 minutes, shows more silver deposited but the image is still somewhat weak.

4. No. 4, developed for 4 minutes, shows a fairly well defined image.

5. No. 5, developed for 5 minutes, shows all essential details, for the maximum practical amount of silver has been deposited on the film. The x-ray exposure was such as to provide a satisfactory image when developed for 5 minutes. The amount of silver deposit with longer development times, however, is not sufficient to justify extension of the development time beyond the basic 5-minute period.

6. Nos. 6-10, developed for 6 to 10 minutes, show little gain in density.

Figure 257. Radiographs manually processed in regular developer solution for 1 to 10 minutes at 68 degrees F. The number of minutes of development time is marked on each film.

Figure 258. (*Top*) Radiographs developed for the same period of time, but with increasing solution temperatures from left to right, showing: (A) 60 degrees, (B) 68 degrees, (C) 75 degrees and (D) 80 degrees. Note increased density due to higher temperatures. (*Bottom*) Radiographs developed at the same temperatures as above, increasing left to right, but with corresponding reductions in development time to compensate: (A) 8.5 minutes, (B) 5 minutes, (C) 3.5 minutes and (D) 2 minutes. Note balancing of densities.

INFLUENCE OF DEVELOPER SOLUTION TEMPERATURE

Chemical reactions are stimulated or retarded with temperature. Since processing is essentially a series of chemical reactions, the temperature of the solutions assumes major importance. Variations in temperature require adjustment in the development time factor so that uniform densities may be maintained. Temperatures should never be estimated and a good thermometer is essential to determine the correct solution temperature.

The influence of developer *temperature* on the density of the radiograph is demonstrated in a series of radiographs of the hand, Figure 258, Top, when times of exposure and development are held constant.

1. Radiograph A was developed for 5 minutes at 60°F. Note the weak image and the lack of silver deposit (density), as well as the low contrast within the image.

2. Radiograph B was correctly developed for 5 minutes at 68°F. Note the satisfactory gradation of densities and contrast of the image.

3. Radiograph C was developed for 5 minutes at 75°F. Note the higher density.

4. Radiograph D was developed for 5 minutes at 80°F. Note the excessive density of the image. The presence of excessive density and fog tends to produce unsatisfactory radiographic quality.

In Figure 258, bottom, radiographs D-F demonstrate that temperature differences require adjustment of the development time to secure comparable densities. These radiographs exhibit approximately the same overall density.

1. Radiograph A was developed at 60°F. for $8^{1}/2$ minutes. Note that density is almost comparable to that of radiograph B.

2. Radiograph B was developed for 5 minutes at 68°F. and exhibits normal density and contrast.

3. Radiograph C was developed for $3^{1}/2$ minutes at 75°F. and is comparable to B.

4. Radiograph D was developed for 2 minutes at 80°F. Note that the image is fairly comparable to B, yet a slightly higher density is present because of the greater activity of the developer at this temperature and, as the solution ages, chemical fog would accrue to increase the density.

TIME COMPENSATION FOR TEMPERATURE CHANGES

Although manual solutions should be maintained at the optimum of 68°F., for the best quality, there are occasions when it is necessary to process films at other temperatures. Some compensation can be made for temperature variations *within limits* by increasing or decreasing the time of development. For higher temperatures, shorter developing times are necessary to maintain uniform radiographic density. The ideal method is to employ the time-temperature system that accurately compensates for temperature differences with the correct time of development. It is true that x-ray film may be manually developed satisfactorily without special treatment at any temperature between 60° and 75° as long as the temperature differences are compensated by appropriate development times. The lower temperatures in this optimum range require longer development times and the higher temperatures, although permitting shorter development times, are closer to the zone where processing defects may begin to appear on the radiograph. Generally, a change of 2° will change the resulting density by 15 per cent.

Figure 259 demonstrates how extreme solution temperatures can melt film emulsion.

INFLUENCE OF DEVELOPER SOLUTION CONCENTRATION

If developer solution is initially mixed to be too weak from excessive dilution with water or from inadequate amounts of active ingredients, the darker black areas of the radiograph will fail to be fully developed in the standard time. Therefore, not only will

Figure 259. Radiograph exhibiting melted emulsion from excessively high temperature processing.

oped, and the finished radiograph has a washed-out, noncontrasty appearance.

At the ideal concentration level, attained by carefully following the manufacturer's directions in mixing the solution components, optimum contrast levels and medium overall density will be achieved.

The solution may become too concentrated from high levels of evaporation of the water when excessive ambient temperatures are present or when it is allowed to sit uncovered for extended periods of time. Hyperconcentration can also occur from improper mixing. A developer solution which is too strong will attack the *unexposed* silver bromide crystals in the film emulsion as well as the exposed crystals, so that areas that should have demonstrated a white or clear shade will develop to a gray shade, and information will be lost from the ensuing lack of contrast.

When the film is overdeveloped because of hyperconcentrated solution, the resultant loss of image contrast is referred to as *chemical fog.* It will be recalled that a fogged film can either appear too light or too dark. Either the failure to develop the very dark areas of the radiograph or the very light areas of the radiograph results in a loss of recorded information. For this reason, optimum concentration levels must be carefully monitored in the darkroom.

insufficient density develop in the image but also image contrast will be low because of the lack of dark black shades. The same effect occurs when solution is weakened due to contamination from fixer solution or other chemicals, or due to exhaustion from air oxidation or unreplenished usage. Only the lighter-gray shades are devel-

FIXING PROCESS

The development process reduces only a portion of the silver bromide emulsion to metallic silver. The remaining unused silver bromide must be removed, for it would impair the diagnostic and photographic character of the silver image. Subsequent chemical treatment known as the fixing process serves to *clear* the film of this unwanted silver bromide without damage

to the image and, to *harden* the gelatin emulsion.

When the film is placed in the fixing solution it is milky in appearance because of the residual unexposed and undeveloped silver bromide crystals but, as it is moderately agitated until both film surfaces are completely bathed by the solution, this milkiness gradually disappears. The action of the acidifier immediately neutralizes the residual alkaline developer and any continuing development action ceases. Since the gelatin is still swollen and porous, the clearing agent dissolves out the unexposed and undeveloped silver bromide crystals, leaving untouched the developed silver image. This is the *clearing action.* As clearing abates, the *hardening action* begins, resulting in shrinking and hardening of the gelatin emulsion containing the silver image. This hardening action is most important, since it prevents swelling of the emulsion to any marked degree in the later washing operation. It is advisable not to turn on the white light in the processing room until the film is entirely clear; otherwise it will become fogged.

INFLUENCE OF FIXER SOLUTION TEMPERATURE

As with most chemical reactions, the higher the temperature the greater the speed of fixation; the lower the temperature, the slower the speed of fixation. In fixer solutions, however, there is an optimum range of temperatures that should be used. With higher temperatures, a fixing solution tends to sulfurize thereby shortening its life. It must, therefore, be specially treated when high temperatures prevail.

INFLUENCE OF FIXATION TIME

The duration of fixation is dependent upon several factors, such as the strength and nature of the fixer employed; the temperature of the solution; the amount of film agitation; the volume of fixing solution as related to the number or surface area of the films being fixed; and the emulsion thickness. The total *fixing time* is made up of the duration of time needed to *clear* the film and that required to harden the film. For manual processing, the film should remain in the fixing bath at least for *twice* the time necessary to clear the film.

INFLUENCE OF FIXER CONCENTRATION

Alterations in the chemical concentration of the fixer solution have essentially the same effects upon the film as the corresponding changes in fixer solution temperature or fixation time. The fixation process is not a controlling factor over the essential image qualities of density, contrast, and geometrical integrity. The clearing portion of the cycle is necessary for the removal of the image *noise* which would result from failure to strip the unexposed areas of the emulsion from the film, leaving various possible artifacts. The fixing portion of the cycle is exclusively designed to ensure adequate protection and preservation of the permanent image.

Insufficient fixer concentration can result from improper solution mixing, either inadequate amounts of water or too much active ingredients. Exhaustion of the solution can occur from air oxidation when the solution is left uncovered for extended periods of time or from unreplenished usage. Insufficient fixation can leave the film emulsion sticky or wet and thus result in emulsion damage when handled. It can also result in some of the developer solution being left in the emulsion, which may demonstrate a *milky* appearance or turn the emulsion brown or yellow.

Too much fixer concentration, resulting from improper mixing or from evaporation of the water in the solution, can make the film too brittle. The emulsion would then begin to crack and deteriorate with handling and storage.

Optimum fixer concentration must be monitored to ensure a long lifetime for the permanent image. Otherwise, film damage can result which can have serious medical and legal implications.

TYPES OF IMAGE QUALITIES AFFECTED

It should be noted that all of the discussion concerning the effects of developmental variables upon the radiographic image is limited to the *visibility* functions–density, contrast and noise. The entire development process is devoid of geometrical factors. Therefore, the processing of the radiograph cannot and does not have any bearing upon the recognizability functions of the image. It has no effect upon sharpness of recorded detail, magnification or distortion.

SUMMARY

1. Increasing development *time* increases image density. It also increases image contrast to a certain point, beyond which excessive development time will turn the entire film black, destroying contrast.
2. Increasing developer solution *temperature* increases image density. It also increases image contrast to a certain optimum level, beyond which excessive temperatures chemically fog the film, destroying contrast.
3. A 10° temperature change can be *compensated* for by adjusting development time by a factor of 2. A 2° temperature change can be compensated with a 15 per cent adjustment in development time.

4. Increasing chemical *concentration* of the developer solution increases image density. It also increases image contrast to a certain optimum level, beyond which excessive concentration chemically fogs the film, destroying contrast.
5. Insufficient *fixation* time, temperature or chemical concentration can result in emulsion damage and discoloration. Excessive fixation time, temperature or chemical concentration makes the film too brittle. In either case, the archival life of the radiograph is lost and artifacts may result.
6. Film processing has no relation to geometrical or recognizability functions in the image.

REVIEW QUESTIONS

1. How will excessive development time, temperature or concentration (replenishment) affect image *contrast*?
2. The standard development time and temperature for a particular facility is 60 seconds at 68°F. If the solution temperature should climb to 74°F, how long should you develop?
3. Over-fixation (or inadequate washing) will cause what problem in preserving the radiograph?
4. At solution temperatures below 60°F, which reducer fails to function properly?

Chapter 38

AUTOMATIC PROCESSORS

THE FIRST FULLY AUTOMATIC processing systems were announced in 1957. An electromechanical transport system used a series of rollers to immerse the film into and through the development tank so that the time of development became a standard factor based upon the speed at which the rollers turned. The same system then transported the film from one tank to the next and finally through a blow-dryer compartment. An electrical thermostat and heating system allowed for a self-correcting high temperature to be maintained in the solutions so that development time could be dramatically reduced. Because of the high temperatures, the chemical *phenidone* replaced metol or elon as the reducing agent designed to develop the gray scale in the image. Metol and elon become unpredictable at high temperatures. Hydroquinone was still used to develop the maximum densities in the image, so that the automatic developer solution came to be known as *PQ* (phenidone-hydroquinone) developer. The most serious problem to overcome was that the softened emulsion making contact with the rollers would stick to them and be pulled off of the film. This was resolved by adding a precise amount of the hardener *gluteraldehyde* to the automatic developer solution. The gluteraldehyde counterbalances the effect of the activator, so that the emulsion is allowed to swell and soften enough for adequate penetration of the developer chemicals into the emulsion, yet not so much as to stick to the rollers.

With time and temperature both stabilized, replenishment of the solution concentration became the primary variable in controlling image quality. Electromechanical replenishment pumps were connected to reserve solution tanks, allowing a precise rate of replenishment to be established as films were detected passing through the feed rollers. This replenishment rate could be increased or decreased to control image quality.

The resulting advantages of automatic processing were dramatic in magnitude: First, processing time was greatly reduced. While older processors required seven minutes for the entire cycle from development to drying to be completed, modern processors produce dry films in 1-4 minutes, depending on the type. Second, because the processor monitors its own internal environment, maintaining temperature, circulation, concentration and time, the quality control of radiographic images was vastly improved. In short, more consistent results are obtained in much less time.

Although some portions of an automatic processor should not be tampered with by radiographers who have no training in electronics, radiographers should understand enough about automatic processors to be able to diagnose problems and make minor corrections and repairs.

There are five interrelated electromechanical systems in the automatic processor which provide all of the functions of manual processing. They include

Figure 260. Diagram of automatic processor components.

the transport system, the circulation/filtration system, the replenishment system, the tempering system and the drying system.

A diagram of the main components of an automatic processor is provided in Figure 260. The path of the film is shown as it enters from the feed tray and is directed by the various rollers and guide shoes of the transport system through the development tank, the fixing tank, the wash tank and finally the dryer compartment. Parts of the circulation/filtration and tempering systems can be seen at the bottom of the diagram. Also, note the tubes from the replenishment system coming into the developer and fixer tanks at the bottom. You may wish to refer to this diagram frequently as you read the following sections.

THE TRANSPORT SYSTEM

All of the rollers in the automatic processor are interconnected with drive chains, elastic drive belts or intermeshing gears so that all turn at exactly the same rate. The entire transport system is driven by a master drive shaft consisting of several worm-gears (Figure 261). This drive shaft is turned by a small motor, to which it is connected by a drive chain (Figure 262). The rollers are arranged into four different types of racks.

The *detection rack* or *feed rack* is the first rack of rollers that the film comes into contact with as it is slid in from the feed tray (Figure 260). It typically consists of two ribbed detection rollers and a guide shoe plate which turns the film downward into

Figure 261. Automatic processor main drive shaft pointing out worm gears used to turn all of the racks of rollers to transport the film.

Figure 262. Drive motor and chain for automatic processor transport system.

the development tank. As the film is pulled between the detection rollers, it separates them, pushing one upward. The movable roller is connected to a microswitch on each end, so that when the film separates the rollers, the microswitch is also separated from its counterpart on the wall of the processor (Figure 263). When the microswitch is separated, the replenishment system is activated to pump fresh replenisher solution into both the developer and fixer tanks. As soon as the film pass-

es through the detection rollers, the upper one falls back down from gravity plus the magnetic attraction of the microswitch, and the switch closes to shut off the replenishment system. Hence, the longer the film being fed into the processor, the longer the replenishment system will be activated. In this way, the actual replenishment is kept roughly proportional to the total film area being processed on a daily basis. If the detection rollers were flat, the thin film would not be able to separate them sufficiently to activate the microswitch. By using ribbed rollers, the separation effect of the film is exaggerated so that the microswitch will work (Figure 264).

The *deep racks* (used in the developer, fixer and wash tanks) consist of alternating phenolic (compressed paper and resin) rollers designed to smoothly transport the film through the tank. At the bottom of each rack, the film direction is reversed by the use of a large phenolic roller and guide shoes. The guide shoes are ribbed to prevent wet film from sticking to a flat surface and jamming up in the processor. For each deep rack, the large roller at the bottom is frequently called the *solar* roller and the smaller ones are called *planetary* rollers, comparing them with the sun and its smaller planets.

At the end of each deep rack is a set of *squeegee* rollers set flush against each other

and typically consisting of one metallic roller and one rubber roller or two rubber rollers (Figures 260 and 265). The squeegee rollers are necessary to prevent excessive amounts of solution from being carried by the film over into the next tank or, in the case of the wash rack, to prevent excess moisture on the film as it enters the drying system. Thus, the squeegee rollers replace the manual function of draining the films before placing them in the next tank.

Crossover racks consist commonly of a pair of phenolic rollers and two guide shoes (Figures 260 and 266) and are designed to transport the film from one deep tank into the next, making a 180-degree turn.

Finally, the *dryer rollers*, usually phenolic, are alternated to transport the film through the blow-dryer system with maximum surface exposure to the drying air and deposit it in the external catch bin.

Figure 263. Detection rack showing ribbed rollers which separate when film is fed through them to activate replenishment pump microswitch (arrow).

FILM

Figure 264. Diagram of exaggerated separation of ribbed detection rollers when a film is fed into an automatic processor which is necessary to sufficiently move the replenishment microswitch .

Figure 265. Deep solution tank rack showing pair of (lighter colored) squeegee rollers at film exit point.

Figure 266. Crossover rack with ribbed guide shoes to turn film from one deep tank into the next.

THE CIRCULATION/ FILTRATION SYSTEM

Both the developer and the fixer solutions must be constantly circulated through the deep tanks to ensure even coverage across the film emulsion and eliminate air bubbles clinging to the film. The circulation system replaces the manual function of agitation. Further, it ensures consistent development of films run through both the right and the left sides of the tanks by constantly stirring the solution. The proper circulation is provided by separate pumping systems attached to the developer and the fixer tanks (Figure 267). A filter may also be added to the circulation lines for the purpose of cleaning out emulsion gelatin particles, dirt, foreign particles and algae (Figure 268). The thermostat and heater of the tempering system may also be found within the circulation lines (Figure 269).

Figure 260 illustrates only the circulation line for the developer tank, with filter, pump and heater. After heating, the line

Figure 267. Circulation pumps for developer and fixer lines in an automatic processor.

Figure 268. Filter placed in developer line to remove debris.

passes through the bottom of the fixer tank, serving as a heat exchanger so that the fixer solution temperature is maintained slightly less than the developer solution temperature. The fixer tank has its own circulation line, not shown in the diagram, but does not have its own heating element. The circulation system operates continually whenever the processor is turned on.

THE TEMPERING SYSTEM

Most automatic processors utilize a tempering system in which only one chemical solution is physically heated, and then that solution is used to transfer heat to the other tanks. In the most common example, the developer circulation line includes a thermostat and a heating coil surrounding the line. Each time the temperature reaches a minimum allowable, the thermostat activates the heater. Obviously, the temperature does not remain at an exact level but fluctuates up and down within a small range as the heater turns on and off, overcompensating slightly each way. However, this fluctuation is restricted to such a short range that temperature changes are not a

Figure 269.   Thermostat-controlled heater coil surrounding developer line.

significant factor in controlling image quality.

Once a solution is heated, its lines may be passed through the other tanks (Figures 260 and 270) so that the heat is transferred out of its pipes to the other solutions. This is called a *heat exchanger* system. Other variations of this system may initially heat a different specific solution or use a different pipe arrangement, but the principle is the same. It is recommended that the fixer and wash temperatures be maintained slightly less than or equal to the developer but never more than the developer temperature. For this reason, it is best to initially heat the developer and use it in the heat exchanger system.

In addition, thermostatic mixing valves are usually used to control the temperature of incoming water to the wash tank (Figure 271). This water may pass on through and out the drain or it may be recycled and filtered to save costs.

Developer temperature may be set and adjusted by a small screw in the electrical box of the processor, but, as a rule, this should not be tampered with once it has been set at an optimum level. It is better to use replenishment rates to control image quality.

Three- and four-minute processors typically set the developer temperature in a range of 84-86°F., and the faster 90-second processors typically use temperatures of 92-96°F.

THE REPLENISHMENT SYSTEM

As described in the transport system section, the replenishment microswitches are turned on each time a film passes through the detection rollers from the feed tray (Figure 263). These switches activate the replenishment pumps for both the fixer and the developer (Figure 272). The solution is pumped up from external reserve tanks into the bottom of the appropriate deep tank. Older developer at the top of the tank is sloughed off through an overflow funnel to one side of the deep tank and down a drain tube. The circulation system ensures that the solution within the tank remains well mixed. The reserve replenishment tanks should always have solution in them, because the pumping of air through the replenishment lines not only oxidizes the solutions in the deep tanks but can damage the pumps. Floating lids

Figure 270. Heat exchanger pipe (arrow) carrying heated developer solution through fixer tank.

Figure 271. Thermostatic mixing valve on incoming water line.

which sit directly on the solution surface in the replenishment tanks should be used, in addition to the regular tank lids, to help prevent oxidation of the replenishment solution over time.

The replenishment rate is set by a small screw on the side of the replenishment pump cam (Figure 273) which adjusts the position of the pumping diaphragm relative to the cam. Although the specific replenishment rate must be determined either from the manufacturer or sensitometrically, typical replenishment rates for a 14- x -17-inch film fed crosswise range from 50 to 100 cc for developer and from 90 to 150 cc for fixer. Recall that in manual development, the total fixing time is double the developing time when concentration and replenishment are equivalent. Twice as much fixing is required than developing. In automatic processing, the time during which the film is immersed in each solution is equal. For example, in a 90-second processor, it spends about 20 seconds in

Figure 272. Automatic replenishment pumps of diaphragm type which pump developer and fixer solutions from replenishment tanks into deep tanks each time a film passes through the detection rollers.

each deep tank. Since, the time and the temperature are equivalent, the replenishment rate for the fixer must be considerably greater than that for the developer. A high level of fixer concentration allows the solution to both clear and harden the film sufficiently in only 20 seconds. The higher replenishment rates of the fixer require that fresh fixer replenishment solution be added to the reserve tank almost twice as often as the developer.

The specific replenishment rates set are based upon an average width of film passing through the detection rollers, which would be about 11 inches. The only dimension the detection rollers can *measure* is the length of the film being fed. While this procedure is entirely functional for normal work loads in a radiography department, specialized departments must consider adjustments in replenishment rates to account for extremes in film size. For example, in an angiography department with its own processor, most films developed are of the 14-x-14-inch size. Furthermore, whole series of angiography films are processed sequentially. Replen-

Figure 273. Location of replenishment rate adjustment screw on cam of replenishment pump.

ishment rates will most likely need to be adjusted upward in comparison with a gen-

Figure 274. Air blower fro drying system in automatic processor.

Figure 275. Compartment containing heating elements for dryer system showing opening (arrow) for heated air to pass down dryer tubes.

eral diagnostic department.

In the case of the wash tank, one to three gallons of water should pass through the tank per minute to provide adequate replenishment and circulation.

THE DRYER SYSTEM

The drying system is composed of a blower (Figure 274), which takes in external room air and directs it under pressure through a compartment full of heating elements (Figures 260 and 275) The heated air is then directed down a series of tubes which surround both sides of the film as it passes through the dryer rollers. Each of the dryer tubes has a narrow slit along one side, the side facing the film, through which the heated air is forced (Figure 276), as well as an insert which narrows the effective diameter of the tube in a direction away from the blower. The air pressure decreas es with distance away from the blower and would result in uneven drying of the film, with the near side drying long before the far side. By narrowing the inside of the tube away from the blower, the air pressure is maintained equally across the surface of the film.

A thermostat on the side of the processor away from the heating elements adjusts the heating coil to obtain the actual tem-

perature set for the dryer (Figure 277). For a given average work load, the dryer temperature should be set at the minimum necessary to completely dry the films. The most commonly used dryer setting is about 120°F.

An outlet must be provided for the used air as it cools. On the side of the processor away from the heating elements, a duct directs the air out of the processor and preferably out of the building (Figure 278). It should always be remembered that the

Figure 276. Heater tube showing slit through which air is directed toward the film surface, and plastic insert (*bottom*) which gradually narrows air passage toward the far end of the tube in order to maintain equal pressure.

Figure 277. Thermostat at far side of dryer rack assembly.

efficiency of such an exhaust system is lost with every additional bend and turn in the duct, and as direct a route as possible should be provided to the outside.

PROCESSOR MAINTENANCE

Unlike manual processing facilities, the deep tanks in an automatic processor cannot have separate covers, because of the roller arrangement, and share a common lid in the processor cover. Chemicals evaporating upward may precipitate from the lid back into the other tanks and cross-contaminate each other. For this reason, it is recommended that the lid on an automatic processor be opened slightly during periods of nonuse.

Rollers must be cleaned periodically to prevent the buildup of chemical deposits and dirt which cause artifacts as shown in the next section. During periods of nonuse, wash tanks should be drained to prevent the growth of algae. All gears and moving parts should be cleaned often to ensure smooth function. Care must also be taken not to bend or misalign any of the guide shoes or support bars on the deep racks. Even slight misalignments in rollers and guides can lead to film jamups in the processor.

Figure 278. Heater exhaust duct. Replenishment tanks are visible below.

Figure 279. Radiograph exhibiting guide shoe scratches from misalignment of guide shoes in an automatic processor. Scratches run parallel to direction of film travel.

Figure 280. Radiograph exhibiting dark pi lines artifact. Note regular intervals of distance between lines indicative of roller size involved. Pi lines run perpendicular to direction of film travel.

COMMON AUTOMATIC PROCESSING ARTIFACTS

In addition to the fogging, static discharges, reticulation, crescent marks, stains and other artifacts which may be caused on a radiograph from rough handling or improper manual processing, there are a few artifacts that are peculiar to automatic processing.

Scratches appear as clear or *white* lines because emulsion is removed from the film base. When such scratches are straight and run in a direction *parallel* to the travel of the film through an automatic processor (Figure 279) they are indicative of guide shoes that are out of alignment or not properly seated in the processor. Improperly seated dryer tubes or roller racks may also cause parallel scratching. In all of these cases, a sharp corner of metal or plastic is brought into contact with the film as it passes through the processor, damaging the emulsion.

If a guide shoe (Figure 266) is set at too steep an angle, the tips of all of the ribs impressed in it will tear emulsion off of the film. The resulting artifact is a series of scratches that are parallel to the direction of the film travel and at equal intervals across the film.

Pi lines are dark linear densities running across the film *perpendicular* to the direction of film travel through the processor. They occur at regular intervals (Figure 280). Pi lines are the result of chemical or dirt deposits on processor rollers. Each time a

Figure 281. Radiograph exhibiting light hesitation marks on the left side from momentary failure of transport system. Lines run perpendicular to direction of film travel, where contact with rollers protect the emulsion from continued development. Note that some lines have a darker line to either side due to lessened pressure of the roller.

Figure 282. Radiograph exhibiting detection roller marks (*top*) and chemical splashes, caused by pulling film back out of an automatic processor after its leading edge had submerged into the developer solution tank.

cleaned and the deep tank solution levels checked.

Figure 281 is an example of *hesitation marks.* Hesitation marks are one of the most common artifacts in automatic processing. They are caused when there is a pause in the smooth transfer of the film through the various rollers of the transport system. There are several possible causes for the film to stop, including misalignment of guide shoes or rollers, the breaking of a roller gear so that a roller fails to rotate, breaking of the drive chain or a drive shaft gear, transport motor failure, or even an accidental switching off of the processor by personnel. In any case, when the film pauses, lines of altered density are created across the film wherever it is in contact with rollers, because while the developer or fixer solution continues to act upon the rest of the film, the solution cannot get to the areas that are in direct contact with a roller. These lines will always lie *crosswise* to the direction of film travel. But, unlike pi-lines, they are usually at *uneven intervals* because many different rollers may be in contact with the film at the same time, there are different distances between deep rack rollers and crossover rollers, and some of the rollers may be different sizes.

Hesitation lines may be light in color, or, more commonly, they may consist of a triple line–a light line with a dark density line along either side. *Any marks on the film caused by pressure effects, such as hesitation lines, pi lines, or crescent marks (discussed in the next chapter) may be either lighter or darker than the background density of the film. It is the amount of pressure that determines the color of the mark: Slight pressure sensitizes the film emulsion, causing it to turn dark. High pressure compresses and damages the emulsion, leaving a lighter area.* Hesitation marks most commonly show a light area in the middle where the pressure of the roller was great-

dirty roller turns, the pressure of the deposit against the film sensitizes the emulsion and turns it dark. The distance of the intervals between the pi lines is equal to the circumference of the roller causing them. The circumference of a roller is equal to 3.14 (pi) multiplied by the diameter of the roller. Hence, an aid in locating the roller causing the artifact is to divide the interval distance between the pi lines by 3.14 to derive the size of the roller. To eliminate the artifact, the rollers must be thoroughly

Figure 283. Radiograph showing dark streaks caused by dirty developer solution or by spillage of one solution into another while the film was submerged.

Figure 284. Radiograph exhibiting reticulation from excessive changes between processing solutions.

est and where solution was prevented from reaching the film, with a dark line to either side where the pressure of the roller was diminished.

Uneven or streaky sheen on the surface of the film may be caused by uneven drying from dirty or improperly seated dryer tubes or by poor alignment of squeegee rollers, leaving the film excessively waterlogged as it enters the dryer.

Failure to transport may result from overlapping films, broken drive gears, or improperly seated, warped, or dirty roller racks, guide shoes or tubes.

To avoid film jam-ups in the processor, always wait until the buzzer sounds indicating that the previously fed film is fully into the system and the film path is clear; And, alternately use the sides of the feed tray to guide the film straight into the rollers. When a film is fed crooked, students are sometimes tempted to pull a film back out of the processor. If the leading edge of the

film has reached the developer solution, just a couple of inches past the detection rollers, pulling it back out will result in the artifact illustrated in Figure 282, as developer solution is dragged through the detection rollers and splashed onto the feed tray. The feed tray and detection rollers must be cleaned immediately after such an accident.

Figure 283 demonstrates the classic appearance of a radiograph that has been processed in dirty developer or fixer solution. Such a film indicates the need for an immediate cleaning of the processor tanks and the addition of fresh solutions. This is also the appearance caused if one solution is somehow spilled into a different solution tank while the film is in the tank. Figure 284 shows an example of film *reticulation*, a network of fine cracks in the film emulsion. Reticulation is caused when the temperature is quickly and drastically changed during processing, with the film passing either from a very cold solution into a very warm solution or vice versa. In automatic pro-

cessing, this would indicate a failure within the tempering system.

SUMMARY

1. *Automatic processors* reduce total processing time to as little as 90 seconds by using high solution temperatures and ensure consistency in processing.
2. The *transport* system controls development time by its speed, while specialized rollers squeegee the film after it passes through each solution and detect inserted films to trigger the replenishment system.
3. The *circulation/filtration* system ensures uniform chemical distribution across the film and clean solution.
4. The *tempering* system uses thermostat control and heat exchangers to maintain proper solution temperature.
5. The *replenishment* system maintains proper solution concentration by adding new solution each time a film is detected. Since time and temperature are relatively fixed in automatic processing, the primary *control* for development is the replenishment rate set on the replenishment pumps.
6. The *dryer* system shrinks and dries the emulsion for permanence.
7. Parallel scratches, pi lines, and uneven sheen are examples of artifacts specific to automatic processors. Once fed, films should not be pulled back out of the processor.
8. Dark streaks are caused by dirty solutions or solutions contaminated during processing. *Reticulation* is a network of cracks caused by sudden changes in solution temperature.
9. *Hesitation marks* are light lines running *crosswise* to the direction of film travel, which usually have a dark line on either side. Anything which causes the film to temporarily stop during development will leave a lighter lines where the rollers were in contact with the film preventing the solutions from reaching it, with darker lines where the roller pressure was less.
10. *Pressure artifacts* of various types appear dark when pressure is slight and sensitizes the emulsion, and appear light when pressure is great enough to damage the emulsion.

REVIEW QUESTIONS

1. Name the two main advantages of automatic processing over manual.
2. What was the primary variable change that made it possible for automatic film processors to develop radiographs so quickly ?
3. What problem would result if gluteraldehyde were not added to automatic developer solution?
4. Why are detection rollers ribbed?
5. What replaces the function of the "rinse bath," "stop bath," or draining the film in an automatic processor?
6. How does an automatic processor compensate chemical replenishment for different sizes of films?

7. What is the purpose of guide shoes?

8. What automatic processor system replaces the function of agitating films in manual solutions?

9. In what temperature range should the developer solution be maintained for most 90-second automatic processors?

10. What are the typical replenishment rate ranges for developer and fixer in an automatic processor (per 14" film)?

11. What undesirable results occur when replenishment tanks are allowed to run out of solution?

12. In manual processing the fixing time is double the developing time. Why can the automatic processor use 20 seconds for *both*?

13. What replenishment effect would it have on automatic solutions if, at average replenishment rates, dozens of small films were processed in sequence with no large films being run?

14. What is usually the ideal air temperature for drying x-ray films in the automatic processor?

15 What can result if rack braces, guide shoes, tubes or rollers are carelessly bent during cleaning?

16. What causes scratches, at regular intervals, in straight lines parallel to film travel?

17. Which direction do both pi lines and hesitation lines lie in relation to the direction of film travel?

Chapter 39

FILM HANDLING AND DUPLICATION PROCEDURES

X-RAY FILM is a delicate material and it should not be handled carelessly or roughly. It is sensitive to treatment of any kind—and heat, light, x-rays, radium, chemical fumes, pressure, rolling, bending, etc., are capable of adversely affecting the emulsion. Fortunately, it can be handled safely and swiftly in accordance with all the various radiographic needs as long as the radiographer knows what he must do to avoid the production of foreign marks (artifacts) on the film. The increased speed of film in late years has made it a bit more sensitive to handling operations, and greater care must be exercised.

Safety x-ray film is in common use today. It represents no greater hazard in the stock, radiographic, processing or filing rooms than would an equal quantity of paper records. Radiographs made with this film can be stored on open shelves, in manila envelopes. Discarded film boxes may be stood on end and employed for filing radiographs.

PACKING

X-ray film is packed in a hermetically sealed bag and paper wrappings to protect it from light and moisture. Each unit quantity is placed between cardboard and wrapped in black protective plastic. The package is hermetically sealed under conditions that insure approximately 50 per cent humidity *inside* the package. The package is then inserted in a cardboard carton.

STORAGE

Unexposed and unprocessed x-ray film should always be kept in a cool, dry place. It should never be stored in basements or near steam pipes or other sources of heat. In extremely warm climates only small quantities of film should be ordered at one time, so that a rapid turn-over takes place.

HEAT

High temperatures exert injurious effects on the emulsion causing loss of contrast and the production of fog (Figure 285). Unexposed x-ray film should not be expected to be usable more than a few weeks after subjection to temperatures of 90° to 100°F.; or more than a few days at 110° to 120°F. A relatively brief period of excessive heat in transit or storage may ruin the film regardless of how well it is protected during the major portion of its life. Because x-ray film is packed in hermetically sealed containers does not mean that it no longer requires care or protection. Such packing does protect film from moisture, both from humid air or actual water immersion, and from other contaminants— as long as the package is *unbroken.* However, it does *not* provide protection from high temperatures.

An approximate guide to usability of film under various temperature storage conditions and approximately 60 per cent humidity is as follows. If film is to be used in 2 months, it can withstand temperatures up to 75°F. without deterioration. If stored at 60°F., it can be kept 6 months in storage; at 50°F., for 1 year. Ideal storage conditions will prevail at temperatures of 50° to 70°F. and 40 to 60 per cent relative humidity.

X-RADIATION

Film must be suitably protected from the

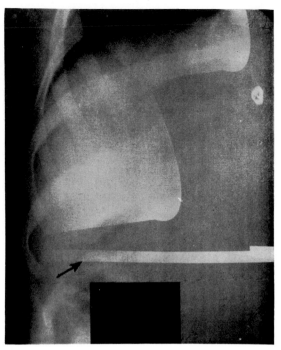

Figure 286. Radiograph made with film from a box that had been exposed to x-rays in a laboratory. Note radiographic image of lead foil band that was incorporated in cardboard box.

unwanted action of x-rays or radium by lead-lined walls or chests (see Figure 286). Film bins located in the processing room should be protected by sheet lead.

FUMES

X-ray film must never be stored in drug rooms or other places containing fumes of any kind. Illuminating gas, formalin, ammonia, volatile oils, sewer gas, etc., will fog film in opened packages if it is stored in an atmosphere containing these substances.

PRESSURE

Film should never be subjected to extreme pressure such as wrinkling, bending, or rolling because changes take place

Figure 285. Radiograph exhibiting fog produced during storage of film in a hot basement.

in the emulsion which, upon development, appear as artifacts on the finished film. To avoid pressure markings, packages of unexposed x-ray film should always be stored on edge; they should never be stacked one upon another.

EXPIRATION DATE

All film should be used before its expiration date because film aging causes loss in speed and contrast.

REFRIGERATION

Storage of unopened packages of x-ray film in refrigerators is satisfactory provided packages are removed 24 to 36 hours before they are used. This procedure is necessary to avoid the production of condensing moisture on the film when each sheet is removed from the package under high atmospheric temperatures. Open boxes of x-ray film should not be stored in refrigerators wherein conditions of high humidity usually prevail. Once a box of film is opened it should be used as soon as possible. If opened boxes of film must be contained in refrigerators, no other materials should be stored therein and some type of dehydrator should be placed in the refrigerator to reduce the humidity.

THE DARK ROOM

The construction of a "dark room" must take into account the necessity for protecting film stored there from heat, radiation, and fumes. If it is located adjacent to radiation exposure areas, the walls must have an appropriate lead equivalency. The room must be well ventilated and temperature-controlled at less than 70 degrees F (21° C), both to protect the film and to assure a healthy working environment for technicians working there. Humidity must be maintained between 40 and 60 per cent to prevent static discharges on film when it is moved across counters, into and out of cassettes and into the processor feed tray.

Of course, the dark room must be made as light-proof as possible. Weatherstripping can be used around the edges of the processor and door, and a rotating door or double door will assure a light-tight entrance. Electrical interlocking systems now available for film bins and are highly recommended when regular entrances are used. These systems either lock the film bin any time the entryway door is not fully closed, or sound a warning buzzer if the door is ajar and the film bin is opened.

In constructing dark rooms, it is a mistake to use colored Formica®, tile, or paint. Loading benches must be white so that films lying on them can be recognized, and all other surfaces should be white so as to reflect the small amount of light coming from the red safelight and maximize general visibility. The loading bench should be removed, preferably opposite, from the processor and any chemical storage.

HANDLING

In handling x-ray film, the radiographer should avoid touching the film surfaces. Film should be held as near the edges as possible with clean dry hands. X-ray film is

Figure 287. Knee radiographs demonstrating crescent (crinkle) marks from rough handling before or after exposure. Marks can be white (A) when pressure is great, or black (B) when less pressure is applied.

very sensitive to almost all forms of energy. When it is properly handled, exposed and processed, a satisfactory image free of artifacts will result.

When films are carelessly handled in loading and unloading cassettes, they may be bent around the tips of the fingers, damaging the emulsion. The resulting artifacts are called *crescent marks* or *crinkle marks* and are semi-circular in shape.

Figure 287 demonstrates that crescent marks can either be light or dark. Dark crescent marks are caused when the pressure applied to the film is slight. In this case, the pressure sensitizes the film emulsion, causing the silver bromide crystals to develop a latent image and process as dark

images. Light marks are caused when greater pressure is applied to the film, so that the emulsion is actually compressed and damaged, such that crystals are pushed to the side.

It is well to remember that any form of white light creeping into a processing room through cracks around the edges of partitions, windows, doors, or open film bins may fog x-ray film. Be sure that all white light is turned off in the processing room when handling film. When white light is on, film bins should be tightly closed and the tops secure on all film boxes. White light should never be turned on while films are developing because films will be fogged in the tank.

Figure 288. Radiograph exhibiting safelight fog because exposed film was laid on loading bench too long and partially covered by a piece of paper (below arrow).

SAFELIGHT ILLUMINATION

X-ray films are sensitive to white light and must be handled either in darkness or under safelight illumination of the proper quality. The processing room should be adequately provided with both white-light and safelight illumination. White-light is necessary to perform many activities such as the mixing of chemicals, cleaning of tanks, caring for intensifying screens, placing films in the dryer, and unloading film hangers. Fixtures for white-light should be properly located to afford general illumination when films are not being developed.

Safelight illumination should be furnished in the working areas by hanging "direct" or "indirect" type lamps. Film exposed with x-ray intensifying screens is approximately 8 times more sensitive to

safelight illumination than unexposed film. Because films are subjected to safelight illumination at the loading bench for a longer period than in any other zone, direct-type safelight lamps over this area are liable to raise the amount of postexposure fog to an undesirable degree. For this reason, the loading bench should be illuminated by an indirect safelight lamp. No film should be exposed to the safelight lamp for a period longer than it takes to unload a film and place it in the processor.

Safelight illumination is designed to give enough visibility in the processing room for the radiographer to accomplish all necessary duties in connection with the handling and processing of x-ray film without harmful effect to any unprocessed film that may be exposed. No safelight is safe if the standards of safety are abused. Film left out under a safelight lamp too long will fog (Figure 288). If film cannot be processed at once, it should be stored in a light-tight container. *Exposed* films being more sensitive to safelight illumination should be set to one side away from the direct beam of a safelight lamp or, better still, placed under or behind a protective screen. If the films cannot be covered, the safelight lamp nearest the stacked films should be turned off.

Improper safelight illumination is a common cause of film fog. Excessive examination of films under a safelight during development as well as holding them too close to the safelight causes aerial fog and/or light fog on film. Therefore, certain considerations must be kept in mind in connection with safelight lamps and safelights.

1. The illumination will be safe only if bulbs of the wattage indicated on each lamp are used.

2. All safelight filters are safe only as long as specific conditions prevail. The standard of safety for all safelights is such that unexposed x-ray film may be safely

Figure 289. Various types of safelight lamps employed in darkrooms, equipped with 6B or GBX filters.

handled in the light at a distance of 3 feet, for 1 minute. These factors apply to the use of safelights with 6B or GBX filters and unexposed film.

Safelight Lamps

Safelight lamps are an indispensable item in every processing room. Safelights, (Figure 289), are lamphouses equipped with filters that provide photographically *safe* illumination in a processing room while handling and developing unprocessed film. The light emitted by a safelight is of such spectral quality and intensity that it does not fog film handled under it for a reasonable handling period and yet the illumination provided by it is as high as possible consistent with safe handling of the film. As far as practicable, the general illumination should be made indirect by suspending from the ceiling one or more safelight lamps of appropriate design and size. If the walls and ceiling are painted with a light colored paint, the entire room will be well lighted with safe illumination. For light in specific sections of the processing room, there are safelight lamps of various designs. The choice and arrangement of safelight lamps should depend upon the amount of illumination desired and the angle at which

it must fall.

Blackout conditions in the permanent processing room are neither necessary from a technical standpoint nor desirable from a psychologic one. A dark colored wall finish will absorb much of the safelight illumination. If the quality of the light from a safelight lamp is "safe," the illumination reflected from any surface is also "safe" regardless of its color. Nor does the reflected light gain in intensity over the direct or incident light beam. The wall finish, should, therefore, reflect the maximum amount of safelight illumination and the color should be pleasant. In order to appear bright, the wall color must reflect rather than absorb light from the safelight lamp.

To avoid an excessive rate of safelight exposure to the film during darkroom handling, light bulbs of greater than 15 watts should never be used in the safelight. For regular film designed for use with calcium tungstate screens, the Wratten Series 6B safelight filter is recommended. This filter allows only those wave lengths of light in the yellow to red portion of the spectrum to be emitted. Since regular x-ray film is most sensitive to the blue-violet end of the light spectrum, this color of light in the darkroom will take a relatively long time to fog the film and is therefore considered *safe*.

Special consideration is needed for departments using the newer rare-earth technologies. Orthochromatic film must be used with rare-earth screens because it is designed for high sensitivity to the green light which these screens emit. Since green light is closer to the red end of the light spectrum than is blue light, orthochromatic films are much more sensitive to the yellow-red light emitted by regular safelight filters and fog much faster. The *GBX* filter has been designed to emit only the darkest red portion of the spectrum and must be used in all darkrooms where orthochromatic film is developed. Maximum reflection under safelight illumination is achieved if the wall finish is either a color within this same spectral range, or a light enough shade of any other color. It is desirable also to have a color that is pleasing under white light as well as safelight illumination. In permanent installations, the ceiling and the upper 18 inches of the side walls should be painted white to provide maximum reflection of white light. For the remainder of the side walls, warm tones such as ivory, cream, or pale shades of any desired color, are generally more pleasing than white, which is apt to be too glaring and shows soil quickly.

Checking Safelight Illumination

A simple method of checking the safety of illumination is to cover part of an unexposed film and expose sections of the remainder for different lengths of time in the place where films will be uncovered in handling. This test film is then given standard development. If no fog shows on the parts that receive a reasonably long exposure, as compared with the covered part, the lighting may be assumed to be safe. If fog does appear, the distance of the safe-lights from the film should be increased. All safelight lamps should be tested periodically for white light leaks, fading of filter, and excess wattage of bulbs.

STATIC DISCHARGES

Every precaution in the manufacture and packing of x-ray film is employed to avoid the accumulation of static electricity on the film surfaces. Whenever two dissimilar surfaces are pressed together and separated, static electric charges develop. The electric charge becomes appreciable when one or both surfaces are nonconductors and when the atmospheric humidity is low. The quantity of the charge depends partly upon the electrical storage capacity possessed by the total surface of the area involved and the spacing of the charged parts and the insulating strength of the intervening medium.

A static electric discharge emits visible light capable of exposing the film, and the resulting artifacts assume various shapes (Figure 290). They are usually treelike or bushlike in appearance (the point of discharge always has the greatest density) with fingerlike processes emanating outward from the point of discharge. Often static marks assume the character of black smudges. Discharges are most likely to occur in cold, dry periods and it is then that particular care must be taken to handle film carefully and avoid friction on its surface. The loading bench in the processing room should be grounded so that in the handling of the cassette any static charges that are built up can be dissipated before the cassette is opened.

Prevention of static sparks can be effected by grounding the location where static charges may develop and by increasing the humidity. To raise the humidity of the air in the x-ray and processing rooms, the use

Figure 290. Radiograph exhibiting "smudge" type artifacts from static electricity discharges during handling. Static artifacts can also appear as "tree" or "crown" marks with branching points.

lead to artifacts on the finished radiograph. The fact that the film is coated and dried in an atmosphere free of dust and at an optimum and constant temperature and humidity, serves to keep the formation and production of static electricity to a minimum.

REMOVAL OF FILM FROM CARTON

When obtaining x-ray film from a new carton, rapid movement should be avoided as a protection against the production of static electricity or pressure artifacts. The box of film is placed on the loading bench, the retaining strip at the edge of the cover is pulled and the cover lifted from the box top. All white light in the processing room is turned off and the safelight illumination provides ample light for opening the film box. When the cover of the box is removed, the edge of the heat sealed bag is exposed. One side of the box near its top is scored so that about one inch of the box can be folded down. This will help to remove the films later. The flap on the bag should be stripped by tearing it and stripping the top away to each side. The film then becomes visible. The two cardboard stiffeners are removed and the film may then be easily removed.

of a commercial humidifier will assist in maintaining a satisfactory humidity level. Remember that the danger point for static production occurs when the humidity is 40 per cent or less. As the humidity gets less and less, static electric accumulations grow.

In the emulsion-coating operation during manufacture, static electricity is removed by ingenious and complicated methods so that static charges have no opportunity to accumulate on the film and

LOADING AND UNLOADING FILM

There are two types of containers in which medical x-ray films can be held during exposure—direct exposure holders and cassettes. The choice depends upon the exposure technic to be employed. In the direct exposure technic, the film is placed in the exposure holder which comprises a light-tight envelope. In the double-intensifying-screen technic, the film is placed

between two x-ray intensifying screens that are mounted in a cassette. In loading and unloading x-ray film, all white light must be extinguished in the processing or loading room.

In loading, the film is placed in the open exposure holder; next, the large flap of the envelope is turned down, then the side flaps are brought over, followed by the end flap. It is most important that this procedure for protection of the film be followed if light-fog is to be avoided. The holder is now ready for use.

LOADING THE CASSETTE

When the film is removed from its carton, it should be held vertically at the middle of the top border with the fingertips of the right hand. It is then placed in the cassette on the front intensifying screen. The lid carrying the back screen is gently closed and locked by means of the back springs. When placing the film in the cassette, care should be exercised to avoid scraping or sliding the film over the edges of the cassette or surface of the screen. Be sure that in this operation the hands are dry and chemically free and that they do not come in contact with the x-ray intensifying screens.

FILM IDENTIFICATION

There are two common types of devices used to print patient identification information onto each radiograph. For both devices, a paper card with patient information is inserted into the device, and a flash of light is projected through the card, exposing the film. Regular typed ink will absorb the light and thus appear as white print on the finished radiograph.

The older *film flasher* is still widely used, but is restricted to the dark room. In the dark room after exposure, each film is removed from its cassette, and the corner of the film must be fully inserted forward and sideways into the flasher slot. The top of the flasher is then depressed, closing the device on the film and activating the light source. When a red indicator light at the top of the flasher turns off, the flash exposure is complete and the film can be fed into the processor.

Many newer cassette systems use *identification cameras* which can be used in the light, and are placed into each radiographic procedures room. These systems require special cassettes with a "window" in a corner on the back cover. The window is covered with a sliding panel. Just prior to or after each exposure, the window corner of the cassette is placed into the camera, with the window facing up. A mechanism in the camera slides the window panel to the side, a flash of light prints the information onto the film, and the panel is closed.

When using identification cameras, the radiographer must be sure to slide the cassette fully into the slot of the camera, and hold it there until the entire cycle is completed, indicated by the cessation of noise from the device. If the cassette is pulled from the camera before this sound stops, the window will be open and the identification area on the film will be completely fogged.

Proper, accurate radiograph identification is essential for both legal and medical reasons. If a film is flashed with the wrong information, it can frequently be corrected by placing the correct card into the flasher and reflashing the film three times. If this procedure results in illegible print, or if the identification area is otherwise fogged, a paper sticker with *all* of the correct information should be applied to the film.

DAYLIGHT LOADING SYSTEMS

Mechanized cassette loading and unloading systems have been developed that are designed to preclude the need for a dark room technician or for the radiographer to perform any functions in the dark. These *daylight processing* systems are particularly useful for small departments frequently staffed by a single radiographer: Processing procedures are reduced to the attachment of a film compartment to the processor, allowing the radiographer to return immediately to the procedures room while films are automatically fed into the processor. Further, cassette loading and unloading devices may be placed in each radiographic procedures room, so that the radiographer never has to leave the room to search for additional cassettes during a procedure.

Disadvantages of daylight systems include the initial installation cost, space required for loaders and unloaders in each room, and possibly expensive breakdowns or malfunctions that can result in the fogging of dozens of films in one event. Most of the "bugs" have been satisfactorily worked out of daylight systems, and their advantages can outweigh the disadvantages, but one must shop carefully when selecting a system.

Figure 291. Daylight cassette loading system. The loader (left) uses gravity to drop a single film through a slot in the end of the special cassette. After exposure, the film is dropped from the cassette through the unloader (right) and into the fabric rolls of a transfer compartment. The transfer compartment can then be attached to automatic processor feed tray to process all of the films. In more modern systems, the cassettes are directly unloaded into a specialized processor.

COMPONENTS OF DAYLIGHT CASSETTE SYSTEMS

Most daylight systems use special end-loading cassettes with which the entire radiology department must be outfitted. Each radiographic room is provided with cassette loaders and cassette unloaders (Figure 291). Prior to use, the end-loading cassette is placed into a cassette loader for the proper film size, and a crank or button activates the system, inserting a single film through a light-proof gate in a slit at the end of the cassette. A malfunction at this stage is critical, because several films can drop and be fogged. After exposure, the cassette is placed into the unloader with the slotted end downward (Figure 291). Gravity causes the film to drop into the unloader and strike a microswitch. This activates a motor that winds the film into a spool of fabric. Dozens of films can be stored in the spool of fabric.

When a procedure is completed, the transfer compartment is detached from the unloader and carried to an automatic processor that has been modified for compatibility with the system. When the transfer compartment is placed onto the feed tray of the processor, it depresses switches that turn on the processor and a motor to turn the spool of fabric in the compartment. Each time films are unloaded from cassettes into the transfer compartment, extra fabric is wound onto the spool, so that the films are spaced at intervals corresponding to the feed time required by the processor. In this manner, enough time is allowed for a film to fully feed into the processor before the next film reaches the detection rollers. When a transfer compartment is placed onto the processor, the radiographer may obtain another empty compartment and use it immediately in the procedures room.

Cassette loaders in the procedures rooms are designed to hold a box of 100 films, and must be reloaded each time they run out. Special identification devices are required with daylight systems. The patient's information card may be placed in a handheld *identification printer* which slides into a slot at the top end of the cassette, or the cassette may be slid into an *identification camera* that opens a door on the back of the cassette and flashes the information onto the film using a light source.

To summarize, cassette daylight systems require the following components:

1. Special cassettes
2. Cassette loaders (film dispensers)
3. Cassette unloaders with detachable film compartments
4. Special film identification system
5. Modifications to the automatic processor so it will accept the film transfer compartments.

The modifications to the processor allow it to still be used for manual film-feeding as needed.

CASSETTELESS DAYLIGHT SYSTEMS

Some radiographic units are provided with conveyor belt systems that retrieve films from a storage compartment and bring them directly into the bucky mechanism of the table. A pressure plate system then closes the (permanently installed) intensifying screens against the film and the exposure is made. Following exposure, the screens are opened and conveyor belts carry the film through a tunnel directly into an adjoining automatic processor.

These units might properly be called *cassetteless daylight* systems, since they, too, preclude the need for a dark room. There is an enhancement of efficiency for the radiographer similar to that for cassette daylight systems, accompanied by similar disadvantages: The conveyor belts result in static electricity discharges along the sides of each film which sometimes impinge upon the useful image, and costly film jam-ups can occur.

DUPLICATION AND SUBTRACTION PROCEDURES

Special film and duplication devices are necessary for the duplication or subtraction of radiographs. Duplication film usually has a violet coloration to it and has emulsion on only one side. The emulsion side can be recognized in three ways: First, it has a flat, low-gloss appearance and does not reflect light well. The nonemulsion side appears very glossy, and this can be seen under safelight illumination. Second, the emulsion side also *feels* rougher than the glossy non-emulsion side. Third, most duplication film manufacturers cut a notch into one side of the film near a corner. When the film is held with this notch at the top edge and toward the right corner, the emulsion side is facing you.

Duplication devices typically use ultraviolet light exposure, to which the duplication film is sensitive. The original radiograph and duplication film are placed on a glass plate over the ultraviolet bulbs and a lid closed over the top of the films (Figure 292). The original radiograph should be placed onto the glass plate first. The duplication film is then placed on top of the radiograph by swinging the bottom edge away from you so that the emulsion side faces downward toward the radiograph and light source. If this is done properly, the notch in the duplication film will then be on the edge closest to you and toward the right corner. The films must be *registered* correctly, that is, all edges must be aligned perfectly. It may be advisable to use tape over the edges so that the films do not slide out of place when closing the lid.

It is important to remember that the exposure process used in duplication is *reversed* as compared to normal radiography. Duplication film is designed so that longer exposure times result in *less* density (Figure 293). A duplication film that was not exposed will come out of the processor pitch black. Where ultraviolet exposure takes place, emulsion crystals are removed in processing and lighter densities result. The duplicator exposure control is marked off in 0.1 second *exposure units*. Although

Figure 292. Radiographic duplicator showing glass plate over ultraviolet light source on which films are placed.

Figure 293. Duplicated radiographs of the cervical spine showing the relationship between duplication exposure time and image density. (A) 15 exposure units, (B) 30 exposure units. Note that density *decreases* with longer exposures.

Figure 294. Positive image mask film produced from scout radiograph of a lateral cerebral arteriogram.

Figure 295. Subtraction radiograph of lateral cerebral arteriogram produced when the mask film in Figure 294 was superimposed over a regular radiograph with contrast media present, and then the subtraction film was exposed through both in a duplicator.

most duplication requires from 8 to 16 exposure units to obtain a density level equal to the original radiograph, the actual value to be used for a given set of equipment and film must be derived by experimentation. Once this base value is found, however, further changes in exposure time can be trusted to follow an inversely proportional relationship with density. An exposure of 2 units duration will produce a duplicate that is twice as dense as an exposure of 4 units. Doubling the exposure units results in one-half the density.

When the lid is closed and the exposure button depressed, an indicator light comes on to indicate exposure. When the light shuts off, the exposure is terminated and the lid may be opened. The duplication film is then processed as any other radiograph.

The great advantage to duplication is its potential for saving additional patient exposure when overexposed radiographs are produced. An overexposed radiograph may be duplicated with the exposure control set to lighten up the density. The resulting duplicate may be of sufficient diagnostic value to preclude the necessity for repeating exposure of the patient. Duplicators can be of no assistance, however, with underexposed radiographs, since no information is available in the original image to be duplicated.

Subtraction Technique

For subtraction radiographs, special subtraction mask film and subtraction print film is required. The emulsion of the subtraction film is located in the same way as for duplication film.

Subtraction is only useful in contrast media procedures. The objective is to subtract or erase all of the background anatomy so that only the bolus of contrast media is seen. This may be helpful to the radiologist at times when contrasty anatomy is superimposing the bolus of contrast media and the visibility of some details of interest is hampered. It should be realized, nonetheless, that subtraction technique cannot add any information to the radiograph which was not already present, and its usefulness is therefore limited to the occasional improvement of the certainty of an already suspected diagnosis.

A scout film must be taken without any contrast media. The patient must not move position for the remainder of the procedure after the scout film is taken. After the procedure is completed, subtraction images may be produced from any of the contrast radiographs taken by following a two-step procedure: First, a *mask* image is made from the *scout* radiograph using subtraction mask film. The scout film is placed onto the duplicator plate first, followed by the subtraction mask film placed with the emulsion side down and carefully registered. After exposure, the mask film is processed. The resulting image will be a positive, with bones appearing dark instead of light. It has been reversed from the negative image of a normal radiograph (Figure 294).

For the second exposure, three films are used. A regular *contrast* radiograph from the procedure is selected to subtract and placed on the duplicator plate first. This is followed by the *mask* film with its reversed image, carefully registered so that all background anatomy is reduced to a medium-gray shade and seems to disappear. A subtraction *print* film is then placed emulsion side down over the other two and an exposure is made. On the processed print film, only the bolus of contrast media will show well, with all other anatomy eliminated by the superimposition of positive and negative images (Figure 295).

Solarization

When duplication or subtraction films are grossly overexposed, a phenomenon called *solarization* may occur, whereby the image is reversed from a negative image to a positive image. In the positive image, bones will appear black instead of white, against a gray background (Figure 131 in Chapter 15). To correct the problem, the repeated duplication must be done at reduced exposure levels.

SILVER RECOVERY

Silver is a very valuable mineral, and radiology departments can recover thousands of dollars in film costs by capturing the silver removed from x-ray films in the fixer solution, rather than allowing the fixer solution to carry this silver down the drain with it. Silver reclaiming attachments can be connected to the fixer drain line for this purpose. There are two basic types of silver reclaiming units: chemical replacement units and electrolytic units.

The chemical replacement unit is a simple canister containing iron in the form of steel wool or other similar metal wools. As the fixer solution passes through the steel wool, the silver atoms are chemically attracted to the iron atoms and they attach to the wool. Later, the heavier silver-iron compounds drop off of the wool and fall to the bottom, forming *sludge*. This silver sludge may then be sold to silver reclaiming companies. Test papers for pH may be used to test solution *leaving* the container for excess silver content, indicating the need to change to a new canister. The efficiency of this method in separating silver out of the fixer solution ranges from 75-90 per cent, and the canisters are replaced at a very low cost. The use of two canisters can increase the efficiency to as much as 95 per cent.

The electrolytic unit utilizes an electrical cathode in the form of a drum which is negatively charged. This drum is immersed into a positively charged canister and is rotated by a motor to ensure even coating. Silver ions, repelled by the canister and attracted by the cathode, attach to the drum forming a fine coating. When the coating of silver exceeds about one-eighth of an inch in thickness, the drum should be removed and allowed to dry. After drying, the silver may be gently tapped off of the drum with a mallet to obtain a very pure silver powder. Care must be taken not to dent the drum, or to use too high of an electrical charge during reclaiming which burns the silver. Although the electrolytic method involves a considerable initial expense, the efficiency of silver recovery is 95-98 per cent and there is no replacement cost once the system is operable.

SUMMARY

1. X-ray *film* should be *stored* at temperatures of 50-70°F., and 40-60 per cent humidity, and protected from fumes, radiation, pressure and rough handling.
2. *Safelights* in the darkroom should not exceed 15 watts, should be filtered with a GBX or 6B filter, and should be at least 3 feet away from the loading counter and film bin. Film should be able to be exposed under these conditions for up to one minute without developing substantial fog.
3. Static discharges and other *artifacts* result from rough film handling in the darkroom.
4. When *duplicating* or subtracting radiographs, longer exposure times in the duplicator result in decreased density.
5. For *subtraction* technique, a mask film must be made from a scout radiograph, using subtraction mask film. This mask is then sandwiched between a contrast radiograph and a subtraction print film in the duplicator to produce a subtraction radiograph.
6. Electrolytic or chemical *silver recovery* systems can save thousands of dollars in reclaiming silver from used fixer solution.
7. The dark room must be light-proof, well ventilated, temperature controlled, and generally white in color.
8. Proper radiograph identification is essential. The two general types of identification devices are film flashers and cassette ID "cameras."
9. Daylight cassette loading systems provide in-room loading and unloading of cassettes and can enhance work efficiency, but cost and malfunctions are disadvantages to these systems. Cassetteless daylight systems convey the film into the Bucky mechanism and into the processor automatically.
10. Solarization is due to overexposure upon duplicating a radiograph.

REVIEW QUESTIONS

1. State the ideal temperature and humidity ranges for x-ray film storage.
2. Describe the cause of dark crinkle marks or crescent marks.
3. What is the maximum wattage recommended for dark room safelight bulbs ?
4. What is the recommended safelight filter for darkrooms storing blue-sensitive film ?
5. What is the most common cause of static electricity artifacts on radiographs?
6. In darkroom lighting, how do you recognize which side of a duplication film is emulsion-coated?
7. When duplicating a film, doubling the exposure units will change the resulting density to _____ the original.
8. Define "mask film" in regard to subtraction.
9. What percentage of silver will be

reclaimed from spent fixer solution using the chemical replacement method?

10. List the order in which the three films are stacked (from bottom up) for producing a subtraction radiograph.

11. State the two different reasons why dark rooms must be well ventilated.

12. What color should the loading bench be?

13. When a film is flashed with the wrong ID information, can it usually be reflashed to correct the information ?

14. List the 5 required components for a daylight cassette loading system.

15. What artifact always appears on films from a cassetteless daylight system?

Chapter 40

SENSITOMETRY AND DARKROOM QUALITY CONTROL

Sensitometry is the quantitative measurement of the response of x-ray film to exposure and processing conditions. Such quantification of image qualities is important, because it allows us to monitor changes in radiographic variables and diagnose equipment problems long *before* they become bad enough to cause repeated exposures to patients. When exposure and processing conditions are ensured to be consistent, sensitometric monitoring will indicate changes in the characteristics of the film being used or of changes in the receptor system as a whole. When film, screens and exposure conditions are maintained as a constant, sensitometric monitoring will indicate changes in processing conditions. Sensitometric equipment is much more sensitive than the human eye, so that trends in processing conditions may be detected and corrected before they create visible changes in radiographic quality.

Sensitometric measurements are limited to the *visibility* functions of the image: density, contrast and noise in the form of fog. All three of these qualities are reflected in a graph of the density response of a film to exposure. Referred to as a *characteristic* curve, a sensitometric curve, or an *H and D* curve (named after Hurter and Driffield who developed it for photographic analysis), this graph may be produced by exposing a film and plotting the various density levels against the logarithm of the various exposure levels that produced them (Figure 298).

A controlled exposure is required for sensitometry. There are three methods of obtaining such an exposure. The simplest and least expensive method is to use a step-wedge penetrometer and a medium exposure. The steps on the image are each measured on a densitometer and plotted on graph paper. The primary disadvantage to this technique is that the results may be affected by variations in the exposure caused by electrical fluctuations in the x-ray machine. For best results, all such variables must be eliminated except the one under study (usually film characteristics or processing conditions).

The *sensitometer* was developed to eliminate exposure variables in sensitometry (Figure 296). The sensitometer is a light-exposure device which automatically adjusts for changes in electrical current to ensure that each exposure made is uniform. It is set to always deliver the same amount of light to the film. If there is a decrease in electrical current, dimming the light emitted, it will extend the exposure time until the proper amount of light strikes the film. An x-ray film is placed in the sensitometer in the same fashion as a cassette. When the exposure button is depressed, a red light indicates that exposure is taking place. After this light is extinguished, the film is removed and processed. The resulting image is similar to that obtained from a step-wedge, but the measurements taken are much more reliable.

A third method of obtaining sensitometry exposures is to use pre-exposed test strips. These film strips are prepared by

Figure 296. Photograph of a sensitometer used to expose films for processor monitoring. Note step-wedge optical attenuator at bottom.

the manufacturer to simply be stored in the film bin and run through the processor when needed. This eliminates the need for a sensitometer, but it must be taken into account that if these strips are stored in the film bin for time periods longer than regular boxes of film are stored, they may accumulate excessive levels of fog from aging and safelight exposure and will then not be reliable as an indicator of *current* conditions.

THE H AND D CURVE

The graph obtained from plotting measured densities against the relative exposure levels (corresponding to the step numbers in the step-wedge image, Figure 297) will show a sigmoid-shaped curve (Figure 298). The ascending portions of the curve are referred to as the *toe, body,* and *shoulder,* respectively.

It will be noted that the toe and shoulder portions of the curve level out to a nearly horizontal line. The *toe* represents the minimum density producible on the radiograph. It is never at zero for two reasons: First, the base of most x-ray film has a blue dye added to it to enhance the visualization of contrast. This blue tint attenuates some of the light passing through the film.

Second, a small level of fog accumulated during the manufacture and storage of x-ray film is inevitable. Hence, all x-ray film has an inherent base density before it is exposed radiographically. This density is called the *base-plus-fog.*

The shoulder portion of the curve represents the maximum density level producible on the radiograph. It levels off because there is a finite amount of silver available in the emulsion of an x-ray film to produce density. When all of the silver crystals in a particular area of the film are used up, no more density can be obtained. This level may vary somewhat from one type of film to another, but it is always well beyond what the human eye perceives as

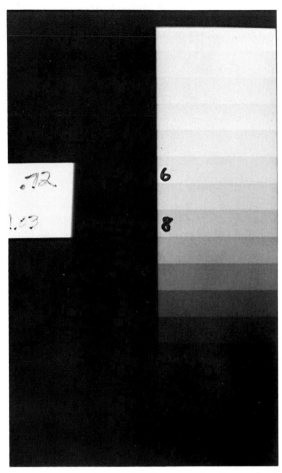

Figure 297. Radiograph of step wedge from which H & D curve measurements are taken. In this case, *speed* would be measured at step number 8 because it is closest to a density of 1.2, while *contrast* would be determined by subtracting step 6 from step 8.

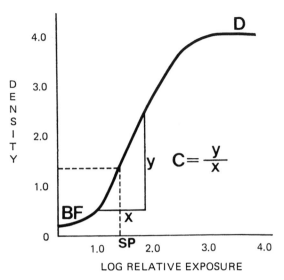

Figure 298. Graph of normal H & D curve showing base-plus-fog (BF), speed (SP), contrast (C) and D-max (D) for an exposure.

around 3.8 on the density scale.

The *slope* of the body portion of the H and D curve is indicative of the *contrast* of the film. This slope is determined by the ratio of the magnitude of a density change over the magnitude of the exposure change which caused it. For example, two exposure levels may be selected along the exposure axis of the graph for comparison. Remembering that these represent different portions of the *remnant* beam of radiation, the lighter exposure might be considered as that occurring under a bone, while the greater exposure would be that occurring under soft tissue (Figure 298). By extending a line upward from these two numbers to the plotted curve and then over to the density axis, the two densities produced on the radiograph for bone and for soft tissue may be obtained. The differences between the two densities and the two exposures are both found by subtracting the lesser from the greater. The density difference is divided by the exposure dif-

pitch black. The level portion of the shoulder of the curve is referred to as the *D-Max*

These two measurements, the base-plus-fog and the D-Max, are simply read off of the density axis of the graph. Normal base-plus-fog values range from 0.18 to 0.22 on the density scale for well-protected film.

The base-plus-fog should generally not exceed 0.25, which would then indicate unacceptable levels of darkroom or storage fogging. Average D-Max levels vary

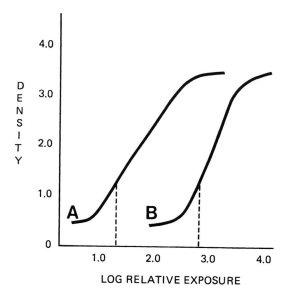

Figure 299. Graph of H & D curves for two different types of radiographic films. Film A is a faster speed film because its speed point is to the left of Film B. However, Film B has higher contrast since the slope of its body is steeper than that of Film A.

ference to obtain a measurement of contrast, as expressed in the formula:

$$\text{Contrast} = \frac{D1 - D2}{E1 - E2}$$

where D is the density and E is the relative exposure. If the body of the H and D curve lay at a 45° angle, the density change would equal the exposure change and the above ratio would come out as 1.0 for the film contrast. If the slope is steep enough so that the density increases by four times when the exposure is doubled, the contrast would be 2.0. *The steeper the slope, the higher the contrast.*

Since the two exposure levels chosen to obtain a contrast measurement are arbitrary, such measurements may be manipulated somewhat. Film manufacturers and sales representatives often refer to the *gamma* of a film as an indicator of contrast. The film gamma is actually the most ideal

contrast measurement that can be obtained from the H and D curve, taken over a small area near the middle of the body. A broader measurement which represents the performance of the film over the entire range of diagnostically useful densities is more valuable to the radiographer. The useful range of densities in diagnostic imaging is considered to be from 0.25 to 2.5. The overall contrast of the film should be measured between the densities 0.25 *plus* base-fog and 2.0 *plus* base-fog. This broader contrast measurement is called the *average gradient* of the film. Typical average gradients range around 2.92.

Film *speed* is obtained in a very different manner. Sensitometrically, speed is defined as the relative exposure required to produce a density of 1.0 *plus* base-fog on the radiograph. Therefore, the density level 1.0 plus base-fog is first found on the graph, and a line is then extended from that point over to the curve and down to the exposure axis. The *less* the relative exposure producing this density level, the *higher* the film speed. To obtain actual film-speed numbers, the log relative exposure number must be inverted algebraically. If a log relative exposure of 1.0 is required, the speed will be 100. If a log relative exposure of 0.5 is required, the speed will be 200. At 0.25, the speed is 400, and so on. Conversely, a log relative exposure of 2.0 translates to a speed of 50.

The primary value of the H and D curve is in comparing different types of films or different types of processing chemicals or conditions. Figure 299 shows two different H and D curves for comparison of film types. Film *A* has greater speed than film *B* because the entire curve, including the body portion at 1.0 plus base-fog, is to the left of the film *B*, indicating that less exposure is required to achieve equivalent densities. However, film *B* has higher inherent contrast than film *A*, because the slope of the curve for film *B* is much steeper. If the same film is used, two such curves could also indicate image changes from processing temperature, time or concentration changes.

On a daily basis, the primary interest in the radiology department in sensitometric quality control is in monitoring the chang-ing *trends* of speed, contrast and base-plus-fog over time. The H and D curve does not provide a *chronological* record of these qualities. The speed, the contrast and the base-plus-fog may be separated into daily measurements and monitored over time by using a different kind of graph called the *processing control chart.*

PROCESSING CONTROL CHARTS

The most valuable application of sensitometric monitoring is found in the use of processing control charts. In effect, these charts break the H and D curve into three separate components so that each one can be individually monitored over time. As long as the same film type is used and there are no drastic variations in electrical equipment factors, these graphs will represent variations in processing conditions. It is important that processing conditions be so monitored because it is in the processor that the greatest degree of variation occurs.

The three sensitometric graphs are for speed, contrast and base-plus-fog (Figure 300). The days of the week or of the month are noted across the graphs. Measurements should be taken each day at the same time after the processor has warmed up and is in regular use.

In the case of processing control charts, the *speed* is measured somewhat differently than with an H and D curve: The density value found at 1.0 plus the base-fog is recorded as a starting point on the speed graph. This value is sometimes called the *medium density,* abbreviated *MD,* and usually falls around 1.22. This value is written at the vertical mid-point on the graph. A heavier line or mark should be made on the graph at density points of 0.1 above and below this value. These are the acceptable limits for speed variation from day to day—

plus or minus 0.1 from the medium density level. Variation upward or downward from day to day is normal. However, when a continuing trend persists over several days, corrective action should be taken *before* the speed crosses over these limits.

The contrast is often called the *density difference* and abbreviated *DD.* When chemistry has been freshly mixed, this value should be measured and recorded at the vertical mid-point of the contrast graph as a starting point for comparison. Like the density, the contrast levels should not surpass plus or minus 0.1 from the initial value. Contrast is actually obtained for processing control charts by subtracting the step with the density closest to 1.0 from the density two steps darker than it (if using a 21-step penetrometer image). On preexposed sensitometry strips, the measurement taken from a labelled *minimum-density* area is subtracted from that of a labelled *maximum-density* area. Typical contrast measurements fall around 1.8.

Base-plus-fog is measured at the thickest step of the wedge or the lightest density area. The initial value is measured and recorded at the vertical mid-point on the graph just after fresh chemistry is mixed. Base-plus-fog should not vary more than plus or minus 0.03 from the initial value without corrective action being taken.

In addition to the three sensitometric

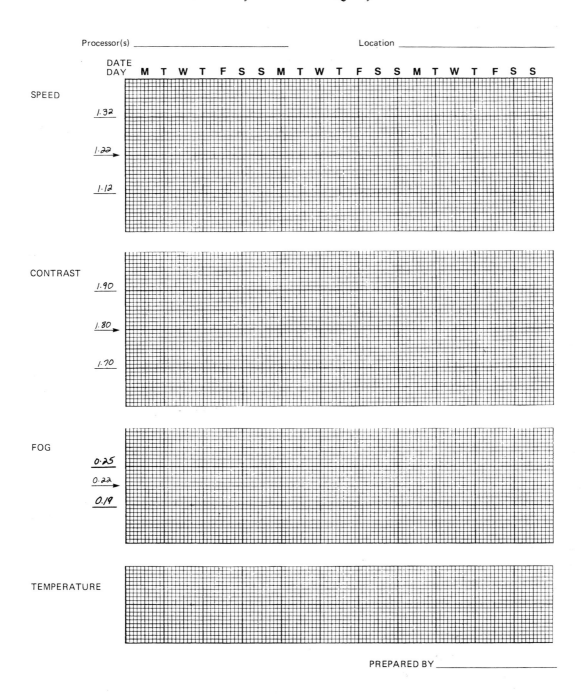

Figure 300. Example of processor control charts for speed, contrast, base-plus-fog and developer solution temperature as they would be set up after an initial test exposure (with fresh chemistry) yielding a speed of 1.22, a contrast of 1.80, a base-plus-fog of 0.22 and an average temperature. Unacceptable deviation limits are set at plus and minus 0.1 for speed and contrast, and at plus and minus 0.03 for base-plus-fog.

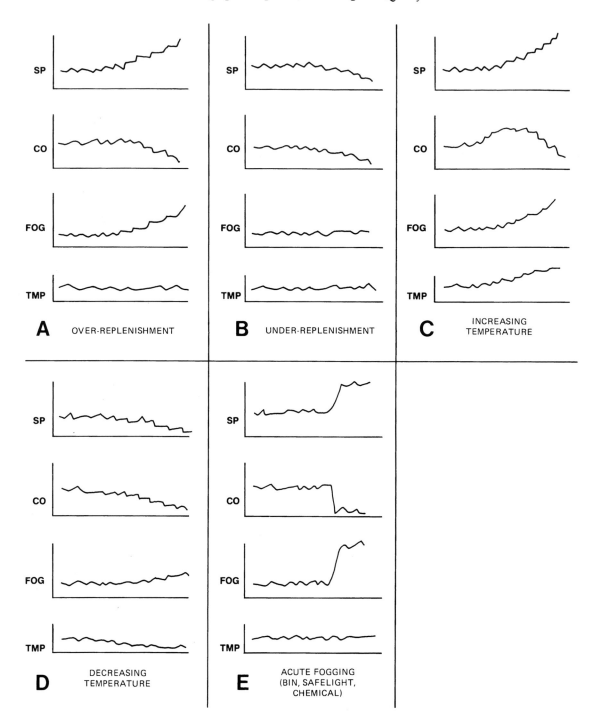

Figure 301. Typical deviation trends on processor control charts for five common problems: (A) over-replenishment; (B) underreplenishment; (C) increasing solution temperature; (D) decreasing solution temperature; (E) fim bin fogging or sudden contamination of solutions.

graphs, a processing solution *temperature* chart should also be used to monitor fluctuations in developer temperature from day to day, (Figure 300). This practice allows any deviations in the other three graphs to be narrowed down to one interpretation and diagnosis, rather than being left with two or three possible problems that might have caused the deviation and having to investigate each of them. Recall that there are three basic variables in processing: time, temperature and concentration. In automatic processing, the time is constant unless mechanical damage occurs to the transport system. For most problems, time may therefore be eliminated as a possible cause, leaving temperature and concentration. By monitoring the developer solution temperature daily, which can be done quickly by using a digital probe thermometer immersed in the developer for only 5-10 seconds, and by plotting the temperature variations along with the other sensitometric plots, temperature can be eliminated at a glance as a possible cause of deviations. That is, if the other sensitometric plots deviate past the acceptable levels and yet the temperature is seen to have remained constant, the problem is almost certainly being caused by improper chemical concentration. Deviation in the concentration of the chemicals could be caused by improper replenishment rates, blocked replenishment lines or broken replenishment pumps, exhaustion or contamination of the solutions.

DIAGNOSING DEVIATIONS

Figure 301 demonstrates the typical trends apparent on control charts for under-replenishment, over-replenishment, increasing or decreasing temperatures, and for sudden contamination of developer solution. When under-replenishment occurs, speed and contrast both tend to decrease while the base-plus-fog and temperature remain constant. For over-replenishment, the speed and fog both increase, the contrast decreases, and the temperature remains constant. When solution temperature is increasing, the speed, fog and temperature charts will all show an increase. The contrast chart will show an increase at first, but as the temperature continues to climb, contrast will reach a peak and begin to decrease. With a loss of heat, the speed, contrast and temperature graphs will show a decrease, while the fog graph may show a slight increase or remain level. When the film bin is light-fogged or when solutions are contaminated due to human error, the graphs will change in the same directions as for over-replenishment, but the change will be acute, spiking suddenly, so that the nature of the problem is obviously human error or complete failure of a processor component such as the heater.

When processing control charts are used faithfully, and deviations are corrected before they exceed the acceptable limits, repeat rates can often be reduced by as much as 35 per cent. Not only does this repeat reduction save almost one-third of all unnecessary patient exposure, but it also can save the radiology department thousands of dollars in film costs. It is to our professional, ecological, and economical advantage to use such a simple and beneficial scientific method of quality control.

SUMMARY

1. *Sensitometry* is the quantitative measurement of film response to exposure and processing conditions.
2. The *H and D curve* is useful in compar-

ing different image receptor systems or processing variables. It shows the base-plus-fog (toe), the D-Max (shoulder), the contrast (slope of body) and the speed points obtained.

3. *Processing control charts* allow deviations in processing conditions to be detected and corrected *before* they cause repeated exposures. Typically, the base-plus-fog should be around 0.2, the speed around 1.2 and the contrast around 1.8. Speed and contrast should not deviate more than 0.1 from the standard, and base-plus-fog should not deviate more than 0.03 from the standard.

4. Since in automatic processing the development time is fixed and the temperature can be monitored, the *combined trends* in processing control charts can be used to diagnose the cause of deviations (replenishment, temperature or acute fogging) with fair accuracy.

5. Quality control of processing can reduce *repeated exposures* by more than 35 per cent.

REVIEW QUESTIONS

1. Define sensitometry:
2. Who were Hurter and Driffield?
3. In monitoring processing conditions, why is it better to use a sensitometer than a penetrometer?
4. What is the typical range for base-plus-fog measurements?
5. What is the typical D-max level of density for most films?
6. Define average gradient:
7. The slope of the H & D curve, measured as either gamma or as average gradient, indicates the level of what image quality?
8. At a density of 1.0 plus the base-fog on an H & D graph, the curve for film B lies to the *right* of the curve for film A. What does this mean in comparing the characteristics of these two films?
9. What is the *formula* for calculating film contrast from an H & D curve?
10. Which portion of the H & D curve would give an indication of the total amount of silver available in the emulsion to produce density in the image?
11. For processing control charts, the start-

ing point for measuring speed is found by taking the density of that step on the "step wedge" which measures closest to what value?
12. For processing control charts, the contrast should not deviate from the base value by more than plus-or-minus _____.
13. What is the maximum allowable deviation for base-plus-fog?
14. On a set of processor control charts, if the measured solution temperature has been stable, yet the contrast, speed and fog all changed, which of the three major processing variables is almost certainly responsible?
15. Over a period of time the speed is seen to be rising, the contrast is dropping and the fog is rising, but the temperature remains steady. What is causing this trend?
16. Describe what the speed, contrast, fog and temperature charts would look like if the solution temperature was gradually decreasing.

APPENDIX I

BLANK TECHNIQUE CHARTS

A. Manual Exposure (2 pp)
B. Automatic Exposure Control

ABBREVIATIONS: GD = Grid
NG = Non-Grid

TORSO / SKULL CHART

Total MAS by PART SIZE

PROCEDURE	Notes	VIEW	kVp	Ave CM	-6cm	-4cm	-2cm	AVE	+2cm	+4cm	+6cm	+8cm	+10cm
GRID CHEST	72"	PA/AP	106	22									
		LAT	116	30									
NON-GRID CHEST	72"	AP	80	22									
		LAT	90	30									
SUPINE CHEST 40" NG		AP	80	22									
RIBS / Sternum	72"	AP↑Diap	60	22									
		OBL↑Dia	64	24									
	72"	AP↓Diap	76	22									
ABDOMEN / IVP	GD	AP/PA	80	22									
		30°OBL	80	24									
PELVIS / HIP	GD	AP	80	22									
HIP (Unil or Groin)	GRID	LAT	80	22									
SACRUM		AP / Coccyx All	76	20									
	GD	LAT	80	28									
LUMBAR SPINE	GD	AP	80	22									
		45°OBL	80	26									
		LAT	80	30									
		L5/S1 SP	*90	30									
THORACIC SPINE	GD	AP	76	22									
	Breathing LAT		60	30									
TWINING C/T	GD	LAT	76	28									
CERVICAL SPINE	40" GD	AP/Odon	76	13									
	72"GD	OBL/LAT	76	13									
	72"NG	OBL/LAT	76	13									
SKULL	GD	PA/Cald	80	19									
		LAT	76	15									
		Townes	80	22									
SINUSES / FACIAL BONES	GD	PA/Cald	76	19									
		Waters	80	20									
		Lat	76	15									
AIR CONTRAST U.G.I. / B.E.	GD	AP/PA	90	22									
		OBL/SIG	90	24									
		LAT	90	30									
SOLID-COLUMN U.G.I. / B.E.	GD	AP/PA	110	22									
		OBL/SIG	110	24									
		LAT	110	30									

EXTREMITY CHART

PROCEDURE	Notes	VIEW	kVp	mAs
HAND		PA /All Fingers	54	
	SFS	OBL	54	
	EXTCAS	Fanned Lat	54	
WRIST	SFS	PA	60	
		OBL	60	
	EXTCAS	LAT	60	
FOREARM	SFS	AP	64	
	EXTCAS	LAT	64	
ELBOW		AP	64	
	SFS	OBL	64	
	EXTCAS	LAT	64	
HUMERUS	SFS	AP	72	
	EXTCAS	LAT	72	
TOES	SFS/EXT	All	60	
FOOT		AP	64	
	SFS	OBL	64	
	EXTCAS	LAT	64	
CALCANEUS	SFS	PD	68	
	EXTCAS	LAT	68	
ANKLE	SFS	AP/OBL	64	
	EXTCAS	LAT	64	
LEG	SFS	AP	68	
	EXTCAS	LAT	68	
TABLETOP KNEE	EXTCAS	AP	70	
		LAT	70	
TBLTOP KNEE REG		All	70	
BUCKY KNEE	GD	AP/OBL	70	
		LAT	70	
FEMUR	GD	AP / LAT	76	
HIP	GRID	FRG/GROIN	80	
SHOULDER	GD	AP/Transax	76	
		Transthoracic	90	
CLAVICLE	GD	AP/PA	74	
SCAPULA	GD	AP	74	
		LAT	74	

ABBREVIATIONS: GD =Grid, NG =Non-Grid. SFS =Small Focal Spot, EXTCAS =Extremity Cassette, REG =Regular Cassette, PIGOST = Pig-O-Stat$_{TM}$

FACIAL CHART

PROCEDURE	Notes	VIEW	kVp	mAs
MANDIBLE	GD	PA	76	
		OBL LAT	66	
	NON-GRID OBL LAT		60	
ORBIT Rheese	GD	PA OBL	76	
SINUSES	GD	SMV	80	
ZYG. ARCH	EXTCAS	SMV	62	
NASAL BONE	EXTCAS	LAT	54	

PEDIATRIC CHART

PROCEDURE	Notes	VIEW	kVp	mAs
"PREMIE" CHEST	40" NG	AP	54	
		LAT	54	
INFANT CHEST	40" NG	AP	60	
		LAT	68	
2-YEAR CHEST	72" PIGOST	PA	66	
		LAT	76	
6-YEAR CHEST	72" NG	PA	70	
		LAT	80	
ABDOMEN / IVP / PELVIS SPINES	INFANT NG		62	
	2-YEAR GD		68	
	6-YEAR GD		74	
CERVIC. SP	2-YEAR	All	64	
SKULL (PA/AP)	INFANT NG		62	
	2-YEAR GD		68	
	6-YEAR GD		74	
UPPER EXTREMITY	INFANT EXTCAS		54	
	2-YEAR EXTCAS		58	
	6-YEAR EXTCAS		62	
LOWER EXTREMITY	INFANT EXTCAS		58	
	2-YEAR EXTCAS		62	
	6-YEAR EXTCAS		66	

A E C TECHNIQUE CHART

PROCEDURE	VIEW	kVp	mA	BACKUP TIME (mAs)	DETECTOR SELECTION	DENSITY SETTING	NOTES
CHEST	PA/AP	106			☐☐☐		
	LAT	116			☐☐☐		
6-YR CHEST	PA	90			☐☐☐		
RIBS ↑DIAPH	AP/OBL	60			☐☐☐		
RIBS ↓DIAPH	AP	76			☐☐☐		
ABDOMEN	AP	80			☐☐☐		
IVP	AP/OBL	80			☐☐☐		
G.B. / Coned	AP/OBL	80			☐☐☐		
PELVIS	AP	80			☐☐☐		
HIP Unilateral	AP/LAT	80			☐☐☐		
LUMBAR SPINE	AP	80			☐☐☐		
	OBL	80			☐☐☐		
	LAT	80			☐☐☐		
	L5/ S1	90			☐☐☐		
THORACIC SPINE	AP	74			☐☐☐		
	LAT	60			☐☐☐		
TWINING C/T	LAT	76			☐☐☐		
CERVICAL SPINE	AP	76			☐☐☐		
	Odontd	76			☐☐☐		
	Lat/Obl	76			☐☐☐		
SKULL (SINUS) (FACIAL)	PA/Cald	80			☐☐☐		
	Waters	80			☐☐☐		
	Townes	80			☐☐☐		
	LAT	76			☐☐☐		
Mastoid/Coned	LAT	76			☐☐☐		
SHOULDER	AP	76			☐☐☐		
FEMUR	AP/LAT	76			☐☐☐		
KNEE / LEG	All	70			☐☐☐		
U.G.I.	All				☐☐☐		
B.E.	AP/OBL				☐☐☐		
	Sigm/Lat				☐☐☐		

APPENDIX II

ANSWERS TO EXERCISES

EXERCISE #1

1.   5 mAs
2.   80 mAs
3.   12.5 mAs
4.   4 mAs
5.   25 mAs
6.   60 mAs
7.   7 mAs
8.   210 mAs
9.   12 mAs
10.   7.5 mAs
11.   1.8 mAs
12.   16 mAs
13.   6.4 mAs
14.   132 mAs
15.   2.8 mAs
16.   15 mAs
17.   350 mAs
18.   62.5 mAs
19.   150 mAs
20.   4.8 mAs

EXERCISE #2

1.   750 milliseconds
2.   300 ms
3.   125 ms
4.   40 ms
5.   83 ms
6.   33.3 ms
7.   5ms
8.   1.2 ms
9.   0.2 second
10.   0.167 sec
11.   0.25 sec
12.   0.035 sec
13.   0.07 sec
14.   0.015 sec
15.   0.008 sec
16.   1.2 sec

EXERCISE #3

1.   2.5 mAs
2.   15 mAs
3.   50 mAs
4.   3.5 mAs
5.   0.8 mAs
6.   40 mAs
7.   25 mAs
8.   7 mAs
9.   9.9 mAs
10.   1.8 mAs
11.   7.5 mAs
12.   100 mAs
13.   32 mAs
14.   2.5 mAs
15.   90 mAs
16.   7.2 mAs

EXERCISE #4

1.   50 mAs
2.   5 mAs
3.   2 mAs
4.   appx. 12 mAs
5.   appx. 8 mAs
6.   appx. .8 mAs
7.   appx. 7 mAs
8.   2.5 mAs
9.   appx. 3.3 mAs
10.   appx. 16 or 17 mAs

EXERCISE #5

1.   appx. 24 or 25 mAs
2.   2.5 mAs
3.   40 mAs
4.   appx. 1.6 or 1.7 mAs

5. appx. .4 mAs
6. 5 mAs
7. appx. 1.6 or 1.7 mAs
8. appx. 3.2 to 3.4 mAs
9. appx. 132 to 134 mAs
10. appx. 30 mAs

EXERCME #6

1. 60 mAs
2. 5 mAs
3. 15 mAs
4. 20 mAs
5. 25 mAs
6. 2.5 mAs
7. 12 mAs
8. 7.5 mAs
9. appx. 3.6 mAs
10. appx. 45 mAs

EXERCISE #7

1. 20 mAs (4 sets of 5)
2. 120 mAs (6 sets of 20)
3. 125 mAs (5 sets of 25)
4. 15 mAs (6 sets of 2.5)
5. 20 mAs (1/3 of 60 or 6 sets of 3.3)
6. appx. 6.4 mAs (4 sets of 1.6)
7. appx. 48-50 mAs (4 sets of 12 or 12.5)
8. appx. 5 mAs (6 sets of .8)
9. appx. 40 mAs (5 sets of 8)
10. appx. 35 mAs (5 sets of 7)

EXERCISE #8

1. 40 mAs
2. appx. 14 mAs (2 sets of 7)
3. 15 mAs (3 sets of 5)
4. 120 mAs
5. appx. 42 mAs (2 x 7 x 3)
6. 70 mAs
7. 160 mAs (2 sets of 80)
8. 240 mAs
9. 45 mAs (3 sets of 15)
10. 60 mAs

EXERCISE #9

1. 0.667

2. 0.2
3. 0.167
4. 0.142
5. 0.125
6. 0.083
7. 0.0667
8. 0.05
9. 0.033
10. 0.025
11. 0.0167
12. 0.0125
13. 0.0083
14. 0.133
15. 0.15
16. 0.4
17. 0.6
18. 0.8
19. 0.2
20. 0.35

EXERCISE #10

1. 1/20
2. 1/30
3. 1/5
4. 3/4
5. 1/40
6. 2/3
7. 1/15
8. 1/500
9. 1/12
10. 1/6
11. 1/8
12. 3/5
13. 1/16
14. 1/120

EXERCISE #11

1. 2 sets of 40
2. 3 sets of 15
3. 2 sets of 33
4. 3 sets of 25
5. 3 sets of 60
6. 3 sets of 40 OR 2 sets of 60
7. 2 sets of 80 OR 4 sets of 40
8. 3 sets of 80 OR 4 sets of 60
9. 3 sets of 30
10. 4 sets of 80

EXERCISE #12

1. 1/40 second
2. 1/15
3. 1/30
4. 1/60
5. 1/80
6. 1/120
7. 2/5 (2 sets of 20)
8. 1/20
9. 1/5 second
10. 3/5 (3 sets of 40)
11. 1/40
12. 2/15 (2 sets of 7)
13. 1/50
14. 1/15
15. 1/120
16. 3/20 (3 sets of 15)
17. 3/5 (3 sets of 60)
18. 4/5 (4 sets of 60)
19. 1/5
20. 3/5 (3 sets of 80)

EXERCISE #13

1. 0.025 second
2. 0.07
3. 0.16
4. 0.033
5. 0017
6. 0.4
7. 0.05
8. 0.025
9. 0.125
10. 0.6
11. 0.025
12. 0.0125
13. 0.7
14. 0.17
15. 0.02
16. 0.07
17. 0.6
18. 0.25
19. 0.2
20. 0.6

EXERCISE #14

1. 4

2. 2.5
3. 10.5
4. 9
5. 16.5
6. 6.75
8. 9
9. 102 kVp
10. 46 kVp
11. 64.5 kVp
12. appx. 58 kVp
13. appx. 118 kVp
14. appx. 37 kVp
15. appx. 87 kVp
16. appx. 65 kVp

EXERCISE #15

1. 24 inches
2. 15
3. 10
4. 4
5. 6
6. 10
7. 30
8. 60
9. 15
10. 18

EXERCISE #16

1. 10 mAs
2. 5
3. 15
4. 7.5
5. 15

EXERCISE #17

1. 1/2
2. 1/5
3. 3/5
4. 3/2 or 1 and 1/2 times
5. 3-4 times
6. 2 times
7. 1/3
8. 2/5
9. 4/5
10. 3/4

EXERCISE #18

1. 1/4
2. 15 x
3. 2x
4. 1/2
5. 6x (6-7)
6. 1/2
7. 1/5
8. 90 x
9. 6x (6-7)
10. a slight decrease
11. 2 x
12. 1/120

EXERCISE #19

1. 0.31
2. 0.69
3. 1.93
4. 0.56

EXERCISE #20

1. 7.2 mAs
2. 8.1 mAs
3. 0.28 mAs
4. 1.17 mAs
5. 4.3 mAs
6. 8. 1 mAs
7. 32 inches
8. 30 inches

EXERCISE #21

1. 75 mAs

2. 30 mAs
3. 30 mAs
4. 30 mAs
5. 15 mAs
6. 10 mAs
7. 15 mAs
8. 25 mAs

EXERCISE #22

1. 16 inches
2. 8 inches
3. 3.3 inches
4. 8 inches
5. 180 inches
6. 24 inches
7. 15 inches
8. 30 inches
9. 1.5 inches
10. 32 inches
11. 40 cm.
12. 7.5 cm.
13. 18 cm.
14. 40 inches
15. 90 inches

EXERCISE #23

Series I:	A.	3x
	B.	2x
	C.	1/2

Series II:	A.	4x
	B.	2x
	C.	1/3

EXERCISE #24

	Density	Contrast	Sharpness	Magnification	Distortion
Increase mA	+	0	0	0	0
Increase Exp. Time	+	0	–	0	0
Increase kVp	+	–	0	0	0
Increase Filtration	–(0)*	–(0)*	0	0	0
From 1-Phase to 3-Phase	+	–(0)*	0	0	0
Increase Field Size	+	–	0	0	0
Increase Motion	0	–	–	0	0
Increase Patient Size	–	–	0(+)**	0(+)**	0
Increase Grid Ratio	–	+	0	0	0
Increase Screen Speed	+	+	–†	0	0
Increase Size of Focal Spot	0	0	–	0	0
Increase FFD	–	0	+	–	0
Increase OFD	–	+	–	+	0
Misalign or Misangle Beam	0	0	0	0	+

*Although a slight decrease in these qualities may be measurable, it is not generally visible (see text).

**Although a decrease in these qualities would occur if larger patient size would inevitably place the part of interest further away from the film, it would make no difference at all if the part was superficial enough to be kept adjacent to the film through proper positioning.

†This is a general rule which applies only when screen emulsion is increasing in thickness, but not when phosphor chemicals are changed to obtain higher speeds.

EXERCISE #25

1. 1 and 1/2 times.
2. Double.
3. Same technique.
4. Double.
5. Four times.
6. Same technique.
7. Double.
8. Same mAs plus about 8–10 kVp.
9. Double.
10. 1/4.
11. Double or increase 8 kVp.
12. Same technique.

Fuchs's Radiographic Exposure, Processing and Quality Control

EXERCISE #26: Explanation: First, complete the even columns of the lumbar spine section using the 4 cm rule to double or halve the mAs values, then simply split the differences to fill in the odd columns. Next, use proportional anatomy to derive the average skull, shoulder and knee techniques as follows: Note that the original 16 mAs for an AP lumbar spine is equal to a Townes skull - The PA skull is 2/3 this technique, yielding about 10 mAs. The lateral skull is ½ the PA, the shoulder is equal to the lateral skull, both at 5 mAs. The knee is 6 kVp less than the shoulder, with the same mAs. Finally, use the 4 cm rule again to complete the remaining skull, shoulder and knee columns.

Procedure	Projection	kVp	Ave CM	MAS						
Lumbar Spine	AP	80	22	18 cm 8	20 cm 12	22 cm 16	24 cm 24	26 cm 32	28 cm 48	30 cm 64
	Oblique	80	26	22 cm 16	24 cm 24	26 cm 32	28 cm 48	30 cm 64	32 cm 96	34 cm 128
	Lateral	80	30	26 cm 32	28 cm 48	30 cm 64	32 cm 96	34 cm 128	36 cm 192	38 cm 256
Skull	PA	76	19	15 cm 5	17 cm 7.5	19 cm 10	21 cm 15			
	Lateral	76	15	11 cm 2.5	13 cm 3.7	15 cm 5	17 cm 7.5			
Shoulder	AP	76	14	10 cm 2.5	12 cm 3.7	14 cm 5	16 cm 7.5			
Knee	AP	70	12	8 cm 2.5	10 cm 3.7	12 cm 5	14 cm 7.5			

VARIABLE TIME CHART:
Divide 200 mA into the original mAs values:

Procedure	KVP	mA	Time for ea. view		
			PA	OBL	LAT
WRIST	60	200	.025	.035	.05

VARIABLE KVP CHART:
Apply the 15 per cent rule:

Procedure	mAs	kVp for each view		
		PA	OBL	LAT
WRIST	5	60	64	68

INDEX